USE OF ANTICONVULSANTS IN PSYCHIATRY: RECENT ADVANCES

EDITED BY

Susan L. McElroy, M.D.

Harrison G. Pope, Jr., M.D.

OXFORD HEALTH CARE, INC. CLIFTON, NEW JERSEY

USE OF ANTICONVULSANTS IN PSYCHIATRY: RECENT ADVANCES

Library of Congress Catalog Card Number: 88-060779

ISBN: 0-945986-00-9

Contents

Introduction

The use of anticonvulsant medications in psychiatric disorders represents a new but growing area in psychopharmacology. Studies of the therapeutic efficacy of this class of compounds are still limited, and only now are controlled investigations beginning to appear. Nevertheless, preliminary experience has accumulated to the point where it seems worthwhile to compile the available data into a book. It is our hope that this book, appearing at an early stage in this evolving field, will stimulate new and expanded research on the efficacy and mechanism of action of anticonvulsants in psychiatric syndromes.

The first section of the book comprises four chapters devoted to general discussions of those anticonvulsant agents which have been studied in psychiatric disorders. The most systematically studied drug, carbamazepine, is discussed by Robert M. Post, M.D. in Chapter 1. Accumulating controlled data support the efficacy of carbamazepine in the acute and prophylactic treatment of bipolar disorder. In Chapter 2, Susan L. McElroy, M.D., Paul E. Keck, Jr., M.D., Harrison G. Pope, Jr., M.D., and James I. Hudson, M.D. discuss the evidence for the usefulness of valproate in psychiatric disorders. There exist many uncontrolled reports of the drug's efficacy in bipolar disorder, but completed controlled studies are very limited. A larger controlled study is just underway. For clonazepam, discussed in Chapter 3 by Guy Chouinard, M.D., there is a body of open data in affective and anxiety disorders but only one controlled study in mania, and another in panic disorder. Larger systematic studies with clonazepam are only now underway. In the last chapter of the section, Rolando Gutierrez-Esteinou, M.D. and Jonathan O. Cole, M.D. discuss phenytoin and ethosuximide—anticonvulsants which have attracted less attention in psychiatry, but which may have a place in certain syndromes. In each of these chapters, safety issues involved in the use of these drugs are discussed.

The next two chapters focus on issues of pharmacology. On a more practical level in Chapter 5, Barry S. Fogel, M.D. discusses general principles for use of anticonvulsants in various neuropsychiatric conditions, with particular attention to the use of these agents in combination with more standard psychotropics. On a more theoretical level in Chapter 6, David Borsook, M.D. discusses research on the effects of anticonvulsants on circadian rhythms, and the implications of these studies for treatment of major affective disorder and primary sleep disorders.

The remaining five chapters of the book review the use of anticonvulsant medications in specific psychiatric syndromes. In Chapter 7, Drs. Keck and McElroy describe the use of anticonvulsants in rapid-cycling bipolar disorder—an illness notoriously difficult to treat with standard agents—in which anticonvulsants, especially carbamazepine and valproate, have shown some encouraging preliminary results. Borderline personality disorder, another syndrome often refractory to both psychosocial and pharmacological treatment, is addressed by David L. Gardner, M.D. and Rex William Cowdry, M.D. in the following chapter. Drs. Gardner and Cowdry present their controlled study comparing carbamazepine, tranylcypromine, alprazolam, and trifluoperazine in patients with borderline personality. In Chapter 9, Drs. Hudson and Pope discuss the use of anticonvulsants in bulimia—a disorder which has been subject to small controlled studies with two anticonvulsants, phenytoin and carbamazepine, and limited anecdotal experience with another, valproate. The use of anticonvulsants in anxiety disorders and drug withdrawal syndromes (the latter sharing many features of anxiety disorders) is then discussed in Chapter 10 by Peter P. Roy-Byrne, M.D. Preliminary findings in this area suggest that carbamazepine and valproate, as well as clonazepam, may merit further study in panic disorder, sedative-hypnotic withdrawal, and alcohol withdrawal. Last, Robert Sovner, M.D. addresses the use of anticonvulsants in patients with mental retardation—another area which has been subject only to preliminary investigation, but is clearly deserving of further study.

If there is a general message to be learned from these chapters, it is that anticonvulsants offer a range of promising new possibilities for both research and treatment in psychiatry. Only further studies, both at the basic and clinical level—the latter using larger, well-defined samples of patients and placebo-controlled designs—can tell us whether this promise will be fulfilled.

Susan L. McElroy, M.D.
Harrison G. Pope, Jr., M.D.
Belmont, Massachusetts
April, 1988

Contributors

David Borsook, M.D.
Fellow in Neurology
Massachusetts General Hospital
Boston, Massachusetts;
Fellow in Neurology
Harvard Medical School
Boston, Massachusetts

Guy Chouinard, M.D.
Director, Clinical Psychopharmacology Unit
Allan Memorial Institute
Royal Victoria Hospital
Montreal, Quebec;
Professor of Psychiatry
McGill University
Montreal, Quebec;
Professor of Research
Psychiatric Research Center
Hôpital Louis-Hippolyte Lafontaine
Montreal, Quebec

Jonathan O. Cole, M.D.
Chief, Psychopharmacology Program
McLean Hospital
Belmont, Massachusetts;
Lecturer in Psychiatry
Harvard Medical School
Boston, Massachusetts

Rex William Cowdry, M.D.
Acting Deputy Director
National Institute of Mental Health
Bethesda, Maryland;
Associate Clinical Professor of Psychiatry
Georgetown University School of Medicine
Washington, D.C.

Barry S. Fogel, M.D.
Director, Psychiatric Medical Program
Rhode Island Hospital
Providence, Rhode Island;
Associate Professor of Psychiatry and Human Behavior
Brown University
Providence, Rhode Island

David L. Gardner, M.D.
Staff Psychiatrist
National Institute of Mental Health
Bethesda, Maryland;
Assistant Clinical Professor
Georgetown University School of Medicine
Washington, D.C.

Rolando Gutierrez-Esteinou, M.D.
Resident in Psychiatry
McLean Hospital
Belmont, Massachusetts;
Fellow in Psychiatry
Harvard Medical School
Boston, Massachusetts

James I. Hudson, M.D.
Associate Chief, Epidemiology Laboratory
Laboratories for Psychiatric Research
McLean Hospital
Belmont, Massachusetts;
Assistant Professor of Psychiatry
Harvard Medical School
Boston, Massachusetts

Paul E. Keck, Jr., M.D.
Assistant Psychiatrist, Epidemiology Laboratory
Laboratories for Psychiatric Research
McLean Hospital
Belmont, Massachusetts;
Instructor in Psychiatry
Harvard Medical School
Boston, Massachusetts

Susan L. McElroy, M.D.
Assistant Psychiatrist, Epidemiology Laboratory
Laboratories for Psychiatric Research
McLean Hospital
Belmont, Massachusetts;
Instructor in Psychiatry
Harvard Medical School
Boston, Massachusetts

Harrison G. Pope, Jr., M.D.
Chief, Epidemiology Laboratory
Laboratories for Psychiatric Research
McLean Hospital
Belmont, Massachusetts;
Associate Professor of Psychiatry
Harvard Medical School
Boston, Massachusetts

Robert M. Post, M.D.
Chief, Biological Psychiatry Branch
National Institute of Mental Health
Bethesda, Maryland

Peter P. Roy-Byrne, M.D.
Director, Anxiety Research
Center for Anxiety and Depression
Harborview Medical Center
Seattle, Washington;
Associate Professor
University of Washington Medical School
Seattle, Washington

Robert Sovner, M.D.
Medical Director
Lutheran Center for Mental Health and Mental Retardation
Watertown, Massachusetts

CHAPTER 1

Effectiveness of Carbamazepine in the Treatment of Bipolar Affective Disorder

Robert M. Post, M.D.
Bethesda, Maryland

INTRODUCTION

Carbamazepine is an agent that is highly effective in the treatment of a variety of seizure disorders, paroxysmal pain syndromes, and disorders of affect regulation. Carbamazepine is particularly effective in the treatment of complex partial seizures and generalized seizures thought to arise from the temporal lobe and limbic systems.[1-5] It is not effective in the treatment of febrile convulsions or absence seizures and may even exacerbate the latter. Similarly, it has a distinctive profile in the treatment of paroxysmal pain syndromes. It is particularly effective in blocking the lancinating component of trigeminal neuralgia and related paroxysmal pain syndromes, but is not effective in more chronic components of these illnesses, nor does it possess efficacy as a typical analgesic. Additionally, carbamazepine is increasingly recognized as an effective alternative to lithium in the treatment of bipolar disorder.

These distinctions are of considerable interest in considering the action of carbamazepine in psychiatric syndromes, particularly bipolar disorder and related excited psychotic states. Because of carbamazepine's diverse profile of clinical effectiveness, it is apparent that one cannot infer a disordered limbic system or an epileptic process in patients with bipolar disorder.[6] Similarly, although carbamazepine is effective in inhibiting seizures kindled from repeated stimulation of limbic structures, its efficacy in a given syndrome cannot be used to infer that a kindling-like process underlies the pathophysiology of that syndrome. This caveat is all the more important in light of recent data indicating that carbamazepine inhibits only some phases of kindling but not others and that the degree of inhibition differs according to the type of kindling model employed, e.g. electrical versus pharmacological.[7,8] For example, carbamazepine does not inhibit the development of electrically-kindled seizures from the amygdala in the rat, while it is highly effective in blocking fully developed seizures kindled from this area.[8] Conversely, chronic oral treatment with carbamazepine is very effective in blocking the development of seizures kindled by the local anesthetics lidocaine or cocaine, but even high doses are ineffective in suppressing these seizures once they are fully developed, or in blocking high-dose cocaine seizures.[7]

Thus, a major question remains to be further delineated, namely, whether the mechanisms of action of carbamazepine's anticonvulsant effects are related to its mechanisms of action in the treatment of paroxysmal pain syndromes and affective disorder. These biochemical and physiological issues are discussed in detail elsewhere,[9] but suffice it to say that there is considerable reason to believe that different properties of the drug may be responsible for its effects in these syndromes, particularly given the differential time course of onset of effect in the different disorders.[10, 11] It is likely that alpha$_2$-noradrenergic, peripheral-type benzodiazepine receptor, and sodium channel mechanisms are involved in the acute anticonvulsant effect of carbamazepine, while

GABA mechanisms are implicated in the antinociceptive effects of the drug. This leaves a host of neurotransmitter, neuromodulator, and peptide candidates as potential mediators of carbamazepine's effects in bipolar disorder. Nonetheless, comparison of the clinical, biochemical, and physiological effects of carbamazepine to the effects of routinely used psychotropic agents, or to other anticonvulsants which either are or are not effective in the treatment of affective disorder,[12] should help clarify which of the components of anticonvulsants' mechanisms of action are more likely responsible for their psychotropic properties.

CARBAMAZEPINE IN ACUTE MANIA

There are numerous reports in the literature of both uncontrolled and double-blind controlled studies that clearly indicate the efficacy of carbamazepine in the treatment of patients suffering from acute mania (Table 1).[13-23] Also, several studies suggest that the time course of the antimanic effects of carbamazepine parallels that achieved with neuroleptics. As illustrated in Figure 1, in equally manic patients studied on a double-blind basis, carbamazepine showed a time course of improvement similar to that of the neuroleptics chlorpromazine, thioridazine, and pimozide.[14]

Moreover, in the study of Okuma and colleagues, not only were the incidence and time course of carbamazepine's antimanic effect comparable to that of chlorpromazine, but there were fewer side effects with carbamazepine.[15] These data are consistent with those in other investigations, indicating that carbamazepine exerts its acute antimanic effect without untoward sedation, extrapyramidal side effects, or other subjective side effects that are often rated as unpleasant by patients treated with neuroleptics. Although a variety of side effects may occur with carbamazepine, including dizziness, ataxia, drowsiness, and diplopia, these are dose-related and can usually be avoided with slow upward titration of dose.

FIGURE 1. Time course of antimanic effects of carbamazepine compared to lithium & neuroleptics (see reference 14)

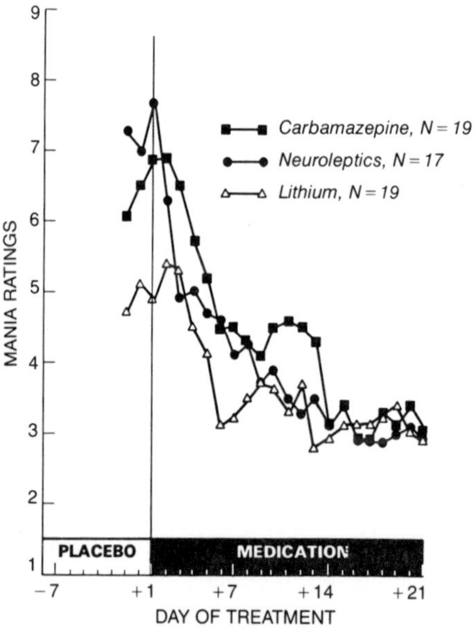

Figure 2 illustrates the differential response of 12 patients who showed excellent improvement during treatment with carbamazepine compared to seven apparent nonresponders in the same study.[14] It is evident that substantial improvement occurred in the first and second week of blind carbamazepine treatment at doses averaging just over 1,000 mg/day. As has been observed previously with response to classical neuroleptics, significant improvement in sleep occurred during the first week of carbamazepine treatment, and excited-hyperactive symptoms tended to improve faster than psychotic symptoms. Of note, during the placebo period prior to active treatment, the responders were significantly more manic than the nonresponders. Also, as summarized in Table 2, responders tended to be more dysphoric, showed a pattern of greater rapid cycling during the year prior to hospitalization as well as over their entire course of illness, and showed a negative family history for major affective disorder in first-degree relatives.[14] Thus, a number of variables that tend to be associated with lithium nonresponse, i.e. greater severity of mania, dysphoric mania, rapid cycling, and a negative family history for affective illness, are also variables that tend to be associated with better response to carbamazepine. Minor electroencephalographic (EEG) abnormalities or a history of epileptic-like psychosensory symptoms were not associated with response to carbamazepine. These data suggest, in addition, the possibility of differential subgroups of patients who may respond better to lithium or carbamazepine.

TABLE 1. Controlled studies of carbamazepine in acute mania

Study	N	Diagnosis	Design	Dose of carbamazepine mg/day (blood level)	Other drugs	Duration	Results
Ballenger & Post, 1978[13] Post et al., 1984; 1987[14]	19	M-D psychosis	Dbl. blind (B-A-B-A)	600-2000 (7-15.5 μg ml)	None	11-56 days	12/19 improved—time course similar to neuroleptics; frequent relapse on placebo substitution
Okuma et al., 1979[15]	32 CBZ 28 CPZ	M-D psychosis	Dbl. blind comparison w/ CPZ 150-450 mg	300-900 (2.7-11.7 μg/ml) (mean = 7.2±3.4)	Bedtime hypnotics	3-5 weeks	21/30 improved on CBZ (marked to moderate) 15/28 improved on CPZ
Klein et al., 1984[16]	27	22 excited mania and 5 excited SA	Blind vs placebo addition to haloperidol	600-1600 (6-18 μg/ml)	Haloperidol (15-45 mg/day) all patients	5 weeks	10/14 improved on CBZ + haloperidol (7/13 improved on placebo + haloperidol)
Müller & Stoll, a) 1984[17]	6	M-D	Blind vs placebo	600-1200	Haloperidol & Hypnotics	3 weeks	?/6; CBZ better than placebo (p<.01)
Müller & Stoll, b) 1984[17]	10	M-D	Blind vs haloperidol (15-50 mg)	600-1200 OXCBZ	Haloperidol & Hypnotics	2 weeks	?/10; OXCBZ = haloperidol
Grossi et al., 1984[18]	15	M-D	Blind vs CPZ randomized	200-1200		3 weeks	10/15 improved on CBZ 13/17 improved on CPZ CBZ = fewer side effects than CPZ
Emrich et al., 1985[19]	7	Manic psychosis	Dbl. blind vs placebo	1800-2100 OXCBZ	None	Variable	6/7 > 25% improvement on IMPS
Lerer et al., 1987[20]	14 CBZ 14 Li	M-D	Blind vs Li randomized	600-2600 (3.3-14 μg/ml)		4 weeks	4/14 improved on CBZ 11/14 improved on Li
Brown et al., 1986[21]	8	Manic	Dbl. blind comparison w/ haloperidol 20-80 mg/day	400-1600	CPZ to 3 pts (only 1 after 2nd day)	6 weeks	4/8 marked improvement on CBZ
Lenzi et al., 1986[22]	11	M-D	Blind vs Li	400-1600	CPZ	19 days	Equal efficacy in CBZ & Li groups. Less CPZ required in CBZ group.
Desai et al., 1987[23]	5	Manic	Blind vs placebo addition to Li	400 fixed dose		4 weeks	CBZ & Li (p<.05) better on BRMS scores than Li alone by second week
TOTAL						68/107 (64%)	moderate to marked improvement

Abbreviations: *CBZ = Carbamazepine; OXCBZ = Oxcarbazepine; CPZ = Chlorpromazine; Li = Lithium; IMPS = Inpatient Multidimensional Psychiatric Scale; BRMS = Bech-Raefelson Mania Scale; M-D = Manic-depressive; SA = Schizoaffective*

FIGURE 2. Time course of antimanic response to carbamazepine in marked responders (see reference 14)

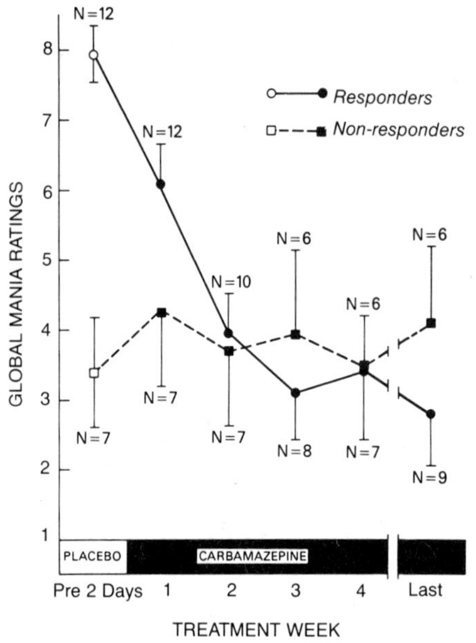

We find that manic patients can be treated with initial doses of carbamazepine of 400 mg/day to 600 mg/day, with daily increments of 200 mg/day until subjective side effects or clinical response is reached. Response is often observed in the dose range of 1,000 mg/day to 1,200 mg/day, although increases to 1,600 mg/day may be indicated in some patients in the absence of side effects. After two or three weeks of administration, carbamazepine induces hepatic enzymes which facilitate metabolism of the drug. Thus, a patient who is unable to tolerate 800 or 1,000 mg/day in the first several weeks of treatment may not experience side effects at these or higher doses after the third or fourth week of treatment.

Although there are occasional reports of neurotoxicity when carbamazepine is used together with lithium, the two drugs appear to be well tolerated in combination in the majority of patients.[24,25] Thus, in the management of the acute severely manic patient, the two drugs may be started simultaneously. When used in this combination, carbamazepine, like a neuroleptic, may help control the extreme elements of excitation and aggression prior to the onset of an adequate response to lithium. If control is not adequate, neuroleptics may be added to this combination. Therefore, it is quite reasonable to treat the most severely manic patient with usual therapeutic doses of several agents together, rather than to resort to extremely high doses of lithium or neuroleptics and the risk of toxicity.

Some patients show a selective response to carbamazepine but not to other anticonvulsants such as valproate or phenytoin (Figure 3).[26]

TABLE 2. Relationship of course-of-illness variables to antimanic response to carbamazepine (see reference 14)

Life history variable	Nonresponders (n=7)	Responders (n=12)	t	p
Age of onset of 1st symptoms	17.9 ± 4.7	20.3 ± 4.9	−1.1	0.30
Duration of illness (years)	15.3 ± 12.1	18.3 ± 11.4	−0.55	0.59
Total no. episodes before current admission	18.2 ± 17.3[a]	42.5 ± 50.3	−1.5	0.15
Total weeks ill before current admission	269.1 ± 275.0[a]	288.8 ± 258.9	−0.15	0.88
Total weeks hospitalized before current admission	61.7 ± 56.6[a]	156.5 ± 297.9	−1.1	0.31
Manic episodes before current admission	10.3 ± 8.6[a]	23.5 ± 29.0	−1.45	0.17
Depressive episodes before current admission	7.8 ± 8.9[a]	19.0 ± 21.7	−1.2	0.25
Episodes/years ill	1.2 ± 0.8[a]	4.4 ± 6.0	−1.8	0.098
Episodes in year before current admission	2.7 ± 2.4	7.0 ± 5.6	−2.3	0.03

Values are presented as means ± SD.
[a] *n=6*

We have also observed patients who responded to valproate when they did not appear to be adequately responsive to carbamazepine alone (Figure 4). Thus, valproate, and perhaps also clonazepam, might be considered as alternatives to carbamazepine in the management of acute severe mania refractory to traditional treatment.[12]

FIGURE 3. Selective response to carbamazepine but not to placebo, lithium, or other anticonvulsants in one acutely manic patient (see reference 26)

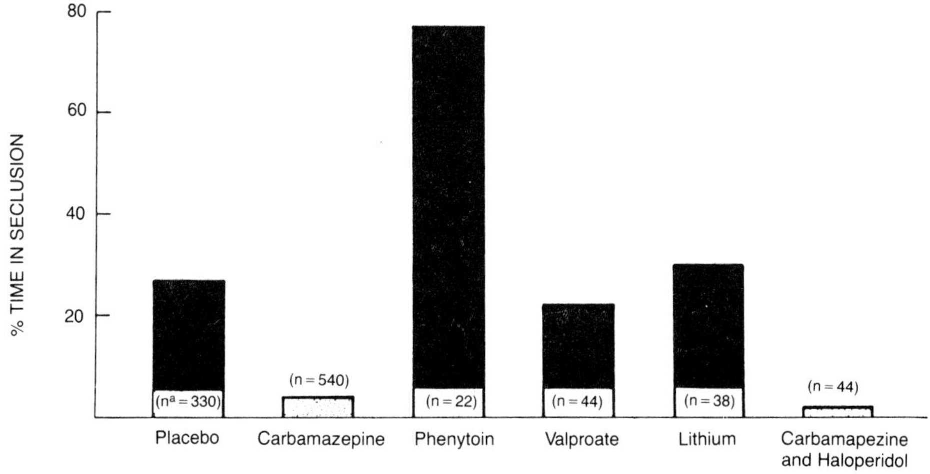

ª *n = Number of days on each treatment in a double-blind fashion. Placebo days were not consecutive, but were interspersed before and in between active trials (see reference 26).*

FIGURE 4. Prophylactic response to valproate in a carbamazepine nonresponder

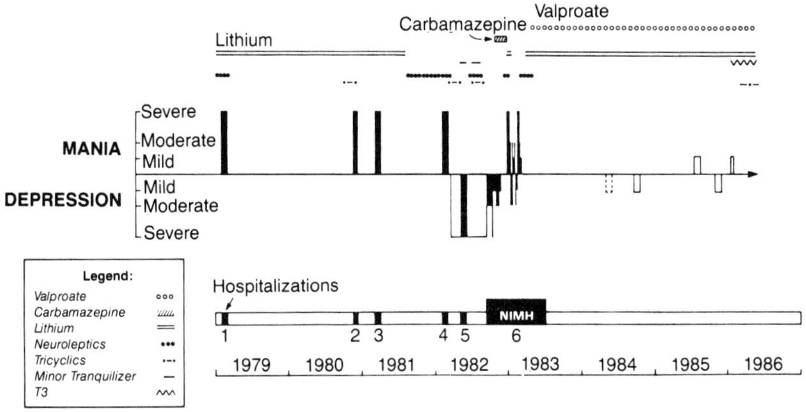

Manic episodes are plotted above and depressive episodes below the mood line. Shaded episodes indicate hospitalizations; dotted lines indicate a mild depression, the timing of which is not precise. This male with bipolar disorder in his early 50's experienced repeated episodes of severe mania which required hospitalization in spite of adequate lithium treatment (1979-1981). At NIMH, he experienced an apparent antidepressant response to carbamazepine, but suffered a breakthrough manic episode on this treatment.

CARBAMAZEPINE IN DEPRESSION

In contrast to the wealth of studies from many different countries indicating the acute antimanic effects of carbamazepine, the effects of this drug in the treatment of acute depression have been less well studied and delineated. In our double-blind study using a B-A-B design, 15 (32%) of the first 47 acutely depressed patients showed a moderate to marked antidepressant response to carbamazepine[27] (and unpublished data, 1987). Substantial clinical change in responders usually began in the second or third week of carbamazepine treatment, with maximal effects not observed until the fourth week of treatment. Observed responses were unlikely to be related to placebo effects, since patients had an extensive period of medication-free evaluation on placebo prior to the initiation of the carbamazepine trial.

While improvement in sleep was noted in the first week of treatment (as assessed by half-hourly checks by nurses who were also blind to the treatment regimen), this initial degree of sleep improvement was unrelated to the subsequent degree of antidepressant response. These findings are consistent with those of a collaborative study with imipramine and amitriptyline revealing that there is little relationship between improvement in sleep and degree of antidepressant response.[28]

The time course of the antidepressant effects of carbamazepine in responders appears to parallel that reported in the literature for more traditional antidepressant agents. However, these antidepressant effects are clearly less rapid in onset than those observed following electroconvulsive therapy or the transient effects observed after one night's sleep deprivation.[29] While good response in approximately one-third of our depressed patients does not appear to be a high antidepressant response rate, it is noteworthy that these patients had previously been relatively refractory to more traditional antidepressant agents. Nonetheless, it is clear that further controlled clinical trials are warranted. These studies should include other methodologies to better assess the relative acute antidepressant efficacy of carbamazepine compared to more traditional treatments in unselected patients.

Of note, initial analysis of responders in the first series of 35 patients suggests that they were more severely ill during the placebo period than were nonresponders. In addition, responders had a history of less chronic depression with a greater number of discrete episodes.[27] We also found that those patients with greater decreases in thyroid indices (T4, free T4) during treatment with carbamazepine showed the best antidepressant response to the drug.[30,31] Family history of major affective disorder in first-degree relatives, minor EEG abnormalities, and the presence of epileptic-like psychosensory symptoms did not predict degree of antidepressant response.

In our studies, the average dose of carbamazepine used for depression was slightly less than 1,000 mg/day. In initiating treatment during euthymic or depressed phases of the illness, it is prudent to start more slowly than when treating the manic phase. Initial doses of 200 mg at night (or less if needed) may be raised by 200 mg increments after several days in order to avoid side effects. Because of the large individual variation in the side effect threshold seen with carbamazepine in the treatment of psychiatric and neurologic patients, dose titration on an individual patient basis is important (Figure 5).[32]

A similar caveat is warranted for blood levels. While levels between 4 μg/ml and 12 μg/ml are generally considered to bracket the therapeutic range for patients with epilepsy, trigeminal neuralgia, and affective illness, there are wide individual differences in blood levels at which patients will experience therapeutic efficacy or side effects. Thus, patients can be managed with dose titration against side effects. However, while routine monitoring of blood levels does not appear mandatory, there is generally a higher incidence of side effects when levels are greater than 12 μg/ml.

FIGURE 5. Interindividual variation in side effect thresholds in five patients treated with carbamazepine (adapted from reference 32)

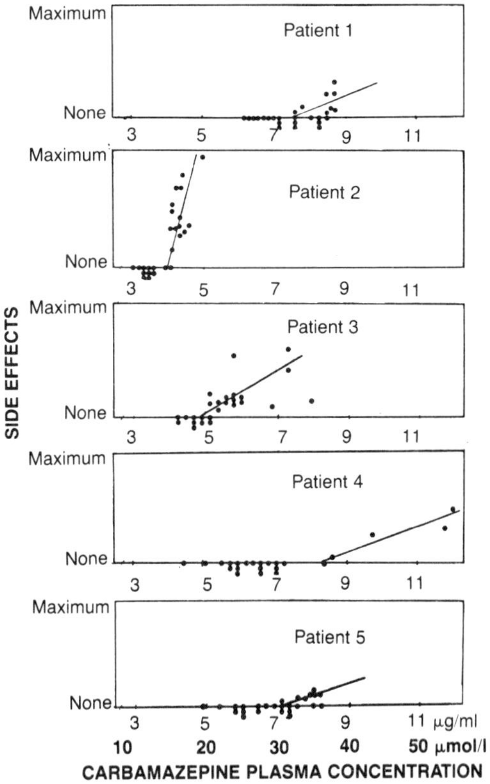

Severity of side effects is measured on the ordinate. These typically include dizziness, ataxia, drowsiness, and diplopia. Blood levels from low (3-4 μg/ml) to high (11-12 μg/ml) therapeutic range are plotted on the abscissa. Each point represents the degree of side effects experienced at a given daily morning (trough) blood level. The diagonal lines represent the approximate slope of best fit for the severity of side effects-blood level relationship. Note the great individual differences in side effect thresholds (i.e. the blood level at which side effects begin to occur or where the slope line intersects the x-axis) and the steepness of the side effects gradient (i.e. as in patient 2 where small increments in blood levels produce large increases in side effect severity, as opposed to patient 5, where similar increases in blood level produce only minor changes in side effects).

Of interest, we did not find a relationship between carbamazepine levels in plasma or cerebrospinal fluid (CSF) and the degree of antidepressant response when blood levels were between 4 μg/ml and 12 μg/ml.[33] However, in our initial series of patients, we found that higher levels of the active metabolite of carbamazepine (its -10,11-epoxide) in plasma or CSF were associated with degree of clinical response.[33] We did not find the relationship of clinical response to plasma levels of the -10,11-epoxide in a larger patient sample, but this parameter warrants further investigation.

PROPHYLACTIC EFFECTS OF CARBAMAZEPINE

Several uncontrolled and controlled studies indicate that carbamazepine is effective in the prevention of both manic and depressive episodes. A controlled evaluation of individual patients was initially reported by Ballenger and Post.[13] Series of such patients were subsequently reported by Post and colleagues[34] and Post and Uhde.[12] An individual case report of a patient responding selectively to carbamazepine but not to valproate or phenytoin has been presented in detail.[26] This patient showed a more notable degree of improvement in her schizoaffective psychosis when carbamazepine was combined with neuroleptics. These data parallel the controlled observations of Okuma and associates[35] and the more recent randomized controlled clinical trial of Placidi and colleagues[36] indicating superior efficacy of carbamazepine when compared to placebo or equal efficacy of carbamazepine when compared to lithium.

Although carbamazepine was added to previously ineffective treatments and patients were not evaluated blindly, the 1973 study by Okuma and associates is interesting in that it suggested that patients responding to lithium and those responding to carbamazepine may not entirely overlap; there was a trend for lithium nonresponders to respond adequately to carbamazepine and vice versa.[37] More recent evidence of Kishimoto and Okuma further supports such a divergence, with rapid and continuously cycling bipolar patients among those who respond best to carbamazepine.[38]

While some rapid cyclers do respond to lithium, a substantial literature indicates that patients with rapid or continuous cycling are often relatively refractory to lithium.[39-45] Joffe and colleagues have also found that rapid-cycling patients are less responsive to lithium but show relatively good responses to long-term treatment with carbamazepine alone[46] (and personal communication, September, 1987). Moreover, a subgroup of patients was identified that responded to a combination of lithium and carbamazepine. These patients exhibited a slower but continuous illness oscillating between periods of mania and depression without a well interval. In summary, the studies in the literature support our findings that rapid cyclers are among those who show the best acute antimanic response to carbamazepine, and that the drug may be a particularly effective adjunctive or alternative agent to lithium in patients showing a pattern of rapid and/or continuous cycling.[35,37,46]

There is the possibility that pharmacological responsiveness in affective illness may differ as a function of the stage of evolution of illness.[8] The preliminary clincial data reveal that many rapid-cycling patients reach this state only after many years of illness. These observations raise the possibility that carbamazepine and other anticonvulsants may be more effective in the latter phases of bipolar disorder, while lithium tends to exert its most robust prophylactic effects in the early and mid-phases. However, because some patients show rapid cycling from the onset of their illness, further studies are required to test this hypothesis more definitively. Moreover, based on the study of Placidi and colleagues[36] and other reports,[20] it is unclear whether carbamazepine would be as effective in the early stages of bipolar disorder as in the later phases.

TABLE 3. Interactions between carbamazepine and other drugs

A. Influence of other drugs on carbamazepine levels

Increased levels associated with toxicity	Increased levels without toxicity
Erythromycin	Valproate (Carbamazepine -10,11-epoxide only)
Josamycin	Propoxyphene
Triacetyloleandomycin	Nicotinamide
Verapamil	Cimetidine (mild acute increases, none after one week)
Diltiazem (not nifedipine)	**Decreased levels**
Isoniazid (not tranylcypromine)	Phenobarbital
Viloxazine	Phenytoin
Nafimidone	Primidone
Danazol	Theophylline

B. Influence of carbamazepine on other drugs

Carbamazepine increases	Carbamazepine decreases
Escape from dexamethasone suppression	Clonazepam
Desmethylclomipramine	Dicoumarol
Clomipramine	Doxycycline
Phenytoin	Valproate
	Theophylline
	Ethosuximide
	Warfarin
	Haloperidol
	Pregnancy tests

Nonetheless, a variety of possible clinical predictors and correlates of clinical response to carbamazepine versus lithium are available for preliminary clinical consideration and subsequent experimental verification. Those favoring response to carbamazepine appear to include severity of illness (greater), quality of illness (dysphoric or mixed), phase of illness (late stages), and genetic subtype (family history negative).

The blood levels of carbamazepine required for long-term prophylaxis have not been adequately delineated but in most studies appear to be similar to those used in treatment of acute episodes. These levels bracket the range used in treatment of trigeminal neuralgia and epilepsy, i.e. between 4 μg/ml and 12 μg/ml. Preliminary observations in our follow-up study, as well as those of Fawcett and Kravitz[47] (and personal communication, October, 1986) suggest that a small percentage of patients, well maintained on carbamazepine for several years, gradually develop apparent loss of efficacy. It is not entirely clear whether this loss is due to development of tolerance to the effects of carbamazepine, to lower blood levels of the drug, or to progressive emergence of the underlying pathophysiological process in spite of adequate treatment.

While there is little evidence for loss of efficacy of carbamazepine in the long-term treatment of patients with seizure disorders, this phenomenon appears to occur in some patients with trigeminal neuralgia.[48] Greater experience with carbamazepine in systematic clinical trials is required to delineate whether loss of efficacy also occurs in affectively ill patients showing therapeutic blood levels of the drug. Data on escape from adequate lithium prophylaxis are not readily available in the literature, despite four decades of experience with this drug. It is our impression from a rather selective view of refractory patients referred to the NIMH clinical research center that a subgroup of patients who were previously well maintained on lithium do develop "breakthrough" episodes in spite of blood levels within the therapeutic range. Many of these patients may again respond to the addition of an anticonvulsant such as carbamazepine, valproate, or clonazepam. Adjunctive treatment with these anticonvulsants may be preferable to the older strategies of adding neuroleptics or antidepressants to deal with manic or depressive "breakthroughs", with their attendant risks of exacerbating the next phase of illness.

PHARMACOKINETIC INTERACTIONS WITH OTHER DRUGS

As summarized in Table 3, carbamazepine has important interactions with a variety of other agents. Most notably, several drugs have been reported to markedly increase levels of carbamazepine, sometimes leading to toxic symptoms in patients otherwise well maintained. These drugs include the commonly used antibiotic erythromycin and its congeners. Isoniazid will produce the same effect, although this has not been reported with other monoamine oxidase inhibitors. Indeed, a clear lack of increase in carbamazepine blood levels has been reported with the monoamine oxidase inhibitor tranylcypromine.[49] Reduction in the dose of carbamazepine is required when it is used in combination with certain calcium channel blockers. Verapamil and diltiazem in particular are capable of significantly increasing carbamazepine blood levels, although nifedipine has not yet been reported to produce this effect. Other drugs that can increase carbamazepine levels to a substantial degree include viloxazine, nafimidone, and danazol.

Minor increases in carbamazepine levels, not associated with significant toxicity, have been reported with nicotinamide, propoxyphene, and the histamine blocker cimetidine (of note, the increases with cimetidine usually occur transiently in the first week of treatment and then return to normal). Valproate produces slight increases in the level of the -10,11-epoxide metabolite, but substantial toxicity is not associated with this combination. Detailed discussion of these findings can be found elsewhere.[50-52]

Carbamazepine induces hepatic microsomal enzymes of the P-450 system, which are involved in the metabolism of a variety of drugs including the barbiturates and oral contraceptives. Thus carbamazepine may decrease the blood levels and efficacy of a variety of compounds (Table 3). For example, carbamazepine has been reported to decrease levels of haloperidol by 40%-60%.[53] While the addition of carbamazepine to preexisting neuroleptics such as haloperidol is generally effective in many refractory excited psychotic patients,[53] occasional exacerbations may be associated with reduction of serum neuroleptic levels to the undetectable range.

SAFETY IN OVERDOSE

In assessing the overall risk-benefit ratio of a medication in affectively ill patients who are at a substantial risk for suicide, the relative safety of the agent in an overdose situation is an important consideration. In this regard, carbamazepine compares favorably with many other more traditional antidepressants, particularly those of the tricyclic class, with which carbamazepine shows many structural similarities. Previous reports have indicated that many patients have survived large overdoses.[54,55] Ten patients survived ingested doses of carbamazepine ranging from 10 to 20 grams, i.e. 50 to 100 capsules.

RELATIVE SAFETY IN USE DURING PREGNANCY

In contrast to lithium, which has been associated with severe cardiac malformations in a small percentage of infants exposed during the first trimester of pregnancy, the literature indicates that there are no consistent or substantial malformations associated with carbamazepine use during pregnancy.[56-65] These clinical trials are further supported by animal toxicology studies which showed that there was no consistent pattern of malformations in the offspring of pregnant mothers taking carbamazepine.[66-70] However, while a recent study revealed that there was not an excess of malformations in infants born to mothers treated with carbamazepine during pregnancy, it found that the newborns had small head circumferences and low body weights.[71] Thus, while the conservative approach to medication during pregnancy should be taken, i.e. no medications unless they are absolutely required, the initial data from the epilepsy literature speak to the relative safety of carbamazepine, particularly in relation to lithium.

TABLE 4. Comparative clinical and side-effect profiles of lithium and carbamazepine

	Lithium	Carbamazepine	Lithium-carbamazepine combination
CLINICAL PROFILE			
Mania	+ +	+ +	+ + +
Dysphoric	+	+	+ +
Rapid-cycling	+	+ +	+ +
Continuous-cycling	+	+	+ +
Family history negative	+	+ +	+ + +
Depression	+	+	+ + +
Prophylaxis of mania and depression	+ +	+ +	+ + +
Epilepsy	0	+ +	?
Pain syndromes	0	+ +	?
SIDE EFFECTS			
White blood count	↑	↓	
Diabetes insipidus	↑	↓	↑, Li*
Thyroid hormones T3, T4	↓	↓	↓ ↓
TSH	↑	—	↑, Li*
Serum calcium	(↑)	↓	
Weight gain	(↑)	—	
Tremor	(↑)	—	
Memory disturbances	(↑)	?	
Diarrhea	(↑)	—	
Teratogenesis	(↑)	—	
Psoriasis	(↑)	—	
Pruritic rash (allergy)	—	↑	
Agranulocytosis	—	(↑)	
Hepatitis	—	(↑)	
Hyponatremia, water intoxication	—	(↑)	
Dizziness, ataxia, diplopia	—	↑	
Hypercortisolism, escape from dexamethasone suppression	—	↑	

Clinical Efficacy	Side Effects
0, *None*	↑, *Increase*
±, *Equivocal*	↓, *Decrease*
+, *Effective*	( ), *Inconsistent or rare*
+ +, *Very effective*	—, *Absent*
+ + +, *Possible synergism*	↓ ↓, *Potentiation*
	Li*, *Effect of lithium predominates*

SIDE EFFECTS OF CARBAMAZEPINE

The side-effect profile of carbamazepine differs considerably from that of lithium (Table 4). Carbamazepine may therefore represent an attractive alternative in patients unable to tolerate lithium. Of importance, the side effects that occur most frequently with carbamazepine tend not to be problematic in their clinical management, while several of those that occur extremely rarely are of considerable concern.

Although carbamazepine causes a mild to moderate decrease in the white blood count in the majority of patients treated, this common mild suppression is usually without clinical impact, as the lowered white count is usually well within the normal range.[72] On occassion, however, it can decrease to 3000 to 4000 white blood cells per ml.

It is of considerable interest that the benign suppression of white count can be totally reversed by concomitant treatment with lithium.[73,74] Lithium increases production of white cells of the granulocytic series as well as platelets, probably by stimulating growth factors such as colony stimulating factors of the granulocytic and megakaryocytic series. Therefore, when lithium is given concomitantly with carbamazepine, not only is the white blood count suppression induced by carbamazepine reversed, but values increase above the baseline observed during placebo administration prior to carbamazepine.[74] Whether lithium would have any protective effect on the more serious hematological reactions to carbamazepine (described below) is unknown, but unlikely.

Reports of agranulocytosis and aplastic anemia associated with carbamazepine have continued to appear in the literature. Pisciotta reviewed the existing literature in 1983 and suggested that the frequency of these events was between one in 10,000 and one in 40,000 patients.[75] Up to that time, those patients with severe hematological reactions tended to be overly represented by older, medically ill individuals treated with a variety of concomitant medications for trigeminal neuralgia or seizure disorders. More recently, several cases in psychiatric patients have been reported, reflecting a rare but continuing incidence of these serious side effects. The most recent estimate of incidence is eight patients per million treated, or approximately one in 125,000.[76]

There is considerable disagreement in the neurological and hematological literatures as to the recommended frequency of hematological monitoring in order to deal adequately with this rare but potentially fatal complication of carbamazepine therapy.[77,78] The most conservative recommendations are weekly or biweekly monitoring for the first four months and monthly thereafter. This monitoring schedule is based in part on the data illustrated in Figure 6, indicating that most of the cases of agranulocytosis and aplastic anemia occur in the first several months of treatment.

However, this apparent early distribution of cases may be an artifact of a greater number of patients exposed to carbamazepine for relatively shorter periods of time. Several cases of serious reactions have been reported in the second part of the first year of treatment or even thereafter.

I have recently become aware of a patient who developed pancytopenia after approximately nine months of treatment with carbamazepine. Her hematological indices were all normal until as late as three weeks prior to the first sign of severe

FIGURE 6. Distribution of cases of aplastic anemia and agranulocytosis as a function of duration of carbamazepine treatment[a] (see reference 75)

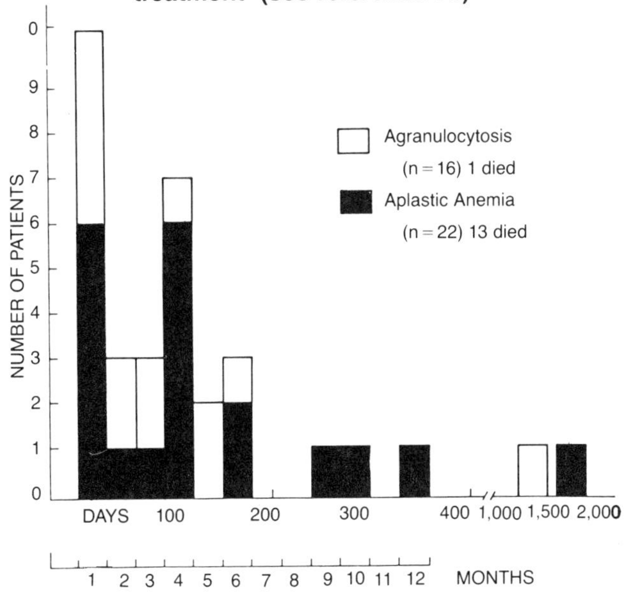

[a] *3 additional cases of agranulocytosis and 2 of aplastic anemia were reported without onset data.*

Data from Pisciotta[75] are plotted to show the temporal distribution of cases of severe hematological reactions to carbamazepine reported prior to 1982. Twenty-eight (85%) of 33 cases where onset was delineated occurred in the first six months of treatment. The most recent estimate of occurrence of these reactions is eight per million patients treated or one in 125,000.[76]

complications—a hemorrhage. A complete blood count then revealed marked suppression of white cells, platelets, and red cells, and the marrow showed complete aplasia.

Although other cases in the literature have not revealed whether consistent monitoring can provide an early warning of an impending aplastic process, this case clearly indicates that even frequent blood monitoring may not be sufficient. This observation tends to support the opinion of many neurological authorities that frequent blood count monitoring of patients on carbamazepine is unwarranted. For example, Trimble and associates, in their epilepsy clinic, alert patients that they should be aware of potential reactions and immediately call their physicians if fever, sore throat, petechiae, or other signs of potentially severe complications develop.[78] They maintain that routine white count monitoring is neither cost effective in detecting the very rare patient with serious hematological problems nor effective as an early warning device, since an idiosyncratic reaction can develop suddenly.

Thus, it would behoove the physician to discuss these issues in some detail prospectively with patients to be placed on carbamazepine, to obtain adequate informed consent, and to decide on a judicious scheme for monitoring hematological indices based on best individual medical judgment. Also, it is important to document normal hematological indices prior to the institution of carbamazepine treatment and to continue monitoring at such a frequency that both patient and physician are satisified that only the benign white count suppression is occurring. The earlier guidelines in the product literature recommending a rigid schedule of frequent monitoring have recently been revised to reflect this more flexible and individualized approach. Although a generally accepted cutoff of 3000 white cells per cubic ml has been indicated as the lower level at which carbamazepine should be discontinued, instances have been reported in which patients have been able to continue on the drug with the white count near or below this level as long as other indices were normal. Since lithium is able to stimulate leukocytes and platelets but unable to stimulate the erythropoietic series, evidence of impairment in red cell production contraindicates the use of lithium as an adjuvant for carbamazepine-induced leukopenia or thrombocytopenia.

Carbamazepine, like lithium, suppresses circulating levels of the thyroid hormones T3 and T4; unlike lithium it is rarely associated with clinical hypothyroidism and the need for thyroid hormone replacement.[10,30] In fact, as noted previously, it appears paradoxically that patients with the greatest suppression of T4 and free T4 are among those who respond best to the acute antidepressant effects of carbamazepine.[31] These data therefore suggest that thyroid suppression may indicate greater potential efficacy of the drug, rather than being a problematic side effect. While carbamazepine alone does not significantly elevate TSH levels, when used in combination with lithium, there is an additive suppression of T3 and T4, and lithium-induced increases in TSH levels may again occur.[74] Whether a greater or lesser degree of lithium-induced hypothroidism is produced with the combination, as compared with lithium alone, remains to be further elucidated.

Based on the drug's ability to stimulate vasopressin receptor function, carbamazepine on occasion has been associated with hyponatremia and, in very rare instances, with water intoxication.[10,79] This retention of water and dilutional hyponatremia is thus an effect opposite to that of lithium, which impairs vasopressin function and is associated with nephrogenic diabetes insipidus. Carbamazepine is therefore an alternative agent to lithium for patients with severe diabetes insipidus. However, carbamazepine does not reverse the effects of lithium-induced diabetes insipidus when the two drugs are used concurrently, since lithium exerts its action at a more primary level by inhibiting adenylate cyclase activity below the vasopressin receptor. In patients on high doses of carbamazepine and in elderly patients who appear more prone to hyponatremia, occasional monitoring of serum electrolytes would appear warranted, as it would with any patient who develops a confusional syndrome or other sign that could be associated with hyponatremia (such as severe weakness or headache). If one assumes that lithium-induced suppression of vasopressin function in the brain accounts for the occasional reports of slowing in subtle aspects of learning and memory, one would not expect carbamazepine to show this side effect because of its opposite effect on vasopressin function. Indeed, initial studies of carbamazepine in normal volunteers and in epileptics suggest that it has little adverse effect on cognitive processes, especially as compared to the anticonvulsants phenytoin and phenobarbital.[78,80,81]

Occasional mild elevations in liver function tests are relatively frequent in many series of psychiatric and neurological patients treated with carbamazepine. They do not appear to warrant special attention or, necessarily, drug discontinuation. With more persistent enzyme elevation, drug discontinuation would appear indicated. In very rare instances, carbamazepine has been associated with severe cases of hepatitis, which on biopsy showed either an inflammatory or a toxic-metabolic picture.

Cardiac toxicities related to carbamazepine occur but are relatively infrequent. Since carbamazepine slows atrial to ventricular conduction, it is relatively contraindicated in patients with preexisting degrees of heart block. The drug has actually been used to treat animals and patients with a variety of arrhythmias, including digitalis-induced arrhythmias and some ventricular tachycardias.

Carbamazepine-induced rashes are very common in psychiatric patients. Although most of the reports in the literature indicate that rashes are observed only in a small percentage of patients treated with carbamazepine, in our psychiatric series[82] and those of Okuma and colleagues[83] and Elphick and colleagues,[84] some 12% to 16% of patients developed a rash. Most authorities recommend discontinuation of carbamazepine with the onset of rash since exfoliative reactions and Stevens-Johnson syndrome can ensue. In our series, onset of the rash has been almost uniformly between the ninth and the twenty-third day of treatment, although an occasional patient can develop a rash after longer periods of time on the drug. Vick reports four cases in which carbamazepine-induced rash was suppressed when prednisone was administered prior to rechallenge with carbamazepine.[85] This strategy should be attempted only in instances where the rash is uncomplicated by other evidence of systemic allergy[86] and in patients who otherwise appear to require treatment with this agent, i.e. are not responsive to alternative modes of therapy.

Other allergic syndromes, reported more rarely, include fever, lymphadenopathy, and a pulmonitis syndrome.

CONCLUSIONS

Emerging evidence indicates that carbamazepine is effective in patients with bipolar disorder who are either refractory or inadequately responsive to treatment with lithium (Table 5). A number of these patients can be successfully maintained on carbamazepine alone or in combination with lithium. The drug appears capable of exerting rapid onset of robust antimanic effects in more than 50% of patients and a more delayed onset of antidepressant effects in a smaller percentage of depressed patients. Positive

TABLE 5. Preliminary indications for individual trials of carbamazepine in affective illness

I. Primary affective illness	
A. Acute and prophylactic treatment of mania	+ +
B. Acute and prophylactic treatment of depression	+
C. Bipolar patients:	
1. Not responsive to lithium	+ +
2. Unable to tolerate lithium side effects including diabetes insipidus, allergy, or tremor	+ +
3. As supplement for lithium partial responder	+ +
D. Schizoaffective illness, especially if cyclic; (use in combination with neuroleptic appears effective and should be further explored)	+
E. Recurrent atypical psychotic syndromes with depressive or confusional features	+
II. Secondary affective illness	
A. Mood and behavioral disturbance of:	
1. Complex partial seizures	+ +
2. Alcohol withdrawal symptoms	+

Further studies are warranted in each area.

+ +: *evidence from controlled studies or several laboratories*
+: *based on few studies or small numbers of patients*

FIGURE 7. Prophylactic efficacy of carbamazepine

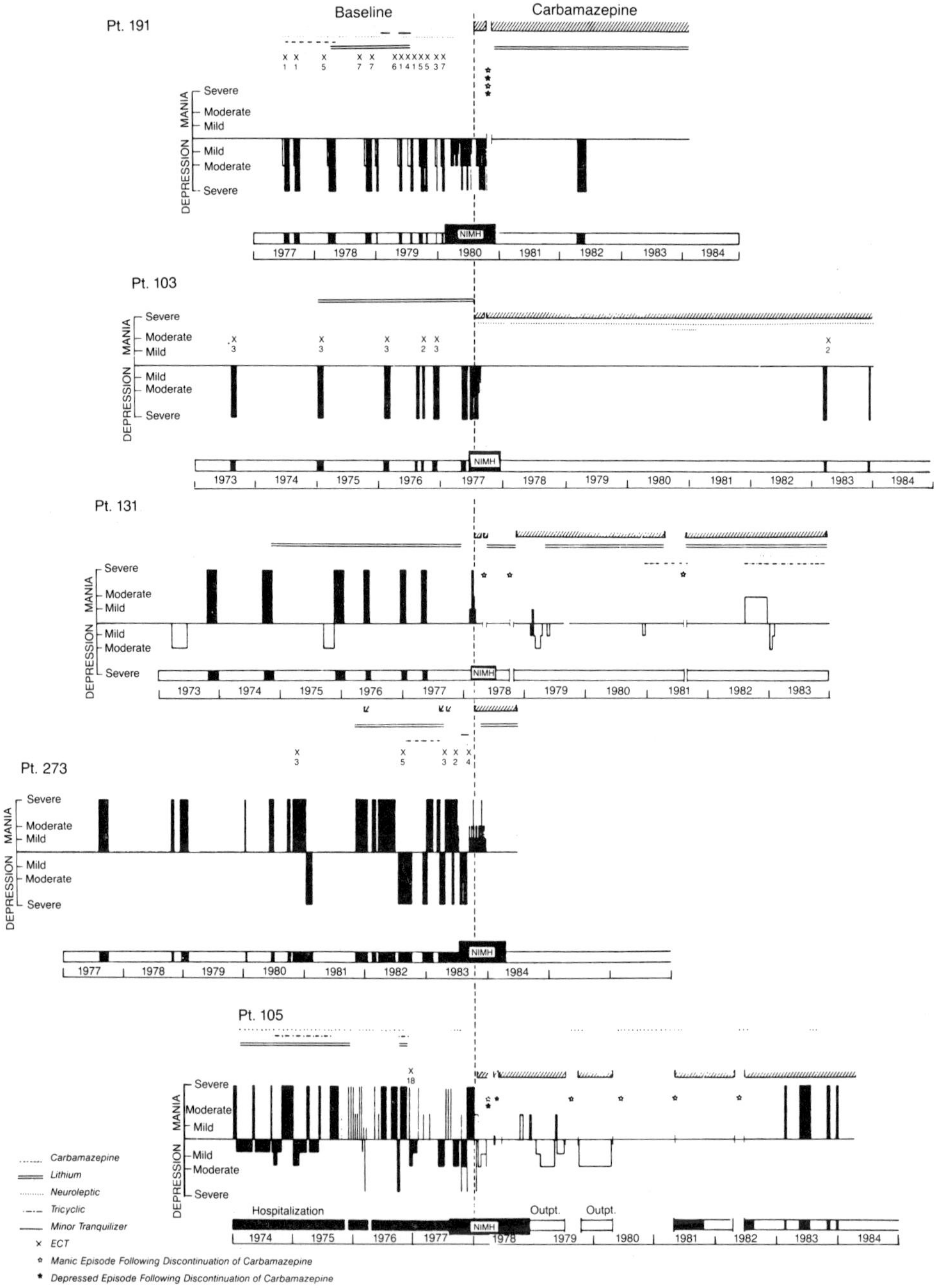

Manic and depressive episodes are plotted above and below the life chart line in five patients with recurrent affective disorder before (left side of dotted line on plot) and after (right side) treatment with carbamazepine. Note the reduction in frequency, severity, and duration of episodes following institution of carbamazepine treatment and the decreased number of hospitalizations (in patients 1-4) and use of ECT (in patients 1-3).

effects in long-term prophylaxis are evident even among the most severely lithium-refractory and most rapidly-cycling patients (Figure 7 and 8). Preliminary evidence suggests that a subgroup of patients may be more responsive to carbamazepine, as compared to those more responsive to the traditional agent lithium.

FIGURE 8. Effect of carbamazepine on percentage of time ill in nine manic-depressive patients (follow-up average = 5.4 yrs). (adapted from references 87 and 88)

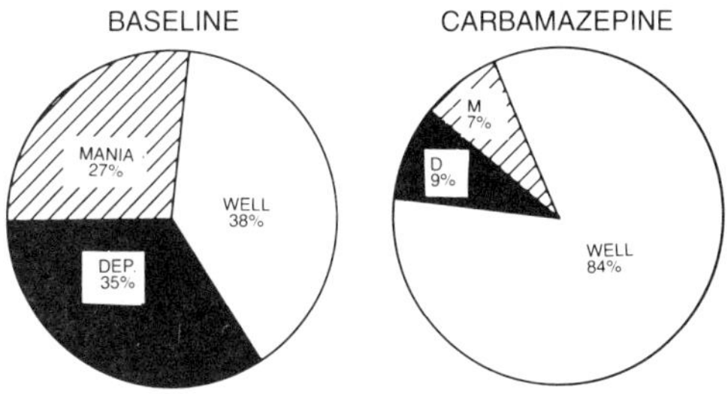

Nine manic-depressive patients (selected for good acute response to carbamazepine) were treated with carbamazepine (right circle) alone or in combination with previously ineffective treatments (such as lithium) used in the baseline period (left circle). Several patients were studied in a double-blind fashion for extended periods at NIMH, but most were followed in the community in an open-label, naturalistic, mirror-image design. That is, manic and depressive episodes were assessed for each patient using systematic life chart criteria during an equal time on drug (average = 2.7 years) and prior to drug initiation (average = 2.7 years). In this severely ill group of treatment-refractory patients, percentage of time ill (defined as moderate or greater severity of depression with functional incapacity or mild or greater mania) decreased from 62% in the baseline period to 16% during carbamazepine prophylaxis.

Compared with the anticonvulsants phenobarbital and phenytoin, carbamazepine appears to have a relatively benign profile in impairing learning and memory. While our initial studies of learning and memory impairment with patients on carbamazepine or lithium suggest few impairments with either drug, how these two drugs compare in this respect needs further investigation.

Like lithium, carbamazepine is associated with a unique profile of side effects, and the clinician should become familiar with the differential side effects of each drug in his approach to the affectively ill patient (Table 4). With appropriate care in prescribing and monitoring this medication, we and others have found that carbamazepine can make a remarkable difference in patients' courses of illness and lives.

We suggest the utility of engaging the patient as an active collaborator in the process of the assessment and treatment of his or her illness, particularly in the systematic assessment of the longitudinal course of illness and of the impact of various psychopharmacological interventions.[87,88] In this way the degree of efficacy of past and current psychotropic interventions can be most accurately assessed, and drug titrations and alternative treatments recommended when appropriate. Use of the life chart may also help in compliance, especially in cases where the recurrent nature of the illness may otherwise be obscured or denied.

Since a subgroup of patients appears to require the combination of lithium and carbamazepine for optimal acute and long-term efficacy, it may be clinically appropriate to assess immediately the maximum degree of clinical benefit from the combination, rather than to pursue the more time-consuming and potentially risky course of discontinuing lithium in order to initiate carbamazepine treatment alone. Once maximum effects are achieved on the combination, the clinician can slowly taper lithium, if clinically warranted, in order to assess whether carbamazepine alone is sufficient to maintain this optimal degree of clinical response. If lithium is being discontinued, it may be advisable to taper the drug slowly over a period of several weeks or longer, in order not to precipitate further affective episodes.

There is recent evidence that rapid discontinuation of lithium may abruptly precipate manic or depressive episodes.[89-93] This reaction can occur in spite of maintenance neuroleptic treatment. While there does not appear to be a substantial withdrawal syndrome following the discontinuation of carbamazepine, we have noted the rapid recrudescence of manic and psychotic symptoms in patients in whom the drug appeared to be exerting a therapeutic action, suggesting that care should be taken in the discontinuation phase with carbamazepine in psychiatrically vulnerable patient populations.[13]

While some patients appear to respond selectively to carbamazepine as oppossed to other anticonvulsant agents, other patients appear to respond to drugs such as clonazepam,[94] valproate,[95-101] or acetazolamide[102] when they may be unresponsive to carbamazepine. Thus it would appear that carbamazepine represents one in a class of anticonvulsants that may be considered in the treatment of affectively ill patients.

Although discussion of the mechanisms of action of carbamazepine and related anticonvulsants is beyond the scope of this chapter, it is of note that these drugs have different anticonvulsant profiles for different epileptic syndromes, as well as different mechanisms of action.[7,9-11] For example, the anticonvulsant clonazepam appears to act at the central-type benzodiazepine receptor, while carbamazepine is inactive at this site and may exert its anticonvulsant effects through the so-called peripheral-type benzodiazepine receptor.[103,104] Valproate, in turn, is not active at either of these receptors per se but appears to exert many of its effects by enhancing GABAergic function through a variety of mechanisms. These different mechanisms of action are evident in the effect of these anticonvulsants in different seizure types. Clonazepam is effective in absence, myclonic, and perhaps complex partial seizures while inactive in tonic-clonic seizures; carbamazepine is effective in complex partial and tonic-clonic seizures but may exacerbate absence seizures; and valproate is effective in a broad spectrum of seizure types.

Thus, on the basis of the differential clinical profiles of these anticonvulsants, as well as on their different mechanisms of action, it appears clinically useful, in the refractory bipolar patient, to consider another anticonvulsant when the first is ineffective. Given the advent of a series of novel agents in addition to lithium in the treatment of affective illness, as well as a variety of traditional agents which are less frequently used, such as electroconvulsive therapy, it is the rare bipolar patient who cannot be substantially helped.[12] Parenthetically, it is of interest that electroconvulsive seizures themselves appear to be capable of exerting substantial anticonvulsant effects such that electroconvulsive therapy, with its dramatic ability to treat both depression and acute mania, may also be included in the group of anticonvulsants.[105]

Several calcium channel blocking drugs have also been reported to be effective in the treatment of acute mania.[106] While these agents generally are not potent anticonvulsants, several of the calcium channel blockers (such as nimodipine and flunarizine) have been shown to possess anticonvulsant activity in various animal model systems. This variety of potential anticonvulsant agents, taken in conjunction with other antimanic drugs that are not potent anticonvulsants—including lithium, neuroleptics, reserpine, beta blockers, and the alpha-2 noradrenergic agonist clonidine—leaves the clinician with a wide array of options in the treatment of the refractory manic patient. An even larger range of potential antidepressant drugs is available for the bipolar patient with refractory depression, again leading to the optimistic view that since many different drugs of different classes are now available, there is an excellent chance for substantial clinical improvement. In addition, recent advances in basic neuroscience and in the understanding of the potential mechanisms of action of carbamazepine and related drugs should eventually lead to the development of newer and more specific agents for the treatment of affective disorder.

REFERENCES

1. Porter RJ, Penry JK. Efficacy and choice of antiepileptic drugs. In: Meinardi H, Rowan AJ, eds. Advances in epileptology, 1977: psychology, pharmacotherapy, and new diagnostic approaches. Amsterdam: Swets & Zeitlinger, 1978:220-30.
2. Ramsey RE, Wilder BJ, Berger JR, et al. A double-blind study comparing carbamazepine with phenytoin as initial seizure therapy in adults. Neurology 1983; 33:904-10.
3. Porter RJ, Theodore WH. Nonsedative regimens in the treatment of epilepsy. Arch Intern Med 1983; 143:945-7.
4. Callaghan N, Kenny RA, O'Neill B, et al. A prospective study between carbamazepine, phenytoin and sodium valproate as monotherapy in previously untreated and recently diagnosed patients with epilepsy. J Neurol Neurosurg Psychiatry 1985; 48:639-44.
5. Mattson RH, Cramer JA, Colling JF, et al. Comparison of carbamazepine, phenobarbital, phenytoin, and primidone in partial and secondarily generalized tonic-clonic seizures. N Engl J Med 1985; 313:145-51.
6. Post RM, Uhde TW. Are the psychotropic effects of carbamazepine in manic-depressive illness mediated through the limbic system? Psychiatr J Univ Ottawa 1985; 10:205-19.
7. Post RM, Weiss SRB. Behavioral pharmacology of carbamazepine: differential effects on kindling. Int J Clin Psychopharmacol (in press).
8. Post RM, Rubinow DR, Ballenger JC. Conditioning and sensitization in the longitudinal course of affective illness. Br J Psychiatry 1986; 149:191-201.
9. Post RM. Mechanisms of action of carbamazepine and related anticonvulsants in affective illness. In: Meltzer HY, ed. Psychopharmacology: a generation of progress. New York: Raven Press, 1987:567-76.
10. Post RM, Ballenger JC, Uhde TW, et al. Efficacy of carbamazepine in manic-depressive illness: implications for underlying mechanisms. In: Post RM, Ballenger JC, eds. Neurobiology of mood disorders. Baltimore: Williams and Wilkins, 1984:777-816.
11. Post RM. Time course of clinical effects of carbamazepine: implications for mechanisms of action. J Clin Psychiatry (in press).
12. Post RM, Uhde TW. Clinical approaches to treatment-resistant bipolar illness. In: Hales RE, Frances AJ, eds. American Psychiatric Association annual review. Vol 6. Washington, DC: American Psychiatric Press, 1987:125-50.
13. Ballenger JC, Post RM. Therapeutic effects of carbamazepine in affective illness: a preliminary report. Comm Psychopharmacol 1978; 2:159-75.
14. Post RM, Uhde TW, Roy-Byrne PP, et al. Correlates of antimanic responses to carbamazepine. Psychiatry Res 1987; 21:71-83.

15. Okuma T, Inanaga K, Otsuki S, et al. Comparison of the antimanic efficacy of carbamazepine and chlorpromazine: a double-blind controlled study. Psychopharmacology 1979; 66:211-7.
16. Klein E, Bental E, Lerer B, et al. Carbamazepine and haloperidol vs. placebo and haloperidol in excited psychoses. Arch Gen Psychiatry 1984; 41:165-70.
17. Müller AA, Stoll KD. Carbamazepine and oxcarbazepine in the treatment of manic syndromes: studies in Germany. In: Emrich HM, Okuma T, Müller AA, eds. Anticonvulsants in affective disorders. Amsterdam: Excerpta Medica, 1984:139-47.
18. Grossi E, Sacchetti E, Vita A, et al. Carbamazepine vs. chlorpromazine in mania: a double-blind trial. In: Emrich HM, Okuma T, Müller AA, eds. Anticonvulsants in affective disorders. Amsterdam: Excerpta Medica, 1984:177-87.
19. Emrich HM, Dose M, von Zerssen D. The use of sodium valproate, carbamazepine and oxcarbazepine in patients with affective disorders. J Affect Dis 1985; 8:243-50.
20. Lerer B, Moore N, Meyendorff E, et al. Carbamazepine versus lithium in mania: a double-blind study. J Clin Psychiatry 1987; 48:89-93.
21. Brown D, Silverstone T, Cookson J. Carbamazepine vs. haloperidol in acute mania. In: Abstracts. Society for Biological Psychiatry. Washington, DC: 1986:28. abstract #229.
22. Lenzi A, Lazzerini F, Grosse E, et al. Use of carbamazepine in acute psychosis: a controlled study. J Int Med Res 1986; 14:78-84.
23. Desai NG, Gangadhas BN, Channabasavanna SM, et al. Carbamazepine hastens therapeutic action of lithium in mania. In: Proceedings of the International Conference on New Directions in Affective Disorders. Jerusalem, April 5-9, 1987:97. abstract.
24. Brewerton T, Kramlinger KG, Post RM. Combination therapy with lithium and carbamazepine. In: Proceedings of the 2nd British Lithium Congress, Wolverhampton, England, September 6-9, 1987. Oxford: IRL Press Ltd. (in press).
25. Kramlinger KG, Post RM. The addition of lithium carbonate to carbamazepine: antidepressant efficacy in treatment-resistant depression. Arch Gen Psychiatry (in press).
26. Post RM, Berettini W, Uhde TW, et al. Selective response to the anticonvulsant carbamazepine in manic-depressive illness: a case study. J Clin Psychopharmacol 1984; 4:178-85.
27. Post RM, Uhde TW, Roy-Byrne PP, et al. Antidepressant effects of carbamazepine. Am J Psychiatry 1986; 143:29-34.
28. Katz MM, Koslow SH, Maas JW, et al. The timing, specificity and clinical prediction of tricyclic drug effects in depression. Psychol Med 1987; 17:297-309.
29. Post RM, Rubinow DR, Huggins T. Differential time course of antidepressant effects following sleep deprivation, ECT, and carbamazepine: clinical and theoretical implications. Psychiatry Res 1987; 22:11-9.
30. Roy-Byrne PP, Joffe R, Uhde TW, et al. Carbamazepine and thyroid function in affectively ill patients. Arch Gen Psychiatry 1984; 41:1150-3.
31. Post RM, Kramlinger KG, Joffe RT, et al. Effects of carbamazepine on thyroid function. Presented at the 140th annual meeting of the American Psychiatric Association, Chicago, May 9-15, 1987. In: Scientific proceedings of the American Psychiatric Association. 140:190. abstract #104D.
32. Tomson T. Interdosage fluctuations in plasma carbamazepine concentration determine intermittent side effects. Arch Neurol 1984; 41:830-4.
33. Post RM, Uhde TW, Ballenger JC, et al. CSF carbamazepine and its -10,11-epoxide metabolite in manic-depressive patients: relationship to clinical response. Arch Gen Psychiatry 1983; 40:673-6.
34. Post RM, Uhde TW, Ballenger JC, et al. Prophylactic efficacy of carbamazepine in manic-depressive illness. Am J Psychiatry 1983; 140:1602-4.
35. Okuma T, Inanaga K, Otsuki S, et al. A preliminary double-blind study of the efficacy of carbamazepine in prophylaxis of manic-depressive illness. Psychopharmacology 1981; 73:95-6.
36. Placidi GF, Lenzi A, Lazzerini F, et al. The comparative efficacy and safety of carbamazepine versus lithium: a randomized, double-blind 3-year trial in 83 patients. J Clin Psychiatry 1986; 47:490-4.

37. Okuma T, Kishimoto A, Inoue K, et al. Antimanic prophylactic effects of carbamazepine on manic-depressive psychosis. Folia Psychiatr Neurol Japon 1973; 27:283-97.
38. Kishimoto A, Okuma T. Antimanic and prophylactic effects of carbamazepine in affective disorders. In: Abstracts of the IVth World Congress of Biological Psychiatry. Philadelphia, Sept. 8-13, 1985:363. abstract #506.4.
39. Dunner DL, Fleiss JL, Fieve RR. Lithium carbonate prophylaxis failure. Br J Psychiatry 1976; 129:40-4.
40. Kukopulos A, Reginaldi D, Laddomada P, et al. Course of the manic-depressive cycle and changes caused by treatment. Pharmakopsychiatria 1980; 13:156-67.
41. Prien RF. Five-center study clarifies use of lithium, imipramine for recurrent affective disorders. Hosp Comm Psychiatry 1984; 35:1097-8.
42. Prien RF. Long-term maintenance drug treatment of mixed mania. In: Abstracts. Annual meeting of the American College of Neuropsychopharmacology. Maui, Dec. 9-13, 1985:19. abstract.
43. Secunda S, Kety M, Berman N, et al. Quantitative measures of clinical subtypes of mania. Clin Neuropharmacol 1984; 7:828.
44. Hanus H, Zapletálek M. The prophylactic lithium treatment in affective disorders and the possibilities of the outcome prediction. Sb Ved Pr Lek Fak Univ Karlovy. 1984; 27:5-75.
45. Himmelhoch JM. Sources of lithium resistance in mixed mania. In: Abstracts. Annual meeting of the American College of Neuropsychopharmacology. Maui, Dec. 9-13, 1985:18.
46. Joffe RT. Lithium and carbamazepine in manic-depressive illness: a clinical evaluation. Pharmacopsychiatry (in press).
47. Fawcett J, Kravitz HM. The long-term management of bipolar disorders with lithium, carbamazepine, and antidepressants. J Clin Psychiatry 1985; 46:58-60.
48. Fromm GH, Killian JM. Effect of some anticonvulsant drugs on the spinal trigeminal nucleus. Neurology 1967; 17:275-80.
49. Joffe RT, Post RM, Uhde TW. Lack of pharmacokinetic interaction of carbamazepine with tranylcypromine (letter). Arch Gen Psychiatry 1985; 42:738.
50. Post RM, Uhde TW. The use of carbamazepine in mania. In: Burrows GD, Norman TR, Davies D, eds. Antimanics, anticonvulsants, and other drugs in psychiatry (Drugs in psychiatry, Vol. 4). Amsterdam: Elsevier/North Holland Biomedical Press, 1988:49-79.
51. Post RM, Uhde TW. Refractory manias and alternatives to lithium treatment. In: Georgotas A, Cancro R, eds. Textbook of depression and mania. Amsterdam: Elsevier Science Publishing Co., 1988:410-38.
52. Post RM. Clinical approaches to the treatment-resistant manic-depressive patient: focus on the combination of carbamazepine and lithium. Presented at the Foundation for Advanced Education in the Sciences Symposium, Psychopharmacology in practice: clinical and research update, Bethesda, MD, October 10, 1987.
53. Post RM, Uhde TW. Anticonvulsants in non-epileptic psychosis. In: Bolwig TG, Trimble MR, eds. Epilepsy in psychiatry. Chichester: John Wiley and Sons, 1986:177-212.
54. Post RM, Uhde TW. Carbamazepine as a treatment for refractory depressive illness and rapidly cycling manic-depressive illness. In: Zohar J, Belmaker RH, eds. Special treatments for resistant depression. New York: Spectrum Press, 1986:281-7.
55. Masland RL. Carbamazepine: neurotoxicity. In: Woodbury DM, Penry JK, Pippenger CE, eds. Antiepileptic drugs. New York: Raven Press, 1982:521-31.
56. Philbert A, Dam M, Benke T, et al. The epileptic mother and her child. Wien Klin Wochenschr 1984; 96:786-90.
57. Kuoppala T, Tuimala R, Koskinen T. The effects of long-term anticonvulsant drug therapy on vitamin D metabolites and mineral homeostasis in pregnant epileptic women and their newborns. Ann Chir Gynaecol 1985; 197:37S-41S.
58. Dalessio DJ. Current concepts: seizure disorders and pregnancy. N Engl J Med 1985; 28:559-63.
59. Niebyl JR, Blake DA, Freeman JM, et al. Carbamazepine levels in pregnancy and lactation. Obstet Gynecol 1979; 53:139-40.

60. Nakane Y, Okuma T, Takahashi R, et al. Multi-institutional study on the teratogenicity and fetal toxicity of antiepileptic drugs: a report of a collaborative study group in Japan. Epilepsia 1980; 21:663-80.
61. Friis ML. Antiepileptic drugs and teratogenesis: how should patients, doctors and health authorities be counselled? Acta Neurol Scand 1983; 94:39S-43S.
62. Butler CD. Carbamazepine, seizure disorders, and pregnancy (letter). JAMA 1983; 250:3164.
63. Colo JA, Chavaz FDJ, Gutierrez JN. Tratamiento de la gestante epileptica con carbamacepina: informe preliminar. Ginecol Obstetr Mexicana 1984; 52:231-5.
64. Kelly TE. Teratogenicity of anticonvulsant drugs. I. Review of the literature. Am J Med Genet 1984; 19:413-34.
65. Lindhout D, Meinardi M, Barth PG. Hazards of fetal exposure to drug combinations. In: Janz D, Bossi L, Dam M, et al., eds. Epilepsy, pregnancy, and the child. New York: Raven Press, 1982:275-80.
66. Sullivan FM, McElhatton PR. A comparison of the antiepileptic drugs carbamazepine, clonazepam, ethosuximide, phenobarbital, phenytoin and primidone in mice. Toxicity Appl Pharmacol 1977; 40:365-78.
67. Wray SD, Hassell TM, Phillips C, et al. Preliminary study of the effects of carbamazepine in congenital orofacial defects in offspring of A/J mice. Epilepsia 1982; 23:101-10.
68. El-Sayed MG, Aly AE, Kadri M, et al. Comparative study on the teratogenicity of some antiepileptics in the rat. East Afr Med J 1983; 60:407-15.
69. Eluma FO, Sucheston ME, Hayes TG, et al. Teratogenic effects of dosage levels and time of administration of carbamazepine, sodium valproate, and diphenylhydantoin on craniofacial development in the CD-1 mouse fetus. J Craniofacial Genet Devel Biol 1984; 4:191-210.
70. Chatot CL, Klein NW, Clapper ML, et al. Human serum teratogenicity studied by rat embryo culture: epilepsy, anticonvulsant drugs, and nutrition. Epilepsia 1984; 25:205-16.
71. Bertollini R, Kallen B, Mastroiacovo P, et al. Anticonvulsant drugs in monotherapy: effect on the fetus. Eur J Epidemiol 1987; 3:164-71.
72. Joffe RT, Post RM, Roy-Byrne PP, et al. Hematological effects of carbamazepine in patients with affective illness. Am J Psychiatry 1985; 142:1196-9.
73. Brewerton TD. Lithium counteracts carbamazepine-induced leukopenia while increasing its therapeutic effect: a case report. Biol Psychiatry 1986; 21:677-85.
74. Kramlinger KG, Post RM. Addition of lithium carbonate to carbamazepine: hematologic, thyroid, and electrolyte effects. Submitted for publication.
75. Pisciotta AV. Carbamazepine: hematologic toxicity. In: Woodbury DM, Penry JK, Pippenger C, eds. Antiepileptic drugs. New York: Raven Press, 1982:533-41.
76. Pellock JM. Carbamazepine side effects in children and adults. Epilepsia 1987; 28:64S-70S.
77. Hart RG, Easton JD. Carbamazepine and hematological monitoring. Ann Neurol 1982; 11:309-12.
78. Trimble MR. The use of carbamazepine in psychiatric patients with seizure disorders. J Clin Psychiatry (Suppl) (in press).
79. Gold PW, Robertson GL, Ballenger JC, et al. Carbamazepine diminishes sensitivity to the plasma arginine vasopressin response to osmotic stimulation. J Clin Endocrinol Metab 1983; 57:952-6.
80. Dodrill C. Psychological effects of antiepileptic drugs. J Clin Psychiatry (Suppl) (in press).
81. Thompson P, Huppert F, Trimble M. Anticonvulsant drugs, cognitive function and memory. Acta Neurol Scand 1980; 62:75S-81S.
82. Kramlinger KG, Phillips KA, Post RM. Skin rash complicating carbamazepine treatment. Submitted for publication.
83. Okuma T. Therapeutic and prophylactic efficacy of carbamazepine in manic-depressive psychosis. In: Emrich HM, Okuma T, Müller AA, eds. Anticonvulsants in affective disorders. Amsterdam: Excerpta Medica, 1984:76-87.
84. Elphick M, Lyons F, Cowen PJ. Low tolerability of carbamazepine in psychiatric patients may limit its usefulness. Presented at the International Conference on New Directions in Affective Disorders, Jerusalem, April 5-9, 1987.
85. Vick NA. Suppression of carbamazepine-induced skin rash with prednisone (letter). N Engl J Med 1983; 309:1193-4.

86. Hampton KK, Bramley PN, Feeley M. Failure of prednisolone to suppress carbamazepine hypersensitivity (letter). N Engl J Med 1985; 313:959.
87. Squillace K, Post RM, Savard R, et al. Life charting of the longitudinal course of recurrent affective illness. In: Post RM, Ballenger JC, eds. Neurobiology of mood disorders. Baltimore: Williams & Wilkins, 1984:38-59.
88. Roy-Byrne PP, Post RM, Udhe TW, et al. The longitudinal course of recurrent affective illness: life chart data from research patients at the NIMH. Acta Psychiatr Scand 1985; 71:3S-34S.
89. Mander AJ. Is there a lithium withdrawal syndrome? Br J Psychiatry 1986; 149:498-501.
90. Bouman TK, Niemantsverdiet-van Kampen JG, Ormel J, et al. The effectiveness of lithium prophylaxis in bipolar and unipolar depressions and schizo-affective disorders. J Affect Dis 1986; 11:275-80.
91. Lenz G, Lourek A, Thau K, et al. Lithium-withdrawal study in schizoaffective patients. In: Proceedings of the 2nd British Lithium Congress, Wolverhampton, England, Sept. 6-9, 1987. Oxford: IRL Press Ltd. (in press).
92. Tondo L, Floris GF, Burrai C, et al. Lithium withdrawal; an outcome. In: Proceedings of the 2nd British Lithium Congress, Wolverhampton, England, Sept. 6-9, 1987. Oxford: IRL Press Ltd. (in press).
93. Greil W, Schmidt ST. Terminating lithium long-term treatment. In: Proceedings of the 2nd British Lithium Congress, Wolverhampton, England, Sept. 6-9, 1987. Oxford: IRL Press Ltd. (in press).
94. Chouinard G, Young S, Annable L. et al. Antimanic effects of clonazepam. Biol Psychiatry 1983; 18:451-66.
95. Lambert P-A. Acute and prophylactic therapies of patients with affective disorders using valpromide (dipropylacetamide). In: Emrich HM, Okuma T, Müller AA, eds. Anticonvulsants in affective disorders. Amsterdam: Excerpta Medica, 1984:33-44.
96. Emrich HM, Dose M, von Zerssen D. Action of sodium-valproate and of oxcarbazepine in patients with affective disorders. In: Emrich HM, Okuma T, Müller AA, eds. Anticonvulsants in affective disorders. Amsterdam: Excerpta Medica, 1984:45-55.
97. Puzynski S, Klosiewicz L. Valproic acid amide as a prophylactic agent in affective and schizoaffective disorders. In: Emrich HM, Okuma T, Müller AA, eds. Anticonvulsants in affective disorders. Amsterdam: Excerpta Medica, 1984:68-75.
98. Vencovsky E, Soucek K, Kabes J. Prophylactic effect of dipropylacetamide in patients with bipolar affective disorder—short communication. In: Emrich HM, Okuma T, Müller AA, eds. Anticonvulsants in affective disorders. Amsterdam: Excerpta Medica, 1984:66-7.
99. Brennan MJW, Sandyk R, Borsook D. Use of sodium-valproate in the management of affective disorders: basic and clinical aspects. In: Emrich HM, Okuma T, Müller AA, eds. Anticonvulsants in affective disorders. Amsterdam: Excerpta Medica, 1984:56-65.
100. Prasad AJ. The role of sodium valproate as an anti-manic agent. Pharmatherapeutica 1984; 4:6-8.
101. McElroy SL, Keck PE, Jr, Pope HG, Jr. Sodium valproate: its use in primary psychiatric disorders. J Clin Psychopharmacol 1987; 7:16-24.
102. Inoue H, Hazama H, Hamazoe K, et al. Antipsychotic and prophylactic effects of acetazolamide (Diamox) on atypical psychosis. Folia Psychiatr Neurol Japon 1984; 38:425-36.
103. Weiss SRB, Post RM, Patel J, et al. Differential mediation of the anticonvulsant effects of carbamazepine and diazepam. Life Sci 1985; 36:2413-9.
104. Weiss SRB, Post RM, Marangos PJ, et al. Peripheral-type benzodiazepines: behavorial effects and interactions with the anticonvulsant effects of carbamazepine. In: Wada J, ed. Kindling III. New York: Raven Press, 1986:375-91.
105. Post RM, Putman F, Uhde TW, et al. ECT as an anticonvulsant: implications for its mechanism of action in affective illness. Ann NY Acad Sci 1986; 462:376-88.
106. Dubovsky SL, Franks RD, Allen S, et al. Calcium antagonists in mania: a double-blind study of verapamil. Psychiatry Res 1986; 18:309-20.

CHAPTER 2

Valproate in Primary Psychiatric Disorders: Literature Review and Clinical Experience in a Private Psychiatric Hospital

Susan L. McElroy, M.D. *Paul E. Keck, Jr., M.D.*
Harrison G. Pope, Jr., M.D. *James I. Hudson, M.D.*
Belmont, Massachusetts

INTRODUCTION

Valproate, a GABAergic anticonvulsant effective in primary generalized and partial epilepsies, is rarely used in the United States in the treatment of primary psychiatric disorders. However, a substantial European literature dating back to the 1960's, together with several recent American studies, has suggested a role for valproate in the treatment of major affective disorder, particularly bipolar and schizoaffective disorder, and possibly schizophrenia and panic disorder.[1-30] It should be noted that some of these studies involved valpromide (a drug not available in the United States) which is quickly and almost completely metabolized into valproate *in vivo*.[31,32] Throughout this chapter the term "valproate" will be used to denote both drugs. However, some investigators, particularly in France, have argued that valpromide may have effects beyond those of its metabolite. Hence studies using valpromide may not be strictly comparable to those using valproate. This issue is addressed in greater detail later in this chapter.

Valproic acid (n-dipropylacetic acid) is a simple branched chain carboxylic acid and is therefore chemically quite different from other anticonvulsants.[33,34] The drug is commercially available in three preparations: as valproic acid (available in 250 mg capsules), as sodium valproate (available as 250 mg per 5 ml of syrup), and as the enteric-coated divalproex sodium, a stable coordination compound containing equal proportions of valproic acid and sodium valproate (available in 250 mg and 500 mg capsules). Divalproex sodium has been reported to cause a lower incidence of gastrointestinal side effects when compared with valproic acid.[35] There are only minor differences in the pharmacokinetics of these preparations, and the common compound in plasma is valproic acid.

Valproate is rapidly and nearly completely absorbed after ingestion. Peak serum concentrations occur in one to four hours, although absorption may be delayed approximately two hours if the drug is taken with food or if the enteric-coated preparation is administered. Valproate is rapidly distributed (reaching the central nervous system within minutes of administration) and highly bound (90%) to plasma proteins, mainly albumin. Concentrations in cerebrospinal fluid suggest equilibration with free drug in the plasma.

The half-life of valproate is six to 16 hours. Concomitant administration of hepatic enzyme-inducing drugs such as phenytoin, phenobarbital, or carbamazepine shortens valproate's half-life. Less than 3% of valproate is excreted unchanged in the urine or feces. Most of the drug is metabolized by the liver where it undergoes conjugation (primarily) as well as beta, omega, and omega-1 oxidation to a large number of metabolites, some of which (notably 2-propyl-2-pentanoic acid and 2-propyl-3-oxo-pentanoic acid) have anticonvulsant activity. In contrast to phenytoin, phenobarbital, and carbamazepine, valproate does not induce its own metabolism or hepatic metabolism in general. Rather the drug appears to act as a nonspecific inhibitor of the metabolism of other drugs and has been reported to increase plasma levels of phenobarbital and ethosuximide. The interactions between valproate and phenytoin and valproate and carbamazepine appear to be more complex. Because valproate does not induce hepatic enzymes, it can be used by women concurrently taking birth control pills.

Valproate is an effective anticonvulsant with antiepileptic activity in a wide variety of seizure types.[33, 34, 36] At present, it is approved by the United States Food and Drug Administration for use in the treatment of simple and complex absence seizures. In addition, valproate is effective in other primary generalized epilepsies including tonic-clonic and myoclonic seizures as well as in secondarily generalized convulsions. The drug has also been reported to be useful in the treatment of infantile spasms, the prophylaxis of febrile convulsions and post-traumatic epilepsy, and the treatment of status epilepticus refractory to usual therapy. It is the treatment of choice for photosensitive epilepsy. Valproate also has some efficacy in complex partial seizures, although not as much as in primary generalized epilepsies. Complex partial seizures, however, are generally more resistant to anticonvulsant treatment.

The plasma concentration of valproate apparently required for anticonvulsant effects is approximately 50 μg/ml to 100 μg/ml, although the correlation between this concentration range and response is poor.[33,34] Some patients exhibit an anticonvulsant response with plasma levels below this range while others[37] respond only with levels well above 100 μg/ml. However, it does seem clear that serum concentrations greater than 50 μg/ml are associated with better clinical effect compared with lower concentrations. Interestingly, 50 μg/ml is the approximate concentration at which the binding sites on plasma albumin start to become saturated. Thus there appears to be a response threshold at 50 μg/ml.[38]

The mechanism of valproate's anticonvulsant action is unknown but is presumed to be related to the drug's GABAergic effects. Gamma-aminobutyric acid (GABA) is an inhibitory amino acid neurotransmitter found throughout the mammalian central nervous system (CNS). GABA and GABAmimetics are anticonvulsant while agents that reduce or antagonize GABA are proconvulsant. As will be discussed later in this chapter, valproate elevates or facilitates GABA within the brain by inhibiting its catabolism, activating its synthesis, and directly enhancing its postsynaptic effects. Other potential mechanisms of valproate's antiepileptic efficacy include direct effects on neuronal membranes, reduction of excitatory transmission by aspartate, and suppression of kindling. For a thorough discussion of valproate's pharmacokinetics, mechanism of action, therapeutic indications, and side effects, the reader is referred to the exhaustive review of Rimmer and Richens.[34] The side effects of valproate will be discussed in greater detail at the end of this chapter.

VALPROATE IN PRIMARY PSYCHIATRIC DISORDERS: A REVIEW OF THE LITERATURE

Of the available studies of valproate in primary psychiatric disorders, 19 reports (several of which represent updates of series published earlier) provide sufficient data for analysis (Table 1). Ten studies examined valproate in bipolar or schizoaffective disorder.[6,7,12-14,17,19-22] In these studies 280 patients received the drug on an open basis and 14 under blind and placebo-controlled conditions. At least one third of the patients studied had failed or were unable to tolerate previous treatment with lithium salts, neuroleptics, or other drugs and combinations. Nevertheless, 158 (56%) patients of the total group displayed significant improvement with valproate and some of these patients were maintained on the drug over follow-up periods ranging from several months to many years. Few patients, however, received valproate alone. Many received either concurrent prophylactic lithium or temporary treatment with concomitant antidepressants or neuroleptics during relapses of depression or mania.In the three double-blind trials, 10 (72%) of 14 acutely manic patients displayed a marked response to valproate alone (Table 2).[12,13,19]

This literature therefore suggests that valproate may be an effective treatment for bipolar and perhaps schizoaffective disorder, both acutely and as a prophylactic agent. Several other impressions can be drawn from the data. First, valproate may be more effective for mania than depression. In the only study which examined large separate cohorts of patients with manic and major depressive syndromes (in this instance using valpromide), 58 (41%) of 141 manic patients showed a significant response compared to 26 (25%) of 103 depressed patients.[6] Second, several authors comment that valproate may be more effective in the prophylaxis of mania than depression, although this impression is based only on uncontrolled or anecdotal observations.[6,12,14] Third, these same investigators note anecdotally that valproate appears to act synergistically with lithium in the prophylactic treatment of some bipolar and schizoaffective patients.[6,12] While this observation remains impressionistic, there appears to be no known contraindication to administration of the drugs together over extended periods of time, and most patients were found to tolerate the combination well.

The eight available studies of valproate in schizophrenia (involving 103 patients) are less compelling.[22-29] Two of the studies, designed to examine the effect of valproate on tardive dyskinesia, incidentally found significant decreases in psychiatric symptoms.[23,24] A third found decreases in paranoid ideation and hallucinations in seven out of 10 patients.[26] A fourth reported improvement in BPRS scores in five out of 14 patients, while in five other patients the score deteriorated. For the total sample of patients, the mean change in BPRS scores was nonsignificant.[27] In the other four studies, three of which used operational criteria for the diagnosis of schizophrenia, valproate appeared to be either ineffective or even deleterious.[22,25,28,29] In all, approximately 32 (31%) of the 103 schizophrenic patients showed a response to valproate. However, since none of the three positive studies used specific diagnostic criteria for schizophrenia, one cannot exclude the possibility that the optimistic results of these three studies may

TABLE 1. Studies of valproate (and valpromide) in psychiatric disorders

Study	Patient population (diagnostic criteria)	Design	Dosage (mg/day);[a] other medications	Plasma levels (μg/ml)	Response
Lambert[6]	(1) 141 bipolar (2) 103 depressed (including 18 schizoaffective) (unspecified)	Open trial, less than 6-163 month follow-up	900-1,800*	NR	(1) 13/141 marked response 45/141 partial response (2) 2/103 marked response 23/103 partial response
Semadeni[7]	32 bipolar, 16/32 lithium-refractory (unspecified)	Open trial, 6-48 month follow-up	900-2,400;* intermittent neuroleptics and antidepressants in 66%	NR	16/32 no relapses, euthymia 7/32 marked improvement 3/32 slight response 6/32 no response
Emrich et al.[12]	(1) 5 bipolar, acutely manic (2) 12 lithium-refractory bipolar schizoaffective (ICD)	(1) Double-blind ABA placebo-controlled trial (2) Open trial, 18-78 month follow-up	(1) 1,800-3,800 (2) NR; eleven with low-dose lithium	50-102 NR	(1) 4/5 marked response 1/5 no response (2) 10/12 no recurrence of affective episodes
Brennan et al.[13]	(1) 8 bipolar, acutely manic (2) 4 lithium-refractory bipolar (DSM-III)	(1) Double-blind ABA placebo-controlled trial (2) Open trial, 9-33 month follow-up	(1) 900-3,600 (2) 900-1,500	NR	(1) 6/8 marked response 2/8 no response (2) 4/4 no recurrence of affective episodes
Puzynski and Klosiewicz[14]	10 bipolar; 5 schizoaffective; 12/15 lithium-refractory (DSM-III)	Open trial, 26-51 month follow-up	900-1,800;* intermittent neuroleptics and tricyclics in all patients	NR	Number of affective episodes decreased by 46%; response in mania better than in depression
Vencovsky et al.[17]	27 bipolar (unspecified)	Open trial, 6-26 month follow-up	900*	NR	Not quantitatively documented, but indicated that drug effective in 25 patients; the other 2 patients dropped out secondary to side effects
Post et al.[19]	1 bipolar, acutely manic (unspecified)	Double-blind crossover to placebo, carbamazepine, phenytoin, and valproate; 30-day trials	2,500	89	No response to placebo, phenytoin, or valproate; marked response to carbamazepine
Prasad[20]	8 lithium- and neuroleptic-refractory bipolar, acutely manic (Feighner et al.)	Open trial, 6 weeks	800-1,500	NR	5/7 definite response; 1 patient dropped out after two weeks (reason not documented)
Lovett et al.[21]	2 lithium-refractory bipolar (unspecified)	Open trial, 24-month follow-up	NR; one with lithium	350-700 μmol/l	1/2 (valproate alone) complete remission 1/2 (with lithium) poor response

TABLE 1. Continued

McElroy et al.[22]	(1) 25 lithium-refractory bipolar and schizoaffective (2) 4 neuroleptic-refractory schizophrenic (3) 2 depressed (DSM-III)	Open trial, 2 weeks minimum	750-3,000; majority with lithium and/or neuroleptic	41-120	(1) 6/25 marked response 9/25 moderate response (2) 4/4 no response (3) 2/2 no response
Linnoila et al.[23]	32 chronic psychiatric with tardive dyskinesia (unspecified)	Double-blind crossover, 14 days	900; maintenance neuroleptics	NR	14/32 had decreased BPRS on valproate vs. placebo ($p = .01$) 4/32 had increased BPRS scores
Nagao et al.[24]	7 schizophrenic with tardive dyskinesia (unspecified)	Open trial, 3 weeks	600; maintenance medications (unspecified)	NR	BPRS cumulative scores decreased by 2.5 ($p = .025$)
Lautin et al.[25]	8 schizophrenic (RDC)	Open trial, 2-31 days	750-3,000; neuroleptics discontinued 3-12 days earlier	53-88	5/18 had qualitative worsening of symptoms 1/8 had minimal response
Gundurewa et al.[26]	10 schizophrenic (unspecified)	Open trial	To 2,100	NR	Unquantitated decrease in paranoid ideation and hallucinations in 7/10 completing trial
Kausen et al.[27]	14 schizophrenic (unspecified)	Open trial, 3 months	900; clozapine	NR	5/14 improved 5/14 deteriorated; overall, no significant changes on BPRS before and after valproate
Ko et al.[28]	6 schizophrenic (RDC)	Double-blind controlled trial, 4 weeks	1,600-2,400; maintenance neuroleptics	NR	No significant change in BPRS scores
Fisk and York[29]	22 chronic psychotic with tardive dyskinesia (unspecified)	Double-blind placebo-controlled trial, 12 weeks	1,200-1,500; neuroleptics	NR	3/22 improved; overall, no significant change
Primeau et al.[30]	10 panic disorder (DSM-III)	Open trial, 7 weeks	NR	NR	Significant improvement on CGI of panic severity, Hamilton Anxiety Scale, and panic inventory self-ratings

[a] *Asterisk denotes use of valpromide. Otherwise, valproate was used.*
NR–Not reported.

TABLE 2. Controlled studies of valproate in acutely manic patients

Investigators	Patient population	Valproate dosage mg/day	Plasma levels (μg/ml)	Response
Emrich et al.[12]	5 bipolar, acutely manic	1,800-3,800	50-102	4/5 marked response 1/5 no response
Brennan et al.[13]	8 bipolar, acutely manic	900-3,600	NR	6/8 marked response 2/8 no response
Post et al.[19]	1 bipolar, acutely manic	2,500	89	1/1 no response
Total				10/14 marked response (72%)

have been partially due to the inclusion of patients with affective or neuropsychiatric syndromes.

Recently, a report appeared describing the use of valproate in 10 outpatients with panic disorder, diagnosed by DSM-III criteria, on an open-label basis.[30] After seven weeks of treatment significant improvement was found on the Clinical Global Impression Scale (CGI) of panic severity ($p<.001$), the Hamilton Rating Scale for Anxiety ($p<.001$), and the panic inventory self ratings of the SCL-90 ($p<.05$). Six (60%) of the 10 patients demonstrated at least moderate improvement. Response occurred rapidly over the first week of treatment, and then more gradually during the last six weeks of the trial.

It is encouraging that none of the above studies reported serious adverse effects with valproate. Gastrointestinal complaints were noted most frequently. Lethargy, increased serum levels of hepatic transaminases, and mild alopecia were found less frequently. In the total group of patients, there were no reports of acute hemorrhagic pancreatitis, severe hepatic dysfunction, or fatal hepatic necrosis—serious problems rarely associated with valproate.

At this point, it should again be noted that some of the above studies utilized the drug valpromide rather than valproic acid. Valpromide, created by the amidification of the carboxyl group of valproic acid, has a shorter half-life, a higher clearance value, and a larger volume of distribution than valproic acid.[31] Because valpromide is rapidly and nearly completely biotransformed into valproic acid in humans after oral or intravenous administration, some investigators have concluded that valpromide is simply the "pro-drug" of valproic acid;[31,32] this would seem consistent with the general impression, upon reviewing studies of these drugs in psychiatric patients, that they are approximately equally effective. However, controversy exists as to whether valpromide may have therapeutic benefits, particularly psychotropic effects, beyond those of its principal metabolite. In particular, French investigators have suggested that valpromide may be more effective than valproic acid in psychiatric disorders in general and bipolar disorder in particular.[6] If in fact valpromide does possess greater psychotropic efficacy, this may be due to: (1) its possessing a nitrogen-containing amide group rather than a free carboxyl group; (2) the fact that small amounts of unchanged valpromide cross the blood-brain barrier; and (3) the ratio of cerebrospinal fluid levels to plasma levels being higher for valpromide than valproic acid.[6] However, we have not been able to locate any human studies directly comparing the two drugs. Therefore, while it must be acknowledged that controversy exists over the relative psychotropic efficacies of these two agents, it is certainly true that valpromide is nearly completely transformed into valproic acid, that valpromide therefore possesses the pharmacologic actions of valproic acid, and that valproic acid itself appears to have significant psychotherapeutic effects.

In summary, the above literature suggests that valproate may be effective in the treatment of bipolar and schizoaffective disorder. The drug may be particularly beneficial in the short-term and maintenance treatment of mania, where it can be used alone or in combination with neuroleptics and/or lithium salts. In such patients, valproate may exert a synergistic effect with lithium. Valproate's efficacy in schizophrenia —especially schizophrenia defined by rigorous diagnostic criteria—remains unproved and poorly supported by the above studies. However, preliminary data suggest that it may be a promising treatment for panic disorder. Finally, valproate appears to be well tolerated and safe, with no instances of fatal hepatic dysfunction yet reported in psychiatric patients.

Despite the encouraging findings of these studies, it should be noted that most have serious methodological flaws which limit interpretation of their data. Most studies were nonblind; most failed to provide specific inclusion and exclusion criteria; many used unspecified diagnostic criteria; none documented neurological status; and the majority did not record serum valproate levels. Therefore, the conclusions drawn from these studies must be considered impressionistic and in need of verification by double-blind placebo-controlled investigations.

EXPERIENCE WITH VALPROATE AT McLEAN HOSPITAL

To augment the clinical data on valproate in psychiatric disorders, while addressing some of the above methodological issues, we retrospectively analyzed the effects of valproate in consecutive patients who received the drug for a primary psychiatric disorder at our center over a five-and-one-half-year period between August, 1981 and February, 1987. We paid particular attention to specific diagnostic and exclusion criteria and documentation of adequacy of valproate trials. Two cohorts were identified. The first included those 36 patients in the entire hospital who received the drug for a primary psychiatric disorder between August, 1981 and August, 1985.[22] The second group, consisting of 41 patients, was restricted to three of the hospital's 12 inpatient units for the period from September, 1985 through February, 1987.[39] The larger number of cases in the second cohort, although it was drawn from only a portion of the hospital and for a shorter time period, indicates an increase in the use of valproate at our center.

Full details of the methods are presented in our earlier reports.[22,39,40] Briefly, we included all patients who received valproate except those who displayed: (1) a concurrent neurologic disorder (e.g. a seizure disorder of any kind, demyelinating disease, cerebrovascular disease, or structural brain damage from trauma); (2) a focally abnormal neurological examination (i.e. a hemiparesis or a Babinski reflex); (3) paroxysmal electroencephalographic (EEG) activity; or (4) gross structural abnormalities on brain computerized tomography (CT) scan. Patients were not excluded if they displayed only "soft" neurologic signs, nonparoxysmal EEG abnormalities, or nonspecific CT scan abnormalities. Patients were excluded if valproate was begun within four weeks before or after any other major changes in their medication regimens. Patients were also excluded if the valproate trial was inadequate (defined as maximum plasma levels of less than 50 μg/ml or duration less than 14 days).

Thirty-four patients were excluded on the basis on these criteria: 12 had seizure disorders or paroxysmal EEG activity; nine received inadequate trials; seven displayed more than "soft" neurological abnormalities (two with structural brain damage secondary to trauma, one with multiple sclerosis, one who had suffered a left hemispheric stroke, one with mental retardation secondary to anoxia at birth, one with pervasive developmental disorder, and one with communicating hydrocephalus); three were begun on valproate prior to hospitalization; two were started on valproate and another psychotropic simultaneously; and one began to improve prior to valproate administration. Finally, one other patient was excluded because records were not available for analysis. Of note, two of the excluded patients were apparent valproate responders: one schizoaffective patient (manic phase), excluded because of an inadequate trial, showed a moderate response with a maximum serum valproate level of 49 μg/ml; the second, a rapid-cycling bipolar patient in the depressed phase, in whom valproate and doxepin were begun simultaneously, demonstrated a marked response, and has remained euthymic for nine months on valproate and lithium without doxepin.[41]

Seventy-three remaining cases qualified for analysis. (Although the two cohorts originally totalled 77 cases, we later excluded four cases from the first cohort because they did not meet the somewhat stricter inclusion and exclusion criteria developed for the second cohort [see reports for details]).[22,39,40] For all cases we recorded, from the chart, the patient's age, sex, psychiatric diagnosis, current affective and psychotic symptoms, duration of illness, previous and concurrent medications, neurologic findings, EEG results, brain CT scan findings, history of head trauma prior to onset of psychiatric illness, valproate dose, maximum level, trial duration, response, and side effects. For cases from the first cohort, family history of affective and neurologic disorder was also recorded. Diagnoses recorded were those made by the administrative ward psychiatrist according to DSM-III criteria.[42] Response was rated using the following scale: 0 = no response; 1 = minimal improvement such that the patient had slight symptomatic improvement, but not enough to warrant continued treatment with valproate; 2 = moderate improvement, such that the patient had significant reduction of symptoms, allowing clearly improved social or vocational functioning; and 3 = marked improvement, with virtual or complete remission of symptoms. The baseline for rating improvement was defined as the patient's condition immediately prior to starting valproate, and response was scored as the difference between baseline and the maximum level of functioning attained within the four-week period after therapeutic valproate levels (50 μg/ml to 100 μg/ml) were documented. The rater was nonblind to diagnosis when rating response. The following is a summary of the most important findings.

All 73 inpatients were symptomatic and highly impaired at the time of valproate administration. In the majority (67 [92%] out of 73), valproate was added to a preexisting, stable medical regimen. In all cases, valproate was added because disabling psychiatric symptoms had proven refractory or only partially responsive to more conventional somatic treatments, including lithium salts, neuroleptics, antidepressants, carbamazepine, various combinations of these drugs, or ECT. Nonetheless, 33 (45%) of the 73 patients showed a moderate or marked response to valproate. Patients who responded tended to do so within one to two weeks, and often within several days, of achieving a serum valproate level greater than or equal to 50 μg/ml.

Although there were no consistent criteria for valproate administration, except for the presence of persistent, severe psychiatric symptoms, the drug was most commonly used in bipolar and schizoaffective patients in the manic, hypomanic, or mixed phase of their illness. Of the 73 patients treated with valproate, 56 (60%) displayed manic symptoms. Thirty-six (64%) of these were bipolar and 20 (36%) schizoaffective.

TABLE 3. Response of various diagnostic groups to valproate (see reference 39)

	Total N	Response (%)			
		None	Minimal	Moderate	Marked
FIRST COHORT (1981-1985)	36				
Bipolar disorder, manic or mixed	17	4 (24)	2 (12)	5 (29)	6 (35)
Schizoaffective disorder, manic or mixed	9	5 (56)	0	4 (44)	0
Major depression	2	2 (100)	0	0	0
Schizophrenia	4	4 (100)	0	0	0
Panic disorder	1	0	0	0	1 (100)
Obsessive compulsive disorder	1	1 (100)	0	0	0
Borderline personality disorder	2	2 (100)	0	0	0
SECOND COHORT (1985-1987)	41				
Bipolar disorder, manic, hypomanic, or mixed	21	2 (10)	5 (24)	7 (33)	7 (33)
Schizoaffective disorder, manic or mixed	11	5 (45)	1 (9)	5 (45)	0
Bipolar disorder, depressed	1	1 (100)	0	0	0
Schizoaffective disorder, depressed	2	1 (50)	1 (50)	0	0
Schizophrenia	5	4 (80)	1 (20)	0	0
Obsessive compulsive disorder	1	1 (100)	0	0	0
COMBINED COHORTS[a]	73				
Bipolar disorder, manic, hypomanic, or mixed	36	5 (14)	7 (19)	11 (31)	13 (36)
Schizoaffective disorder, manic or mixed	20	10 (50)	1 (5)	9 (45)	0
All depression (2 major depression; 1 bipolar, depressed; and 2 schizoaffective, depressed)	5	4 (80)	1 (20)	0	0
Schizophrenia	8	7 (88)	1 (13)	0	0
All other cases	4	4 (100)	0	0	0

[a] *Four patients from the first cohort have been excluded from the combined cohort because of inadequate valproate trials (valproate levels not drawn or subtherapeutic), including one responder with panic disorder, one responder with bipolar disorder, manic phase, one nonresponder with bipolar disorder, manic phase, and one nonresponder with schizophrenia.*

Table 3 displays the various diagnoses of patients receiving valproate as well as the responses of different diagnostic groups to the drug for both the 1981-1985 cohort and the 1985-1987 cohort. For each diagnostic category, response rates were remarkably similar between the two cohorts; hence the cohorts were combined for subsequent analysis. (In combining the cohorts, as noted earlier, we excluded four patients from the first cohort because they did not meet the revised exclusion criteria used for the second cohort. See Table 3 for details.)

The best results were observed in bipolar patients in the manic, hypomanic, or mixed phase of their illness. Bipolar schizoaffective patients also showed some response, though not as robust as that of the "pure" bipolars. More specifically, all 33 responders were among the 56 patients with bipolar or schizoaffective disorder who displayed a manic, hypomanic, or mixed affective syndrome at the time of valproate administration. Twenty-four (67%) of 36 bipolar (manic or mixed) patients responded (i.e. were scored as "2" or "3"); and nine (45%) of 20 schizoaffective patients responded. The one patient with panic disorder in the original cohort of 36, but excluded from the final cohort of 73 for the above mentioned reasons, also displayed a complete response to valproate (see Chapter 10 in this volume for details). However, valproate did not appear effective in other psychiatric disorders. Of eight patients with schizophrenia, five with depression (one with bipolar depression, two with schizoaffective depression, and two with major depression with psychotic features), two with obsessive compulsive disorder, and two with borderline personality disorder, none responded. Since valproate appeared to be effective primarily in bipolar and schizoaffective patients in the manic phase of their illness, we further analyzed this group to see which variables (in addition to the presence of manic symptoms) predicted response to valproate.

TABLE 4. Response to valproate by presence of nonparoxysmal EEG abnormalities (see reference 39)

Response to VPA	Total N receiving an EEG	Nonparoxysmal EEG abnormalities Present	Nonparoxysmal EEG abnormalities Absent
Moderate or marked	27	15[a]	12
None or minimal	22	5[b]	17

Difference significant at p = .04 by Fisher's exact test, two-tailed.

[a] *Includes seven cases with localized slowing, four with generalized slowing, three with brief bursts of higher voltage sharp and slow activity, and one with intermittent background slowing.*

[b] *Includes one case with localized slowing, two with intermittent background slowing, one with persistent background slowing, and one with disorganization of background and generalized slowing.*

Age, sex, duration of illness, presence or absence of psychotic symptoms, family history of affective or neurological disorder, neurologic soft signs, and nonspecific brain CT scan abnormalities were not associated with response. However, the presence or nonparoxysmal EEG abnormalities showed a modest but significant association ($p = .04$ by Fisher's exact test, two-tailed) with response to valproate (Table 4). Eight (14%) of the 56 bipolar and schizoaffective patients with manic symptoms had a history of closed head trauma prior to onset of psychiatric illness. Although all eight of these patients responded inadequately to lithium salts and neuroleptics, seven (88%) responded when valproate was added to their regimens. In contrast, 22 (46%) of the 48 remaining patients (those without histories of head injury) responded to the drug—a difference in response rates which approaches statistical significance ($p = .065$ by Fisher's exact test, two-tailed).[40] Interestingly, five (14%) of the 37 bipolar patients were rapid cyclers, experiencing four or more affective episodes per year. All five of these patients responded to valproate. (The case of one has been previously reported in detail.[43]) One additional rapid cycler, excluded from the cohort of 73 because of the concurrent initiation of valproate and doxepin, as mentioned earlier, also showed a significant response to the drug. On follow-up of three to 25 months, all six patients remained significantly improved on valproate (two on valproate alone, one requiring intermittent addition of neuroleptic during hypomanic episodes, two on valproate and lithium, and one on valproate, lithium, and neuroleptic). For a more detailed discussion of these cases, the reader is referred to our earlier reports[41,43] and to Chapter 7 in this volume. Finally, it is interesting to note that three of the patients with bipolar disorder (including one rapid cycler) had concurrent bulimia. All three patients displayed marked improvement in their affective and bulimic symptoms in response to valproate. These patients are discussed in greater detail in earlier reports[22,41,43] and in Chapter 9 of this volume.

Maximum valproate doses ranged from 750 mg/day to 3,000 mg/day, and peak serum levels were between 51 μg/ml and 120 μg/ml. The median serum valproate concentrations in responders (75 μg/ml) and nonresponders (73 μg/ml) did not differ significantly. Patients responding generally did so within one to two weeks of achieving a level of 50 μg/ml or greater. The majority of patients tolerated the drug well, most without side effects. Reported side effects included five cases of sedation, five complaints of nausea or abdominal cramps, and one instance each of flushing, diarrhea, worsening of tardive dyskinesia, and ataxia with dysarthria—the latter occurring when valproate was added to carbamazepine. Additionally, there were five cases of serum transaminase elevations (SGOT above the normal range of 0 to 41 units)—to 47, 48, 74, 132, and 318 units. In the first three cases, SGOT normalized despite valproate continuation, and in the latter two cases, normalized upon discontinuation of the drug. Among the patients who were excluded for inadequate trials, however, three had valproate prematurely discontinued because of intolerable side effects, including one instance of severe nausea (on valproic acid) and two cases of confusion. (In one of these cases valproate was added to lithium and carbamazepine and in the other valproate was added to perphenazine and benztropine.) In all three cases, symptoms promptly resolved upon discontinuation of valproate.

Although these results appear consistent with the findings of the previous literature, it must be noted that the present study is subject to many of the same methodologic limitations as the earlier studies, in that data were obtained nonblindly and retrospectively, based on open clinical trials in patients who were not selected in a random manner. In addition, valproate was usually added to an existing (though at best only partially effective) drug regimen. With respect to our cohort, although patients with diagnosed seizure disorders, other neurologic disorders, or paroxysmal EEG activity were carefully excluded, the possibility remains that some of the valproate responders might have had seizure disorders that were undiagnosed. We have discussed each of these limitations in detail in our earlier report.[22]

However, even when all of these considerations are taken into account, the moderate to marked response observed in 33 (59%) of 56 patients in the manic phase of bipolar and schizoaffective disorder, many of them chronic and treatment-refractory, seems difficult to dismiss entirely as an artifact of methodology.

DISCUSSION

A growing literature suggests that valproate may be effective in some psychiatric disorders, particularly bipolar and schizoaffective disorder, even in cases refractory to previous medications. To augment this data, we examined two cohorts of patients, comprising 73 cases. The findings in our two cohorts were strikingly similar to those reported in other centers.

Examining our combined cohort of 73 patients, the principal feature that predicted response to valproate was the presence of manic symptoms: both bipolar and schizoaffective patients with manic, hypomanic, or mixed states responded better than depressed or schizophrenic patients. Our findings therefore appear consistent with the impression from the previous literature that valproate may be effective in bipolar and schizoaffective disorder, but less effective in schizophrenia.

Within our group of 73 patients, there was a slight, but significant association ($p = .04$) between response to valproate and the presence of nonparoxysmal EEG abnormalities. Rapid-cycling illness and to a lesser extent, history of closed head trauma, also appeared to be associated with valproate response. Other variables, including age, sex, duration of illness, family history of affective or neurologic disorder, presence or absence of psychotic symptoms, and presence of neurologic "soft" signs or CT scan abnormalities, showed no significant association with valproate response. The majority of our patients were not followed up, and it is therefore impossible for us to comment on the efficacy of valproate as a prophylactic agent.

The finding that valproate may be effective in mania raises the possibility that the inhibitory neurotransmitter gamma-aminobutyric acid (GABA) may be important in the pathophysiology of bipolar disorder. Although the mechanism of valproate's anticonvulsant activity has not been completely elucidated, it has been attributed to the drug's ability to enhance GABAergic transmission within the CNS. Studies indicate that valproate either increases the levels of or potentiates the action of GABA at both types of postsynaptic GABA receptors in the brain ($GABA_A$ and $GABA_B$) by inhibiting GABA catabolism, probably by directly enhancing GABA's inhibitory effect, and possibly by increasing GABA synthesis and release.[44,45] Also, accumulating evidence from animal and human studies suggests a role for GABA in major affective disorder.[8,44,45] For instance, GABAmimetic agents have been shown to induce behavioral effects similar to those of antidepressant medications in animal models of depression, and low levels of GABA have been reported in the cerebrospinal fluid and plasma of depressed patients.[44,45] Agents apparently useful in the treatment of mania (in addition to valproate), including lithium salts, carbamazepine, and clonazepam, affect GABAergic transmission; the anticonvulsant progabide (a direct $GABA_A$ and $GABA_B$ agonist) may have antidepressant properties; and the discontinuation of baclofen (a direct GABA agonist with specificity for the B receptor) has been associated with induction of mania.[44-46] Furthermore, antidepressants and ECT (which is effective in mania as well as depression) have been found to alter $GABA_B$ receptors, which, in turn, modulate monoaminergic transmission.[44,45]

Evidence also exists to suggest that abnormalities in central noradrenergic activity may be important in the etiology of bipolar disorder.[47,48] That GABA neurons may modulate noradrenergic activity is suggested by the finding that GABA agonists (such as progabide and fengabine) increase norepinephrine turnover.[45]

In addition, it should be noted that patients with bipolar disorder appear to have a desynchronization of circadian rhythms.[13] These rhythms are probably regulated by the suprachiasmatic nucleus of the hypothalamus, an area richly innervated by GABAergic neurons.[49] It has therefore been speculated by Brennan and colleagues that valproate exerts its apparent mood-stabilizing effect by potentiation of GABAergic transmission within the suprachiasmatic nucleus of the hypothalamus.[13] Consistent with this hypothesis is Berrettini and Post's observation that a hypothalamic disturbance of GABA neurotransmission could account for many of the phenomena of affective disorder, including disturbances of appetite (via satiety center function), cortisol hypersecretion (via control of CRF release), and mood dysregulation (via limbic connections).[44]

SIDE EFFECTS

Our finding that valproate is generally well tolerated, with a low incidence of adverse effects, is consistent with the findings from the psychiatric and neurologic literature. The drug has a favorable side effect profile when compared to other anticonvulsants[50] and lithium.[17] The more common side effects reported include gastrointestinal complaints, asymptomatic serum hepatic transaminase elevations, tremor and other neurological symptoms, increased appetite and weight gain, alopecia, and less commonly, rashes.[33,34] Gastrointestinal complaints (e.g. anorexia, dyspepsia, nausea, and vomiting) are typically more common with valproic acid than with the enteric-coated divalproex sodium.[35] Rare, but in some instances potentially serious or fatal side effects include hematologic and clotting abnormalities (most commonly thrombocytopenia and impaired platelet function), acute hemorrhagic pancreatitis, and severe hepatic dysfunction.[34] There are two types of hepatotoxicity associated with valproate: a more common, dose-related elevation of serum transaminases (mentioned above) which typically normalizes spontaneously or upon decrease in dosage or discontinuation of the drug; and a rare, idiosyncratic, potentially fatal hepatotoxicity which tends to occur within the first six months of valproate therapy, shows no clear relation to hepatic enzyme levels, and is marked by anorexia, malaise, lethargy, nausea, vomiting, jaundice, and edema.[34,51] Although the etiology of this latter phenomenon remains unknown, it has been speculated to be due to the generation of a saturated, hepatotoxic valproate metabolite (Δ^4-VPA) by the hepatic cytochrome P-450 system, which has been induced by the concomitant administration of drugs (e.g. phenobarbital) metabolized primarily by the hepatic microsomal enzymes.[52]

After analyzing the 37 cases of fatal hepatotoxicity associated with valproate use occurring in the United States between 1978 and 1984, Dreifuss and colleagues identified specific risk factors for development of this syndrome in epileptics.[51] These are: age two years and under, use of multiple anticonvulsants (particularly phenytoin and phenobarbital), and presence of another neurologic disorder in addition to the seizure disorder. These authors further noted that there have been no reports of hepatic fatalities in patients over the age of 10 who were receiving valproate as their only anticonvulsant. Dreifuss and co-workers reported the rate of hepatic fatality in all ages for valproate monotherapy to be 1/37,000. It therefore appears that adult patients with primary psychiatric disorders are at an extremely low risk for developing valproate-induced fatal hepatic dysfunction. (Of note, in the past 24 months since Dreifuss and colleagues performed their analysis, there still have been no reports of hepatic fatalities in the United States in patients above 10 years of age who have received valproate as their only anticonvulsant [Langer DH, personal communication, January, 1988].)

Emerging data indicate that valproate probably has teratogenic effects, since its use during pregnancy has been associated with congenital malformations in animals (including vertebral and renal anomalies)[53,54] and humans (including neural tube defects).[55] In the latter study, Jeavons reviewed 344 reported pregnancies in women receiving valproate and found 68 (20%) abnormal babies, including nine with neural tube defects.[55] Twenty-eight of the abnormalities occurred in women receiving valproate as their sole anticonvulsant agent. In a 1983 report, the Centers for Disease Control stated that "valproic acid and sodium valproate should be considered human teratogens" and estimated that a pregnant woman exposed to valproate would have a 1% to 2% risk of having an infant with spina bifida.[56] Therefore, women for whom valproate appears indicated should be warned of the drug's potential teratogenicity before receiving it. Those who become pregnant while taking it should be offered serum alpha-fetoprotein determination and amniocentesis.[34]

There have been reports of overdose with valproate resulting in coma and death,[57,58] although recovery has been documented with serum concentrations greater than 2000 µg/ml.[59] Of note, serum valproate concentrations have been lowered by hemodialysis and hemoperfusion,[60] and coma has been reversed with naloxone.[61]

CONCLUSIONS

In summary, valproate appears to be a safe agent for use in adult psychiatric patients and a potentially useful addition to the therapeutic armamentarium in psychiatry. Although most of the available data at present are uncontrolled, evidence suggests that bipolar or schizoaffective patients in the manic phase of their disorder are particularly good candidates for the drug as acute and/or maintenance therapy. In studies with valproate or the related drug, valpromide, a moderate or marked response was observed in 177 (54%) of 326 bipolar and bipolar schizoaffective patients. Valproate appears less effective in depression and schizophrenia. Preliminary observations suggest that it may be combined with lithium salts, neuroleptics, or antidepressants, and that it anecdotally appears to potentiate the action of these agents, although the mechanism of its effect remains speculative.

Clearly, given the promising uncontrolled observations presently available, placebo-controlled evaluations of valproate, particularly in bipolar patients, should be conducted.

REFERENCES

1. Lambert P-A, Cavaz G, Borselli S, et al. Action neuropsychotrope d'un nouvel anti-épileptique: le Dépamide. Ann Méd Psychol 1966; 1:707-10.
2. Lambert P-A, Borselli S, Midenet J, et al. L'action favorable du Dépamide sur l'évolution à long terme des psychoses maniaco-dépressives. Comptes Rendus du Congres de Psychiatrie et de Neurologie de Langue Francaise. 66eme session. Clermont-Ferrand, 16-21 Septembre, 1968: 489-93.
3. Lambert P-A, Borselli S, Marcou G, et al. Action thymo-régulatrice à long terme du Dépamide dans la psychose maniaco-dépressive. Ann Méd Psychol 1971; 2:442-7.
4. Lambert P-A. Un nouveau traitement des dysthymies maniaco-dépressives: le dipropylacétamide ou Dépamide. Acutalités Psychiatriques 1972; 2:15-22.
5. Lambert P-A, Cavaz G, Borselli S, et al. Le dipropylacétamide dans le traitement de la psychose maniaco-dépressive. L'Encephale 1975; 1:25-31.
6. Lambert P-A. Acute and prophylactic therapies of patients with affective disorders using valpromide (dipropylacetamide). In: Emrich HM, Okuma T, Müller AA, eds. Anticonvulsants in affective disorders. Amsterdam: Excerpta Medica, 1984:33-44.
7. Semadeni GW. Etude clinique de l'effet normothymique du dipropylacétamide. Acta Psychiatr Belg 1976; 76:458-66.
8. Emrich HM, von Zerssen D, Kissling W, et al. Effect of sodium valproate on mania: the GABA-hypothesis of affective disorders. Arch Psychiat Nervenkr 1980; 229:1-16.
9. Emrich HM, von Zerssen D, Kissling W, et al. On a possible role of GABA in mania. Therapeutic efficacy of sodium valproate. In: Costa E, DiChiara G, Gessa GL, eds. GABA and benzodiazepine receptors. New York: Raven Press, 1981:287-96.
10. Emrich HM, von Zerssen D, Kissling W, et al. Therapeutic effect of valproate in mania (letter). Am J Psychiatry 1981; 138:256.
11. Emrich HM, Gunther R, Dose M. Current perspectives in the pharmacopsychiatry of depression and mania. Neuropharmacology 1983; 22:385-8.
12. Emrich HM, Dose M, von Zerssen D. The use of sodium valproate, carbamazepine and oxcarbazepine in patients with affective disorders. J Affect Dis 1985; 8:243-50.
13. Brennan M, Sandyk R, Borsook D. Use of sodium valproate in the management of affective disorders: basic and clinical aspects. In: Emrich HM, Okuma T, Müller AA, eds. Anticonvulsants in affective disorders. Amsterdam: Excerpta Medica, 1984:56-65.
14. Puzynski S, Klosiewicz L. Valproic acid amide in the treatment of affective and schizoaffective disorders. J Affect Dis 1984; 6:115-21.
15. Puzynski S, Klosiewicz L. Valproic acid amide as a prophylactic agent in affective and schizoaffective disorders. In: Emrich HM, Okuma T, Müller AA, eds. Anticonvulsants in affective disorders. Amsterdam: Excerpta Medica, 1984:68-75.
16. Puzynski S, Klosiewicz L. Valproic acid amide as a prophylactic agent in affective and schizoaffective disorders. Psychopharmacol Bull 1984; 20:151-9.
17. Vencovsky E, Soucek K, Zatecka I. Comparison of side effects of lithium and dipropylacetamide (Depamide). Cs Psychiat 1983; 4:223-7.
18. Vencovsky E, Soucek K, Kabes J. Prophylactic effect of dipropylacetamide in patients with bipolar affective disorder. In: Emrich HM, Okuma T, Müller AA, eds. Anticonvulsants in affective disorders. Amsterdam: Excerpta Medica, 1984:66-7.

19. Post RM, Berrettini W, Uhde TW, et al. Selective response to the anticonvulsant carbamazepine in manic-depressive illness: a case study. J Clin Psychopharmacol 1984; 4:178-85.
20. Prasad AJ. The role of sodium valproate as an anti-manic agent. Pharmatherapeutica 1984; 4:6-8.
21. Lovett L, Watkins SE, Shaw DM. The use of alternative drug therapy in nine patients with recurrent affective disorder resistant to conventional prophylaxis. Biol Psychiatry 1986; 21:1344-7.
22. McElroy SL, Keck PE, Jr, Pope HG, Jr. Sodium valproate: its use in primary psychiatric disorders. J Clin Psychopharmacol 1987; 7:16-24.
23. Linnoila M, Viukari M, Hietala O. Effect of sodium valproate on tardive dyskinesia. Br J Psychiatry 1976; 129:114-9.
24. Nagao T, Ohshimo T, Mitsunobo T, et al. Cerebral fluid monoamine metabolites and cyclic nucleotides in chronic schizophrenic patients with tardive dyskinesia or drug-induced tremor. Biol Psychiatry 1979; 14:509-23.
25. Lautin A, Angrist B, Gershon S, et al. Sodium valproate in schizophrenia. Some biochemical correlates. Br J Psychiatry 1980; 137:240-4.
26. Gundurewa V, Beckmann H, Zimmer R, et al. Effect of valproic acid on schizophrenic syndromes. Arzneim-forsch Drug Res 1980; 30:1212-3.
27. Kausen J, Zimmermann P, Funfgeld EW, et al. Effects of a GABA-mimetic drug (sodium valproate) on visually evoked potentials in chronic schizophrenics. Neuropsychobiol 1984; 11:59-64.
28. Ko G, Korpi E, Freed W, et al. Effect of valproic acid on behavior and plasma amino acid concentrations in chronic schizophrenic patients. Biol Psychiatry 1985; 20:199-228.
29. Fisk GG, York SM. The effect of sodium valproate on tardive dyskinesia—revisited. Br J Psychiatry 1987; 150:542-6.
30. Primeau F, Beauclair L, Fontaine R, et al. An open-label study of valproic acid in the treatment of panic disorder. Presented at the Society of Biological Psychiatry Annual Meeting, Chicago, May, 1987.
31. Bialer M, Rubinstein A, Dubrovsky J, et al. A comparative pharmacokinetic study of valpromide and valproic acid after intravenous administration in humans. Int J Pharmaceutics 1985; 23:25-33.
32. Pisani F, DiPerri R. Some clinical pharmacological aspects of n-dipropylacetamide. Ital J Neurol Sci 1980; 4:245-9.
33. Rall TW, Schleifer LS. Drugs effective in the therapy of the epilepsies. In: Gilman AG, Goodman LS, Rall TW, et al., eds. The pharmacological basis of therapeutics. New York: Macmillan, 1985:446-72.
34. Rimmer E, Richens A. An update on sodium valproate. Pharmacotherapy 1985; 5:171-84.
35. Wilder BJ, Karas BJ, Penry JK, et al. Gastrointestinal tolerance of divalproex sodium. Neurology 1983; 33:808-11.
36. Chadwick D. Comparison of monotherapy with valproate and other antiepileptic drugs in the treatment of seizure disorders. Am J Med 1988; 84:3S-6S.
37. Hurst DL. Expanded therapeutic range of valproate. Pediatr Neurol 1987; 3:342-4.
38. Chapman A, Keane PE, Meldrum BS, et al. Mechanism of anticonvulsant action of valproate. Prog Neurobiol 1982; 19:315-59.
39. McElroy SL, Pope HG, Jr, Keck PE, Jr, et al. Treatment of psychiatric disorders with valproate: a series of 73 cases. Psychiatr Psychobiol (in press).
40. Pope HG, Jr, McElroy SL, Satlin A, et al. Head injury, bipolar disorder, and response to valproate. Compr Psychiatry 1988; 29:34-8.
41. McElroy SL, Keck PE, Jr, Pope HG, Jr, et al. Valproate in the treatment of rapid-cycling bipolar disorder. J Clin Psychopharmacol (in press).
42. American Psychiatric Association, Task Force on Nomenclature and Statistics. Diagnostic and statistical manual of mental disorders. 3rd ed. Washington, DC: American Psychiatric Association, 1980.
43. Herridge PL, Pope HG, Jr. Treatment of bulimia and rapid-cycling bipolar disorder with sodium valproate: a case report. J Clin Psychopharmacol 1985; 5:229-30.

44. Berrettini WH, Post RM. GABA in affective illness. In: Post RM, Ballenger JC, eds. Neurobiology of mood disorders. Baltimore: Williams & Wilkins, 1984:673-85.
45. Lloyd KG, Morselli PL. Psychopharmacology of GABAergic drugs. In: Meltzer HY, ed. Psychopharmocology: the third generation of progress. New York: Raven Press, 1987:183-95.
46. Chouinard G, Young SN, Annable L. Antimanic effects of clonazepam. Biol Psychiatry 1983; 18:451-66.
47. Post RM, Stoddard FJ, Gillin C, et al. Alterations in motor activity, sleep, and biochemistry in a cycling manic-depressive patient. Arch Gen Psychiatry 1977; 43:470-7.
48. Ostrow D, Halaris A, Dysken M, et al. State dependence of noradrenergic activity in a rapidly cycling bipolar patient. J Clin Psychiatry 1984; 45:306-9.
49. Perez de la Mora M, Possani LD, Tapia R, et al. Demonstration of central gamma-aminobutyrate-containing nerve terminals by means of antibodies against glutamate decarboxylase. Neuroscience 1981; 6:875-95.
50. Beghi E, DiMascio R, Sasanelli F, et al. Adverse reactions to antiepileptic drugs: a multicenter survey of clinical practice. Epilepsia 1986; 27:323-30.
51. Dreifuss FE, Santilli N, Langer DH, et al. Valproic acid hepatic fatalities: a retrospective review. Neurology 1987; 37:379-85.
52. Rettie AE, Rettenmeier AW, Howald WN, et al. Cytochrome P-450 catalyzed formation of Δ^4-VPA, a toxic metabolite of valproic acid. Science 1987; 235:890-3.
53. Whittle BA. Preclinical teratological studies on sodium valproate (Epilim) and other anticonvulsants. In: Legg NJ, ed. Clinical and pharmacological aspects of sodium valproate (Epilim) in the treatment of epilepsy. Tunbridge Wells, England: MCS Consultants, 1976:105-10.
54. Nau H, Spielmann H. Embryotoxicity testing of valproic acid. Lancet 1983; 1:762-4.
55. Jeavons PM. Sodium valproate and neural tube defects. Lancet 1982; 2:1282-3.
56. Centers for Disease Control. Valproate: a new cause of birth defects—report from Italy and follow-up from France. MMWR 1983; 32:438-9.
57. Schnabel R, Rainbeck B, Janssen F. Fatal intoxication with sodium valproate. Lancet 1984; 1:221-2.
58. Tift JP. Valproic acid. N Engl J Med 1980; 303:394.
59. Pedersen B, Juul-Jensen P. Electroencephalographic alterations during intoxication with sodium valproate: a case report. Epilepsia 1984; 25:121-4.
60. Mortensen PB, Hansen HE, Pedersen B, et al. Acute valproate intoxication: biochemical investigations and haemodialysis treatment. Int J Clin Pharmacol Ther Toxicol 1983; 21:64-8.
61. Stelman GS, Woerpel RW, Sherard ES. Treatment of accidental sodium valproate overdose with an opiate antagonist (letter). Ann Neurol 1979; 6:274.

CHAPTER 3

Clonazepam in the Treatment of Psychiatric Disorders

Guy Chouinard, M.D.
Montreal, Quebec

INTRODUCTION

Clonazepam is an antiepileptic drug approved by the United States Food and Drug Administration since 1976 for treatment of the following types of seizures: absence, infantile spasms, atypical absence, myoclonic, and atonic (Table 1).[1] When double-blind clinical trials were conducted to establish its efficacy in the treatment of absence (typical petit mal) seizures, clonazepam was found to be as effective as ethosuximide[2] and significantly ($p<.0001$) more efficacious than diazepam in reducing seizure frequency and 3-Hz spike-wave activity on follow-up electroencephalograms.[3] It may be as effective as valproate in controlling absence seizures.[4] Sharing some antiepileptic properties with valproate, clonazepam remains one of the drugs of choice in seizures with myoclonus.[4] Clonazepam was also found useful in the treatment of a variety of movement disorders including Gilles de la Tourette syndrome, myoclonus, restless leg syndrome, and facial spasm. For many years, the use of clonazepam was restricted to neurological disorders, but its usefulness was limited by its sedative properties, which were not desirable in epileptic patients. More recently, interest arose in clonazepam as a treatment for mania,[5] since it possesses two properties currently under investigation for their antimanic activity: an anticonvulsant effect and an ability to potentiate 5-hydroxytryptamine (5-HT) synthesis.

TABLE 1. Effectiveness of clonazepam in the treatment of seizure disorders (see reference 1)

Type of seizure	Effectiveness
FDA-approved indications	
Absence	+ + +
Infantile spasm	+ +
Atypical absence	+ +
Myoclonic	+ + +
Atonic	+ +
Non-FDA-approved indications	
Tonic-clonic	+
Elementary partial	+ +
Complex partial	+ +

It has been suggested that a disturbance in central 5-HT function plays a role in the pathophysiology of bipolar disorder. One hypothesis suggests that 5-HT function is decreased in both mania and depression.[6] Based on this serotonergic hypothesis, we carried out studies using tryptophan, a 5-HT precursor, in the treatment of acute mania.[7] To achieve even a weak therapeutic effect, however, large doses of tryptophan were needed. In the search for another serotonergic agent that could be taken in smaller doses, clonazepam appeared to be a promising choice.

We subsequently initiated a double-blind crossover trial of clonazepam in the treatment of acutely manic patients and found it to be more effective than lithium.[5] We then treated 12 patients with a diagnosis of panic disorder according to DSM-III criteria. The rationale behind this study was the finding, from a just-completed placebo-controlled trial, that alprazolam was efficacious in the treatment of panic disorder.[8] In 10 of the 12 patients with panic disorder treated with clonazepam, we observed a rapid and marked effect on panic attacks.[9] The antipanic effect of clonazepam was later confirmed in both uncontrolled[10] and controlled studies.[11]

Clonazepam is now also being used for a variety of other psychiatric disorders that could be considered as part of a "manic spectrum" (hyperactivity, agitation, logorrhea, and impulsive behavior).[12] More recently, an open-label study of clonazepam in patients with unipolar and bipolar depression indicated that the drug may also have efficacy as an antidepressant.[13] All of the above studies will be discussed in detail later in this chapter.

PHARMACOLOGY

Clonazepam is a 7-nitrobenzodiazepine derivative. Its chemical structure is illustrated in Figure 1. The structural formula of clonazepam closely resembles that of nitrazepam (a benzodiazepine not available in the United States), differing only by a substitution at position 2 on the benzene ring, a configuration that tends to increase the potency of benzodiazepine derivatives. Interestingly, clonazepam and nitrazepam, both 7-nitro derivatives, are the only benzodiazepines currently given as antiepileptics for absence, myoclonic, and infantile spasm seizures. The clinical pharmacology of clonazepam has been reviewed by Browne[1] and more recently by Greenblatt and colleagues.[14]

FIGURE 1. Chemical structure of clonazepam

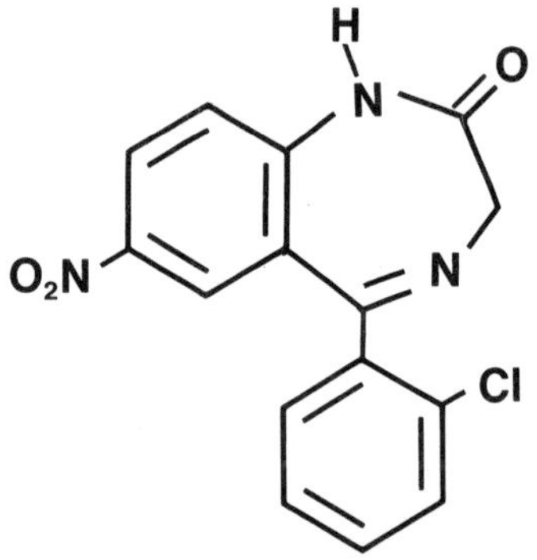

Absorption, distribution, and half-life

Recent data suggest that the bioavailability of oral clonazepam is 85% and its elimination half-life 79 hours. The latter finding would classify the drug as a relatively long half-life benzodiazepine.[14] However, the range of previous half-life estimates varies from 20 to 80 hours.[1,14] Animal studies suggest that clonazepam passes readily across biologic membranes and rapidly from blood to brain. Compared to other benzodiazepines, it has a relatively low lipid solubility.[14] Previously, the drug was estimated to be 47% plasma protein bound, but Greenblatt and colleagues estimated the drug to be at least 80% protein bound.[14] Clonazepam reaches peak serum concentrations one to three hours after oral administration. In some human studies, there was a high correlation between plasma concentration and dose but no correlation between plasma concentration and the antiepileptic effect of the drug.[15,16] Animal data suggest that brain and plasma concentrations are directly proportional to dose.[17] Even though brain concentrations are always higher than those in plasma, the ratio of brain to plasma concentrations remains constant independent of dose.

Metabolism, toxicity, side effects, and precautions

Like nitrazepam, clonazepam is metabolized by nitroreduction, acetylation, and hydroxylation. It undergoes reduction of its nitro group to form a 7-amino metabolite, which is widely distributed in human plasma.[1] This is the major metabolic pathway of clonazepam, and most likely occurs in the liver.The nitroreduction may be slightly impaired by cimetidine but not by old age.[14] Total clearance is likely to be increased in obese patients, thus causing lower blood concentrations.[14] Other antiepileptic drugs, such as carbamazepine, may lower the serum concentration of clonazepam.[18] In contrast, clonazepam does not cause enzyme autoinduction, nor does it decrease serum concentrations of other antiepileptic drugs. Since clonazepam metabolites appear to be pharmacologically inactive, acetylation of its metabolites is not presently believed to have significant therapeutic implications. However, Miller and colleagues suggested that slow acetylators (a trait present in 50% of Caucasians but only 10% of Orientals) generate higher levels of 7-amino clonazepam.[19] It is thus possible that the high concentrations of this metabolite would induce receptor changes, making slow acetylators more likely to develop tolerance and to have withdrawal symptoms upon drug discontinuation. The fact that only 10% of Orientals are slow acetylators may explain the high success rate of clonazepam monotherapy found in previously untreated epileptics in this population: Naito and colleagues noted that 61.3% of 93 patients became seizure-free with a mean duration of follow-up of 32 months.[15] One might, therefore, predict that clonazepam response would be less variable in Oriental psychiatric patients and that the rate of good responders would be higher.

The three most common side effects encountered with the drug are ataxia, drowsiness, and paradoxical behavior changes (including disinhibition). The first two tend to be dose-related, occur early in treatment, and generally subside with chronic administration. Less frequently reported adverse reactions have included treatment-emergent depression and sexual dysfunction.[20] However, it is not clear whether the treatment-emergent depression that has been described with clonazepam[20] was attributable to clonazepam itself or to the withdrawal of alprazolam. Since clonazepam has not been shown to exacerbate depression in bipolar patients (a population which might be expected to be susceptible to this effect), we tend to think that withdrawal of alprazolam may be the more likely explanation. Regarding sexual dysfunction, the incidence with clonazepam, as with other benzodiazepines, appears to be low.

As for teratogenecity, the risks of benzodiazepine use during pregnancy have been the subject of conflicting reports, with earlier reports of increased rates of oral clefts in infants exposed in utero to diazepam not substantiated by subsequent prospective studies.[20] Although one animal study comparing clonazepam with other anticonvulsants suggests that teratogenicity is low with this agent,[21] the 1988 edition of the *Physician's Desk Reference* reports an increased incidence of defects in the infants of rabbits receiving the drug while pregnant. It would thus seem prudent for pregnant women to avoid usage of this agent if at all possible.

Overdosage can cause drowsiness, ataxia, and cyclic coma. In all reported cases of overdose, patients have recovered without sequelae. In this respect, clonazepam appears to be potentially safer than other benzodiazepines, especially if one considers animal studies, where at oral doses exceeding 4,000 mg/kg, no death was observed in rats given clonazepam as opposed to other benzodiazepines.[22]

If patients are taking other psychotropic drugs such as lithium, neuroleptics, or tricyclic antidepressants, monitoring of blood pressure is recommended because of potential additive hypotensive effects when clonazepam therapy is initiated. Clonazepam is contraindicated in patients who are critically intoxicated with alcohol and should be used cautiously in patients who are taking barbiturates.[23] As with any benzodiazepine, patients should be gradually withdrawn from clonazepam, especially when they are taking concomitant psychotropics, such as neuroleptics, antidepressants, or lithium, which may have epileptogenic properties.[24] Of note, a case of clonazepam withdrawal psychosis after an overdose of clonazepam and other psychotherapeutic drugs has been reported.[25]

MECHANISM OF ACTION

The mechanism of action of clonazepam in psychiatric disorders has not been established. It may act by mimicking the effects of the neurotransmitter glycine, by potentiating GABAergic transmission, or by increasing the concentration of 5-HT at synaptic sites.[1] Clonazepam has also been found to be the most specific benzodiazepine for active benzodiazepine receptor sites on the basis of autoradiographic studies.[26] Contrary to ^{3}H-diazepam and ^{3}H-flunitrazepam, ^{3}H-clonazepam has been found to bind only to active benzodiazepine sites, called receptors because they produce a pharmacologic effect, in contrast to benzodiazepine sites where ligand binding occurs without inducing any pharmacologic response.

As for the drug's serotonergic effects, it is well established that clonazepam increases 5-HT synthesis in animals.[27] Furthermore, available clinical data suggest that the drug increases both 5-HT synthesis and function at normal clinical doses in man.[28] Chadwick and colleagues examined the effect of clonazepam and the 5-HT precursor 5-hydroxytryptophan (5-HTP) in patients with myoclonus.[28] They found that (1) those patients who responded to clonazepam were also those who responded to 5-HTP; (2) the patients who responded to these two drugs were those who had low cerebrospinal fluid (CSF) 5-hydroxy-indoleacetic acid (5-HIAA); (3) CSF 5-HIAA increased in one patient who recovered spontaneously, suggesting that low central nervous system (CNS) 5-HT might be involved in the etiology of the disorder; and (4) clonazepam treatment raised CSF 5-HIAA. Thus clonazepam does seem to potentiate 5-HT synthesis and function in man. In a recent study using radioligands, clonazepam was found to specifically increase both $5HT_1$ and $5HT_2$ binding sites in rat frontal cortex.[29]

The beneficial effects of clonazepam, seen in both manic patients and patients with panic disorder, could be related to its anticonvulsant properties. This speculation is supported by the observation that other anticonvulsants appear effective in mania. Carbamazepine, which has the ability to suppress seizure discharges preferentially in limbic regions, has been shown in double-blind studies to be effective in the treatment of acute mania and in the prophylaxis of bipolar disorder[30-32] (and see Chapter 1 in this volume). Valproate has also been reported to have antimanic effects, although to date it has been tested primarily in uncontrolled studies[33] (and see Chapter 2 in this volume).

TREATMENT OF ACUTE MANIA

Clonazepam versus lithium

Our group undertook the first controlled study of clonazepam in acute mania.[5] As mentioned earlier, the rationale behind this study was to give lower doses of a serotonergic drug instead of using high doses of L-tryptophan. Twelve acutely manic patients were treated with clonazepam or lithium carbonate in a double-blind crossover trial. Six patients were randomly assigned to 10 days of clonazepam treatment followed immediately by 10 days of treatment with lithium, while the other six patients received the same treatments in reverse order. A flexible dosage regimen was used (Table 2) with both medications given in an equally divided regimen four times per day. Clonazepam was administered in 2 mg tablets and lithium carbonate in 300 mg tablets. After treatment had begun, no other medications (including hypnotics) were administered except for haloperidol, which, for ethical reasons, was available in cases of agitation that could not be controlled by the study medications. Thus, PRN use of haloperidol served as an indirect measure of efficacy.

Patients ranged in age from 25 to 63 years (median 43 years), and 11 had been hospitalized previously (range 0.1 to 8 years). The study included nine men and three women. None had received depot neuroleptic drugs for at least two weeks prior to the study. The initial severity of mania was measured on a 9-point Clinical Global Impression Scale, and the mean score ± SD was 8.2 ± 0.6.

Table 3 shows the mean scores on the mania items of the Inpatient Multidimensional Psychiatric Scale (IMPS) before treatment and following 10 days of treatment with clonazepam or lithium. There was an overall tendency for clonazepam to be better than lithium on the mania items. It was significantly ($p<.05$) superior to lithium for motor overactivity and tended ($p<.10$) to be superior to lithium for logorrhea. In addition, use of clonazepam was associated with significantly less haloperidol administration. Both the total dose of PRN haloperidol and the number of days that it was needed were significantly ($p<.05$) lower during clonazepam treatment than during lithium treatment (Table 4). Thus patients, as evaluated indirectly by PRN haloperidol administration, did better on clonazepam than on lithium. In fact, it can be argued that use of PRN haloperidol tended to reduce the actual differences between the two treatments on the rating scales because patients were not allowed to deteriorate to the same extent that they would have without the use of PRN's.

Side effects included those generally attributed to lithium (tremor, diarrhea, polydipsia, and polyuria) and, during clonazepam treatment, ataxia and drowsiness. However, the latter tended to remit as treatment continued.

The differences in extrapyramidal symptoms as determined by the physician's examination showed that patients treated with lithium had more parkinsonism than those treated with clonazepam (Table 5). Since lithium-treated patients required more PRN doses of haloperidol, it is not surprising that more akathisia, tremor, and effects on gait and posture were observed in this group (particularly since lithium is known to exacerbate neuroleptic-induced parkinsonism[34]). The scale used to measure extrapyramidal symptoms[35,36] separates the hypokinetic and hyperkinetic movement factors,

TABLE 2. Dosage of clonazepam and lithium (mg/day) (adapted from reference 5)

	Dosage range (mean)	
	Clonazepam	Lithium
Day 1	2-8 (4.2)	900-1500 (1118)
Day 10	4-16 (10.4)	900-2100 (1691)

TABLE 3. Initial and final mean scores on items for mania derived from the Inpatient Multidimensional Psychiatric Scale (adapted from reference 5)

Mania items	Initial mean Score	Final mean score Clonazepam	Lithium
Motor overactivity	5.0	1.8[a]	2.8
Elevated mood	6.1	3.3	3.2
Pressure of speech	5.8	2.3	2.9
Logorrhea	5.3	2.2[b]	2.9
Insight	5.4	2.6	3.4
Total	27.6	12.2	15.2

[a] $p<.05$
[b] $p<.10$

TABLE 4. Haloperidol supplementary medication (PRN) (adapted from reference 5)

	Clonazepam	Lithium	Statistical significance of difference
Phase I			
No. of patients	3	4	
Total dose (mg)	55	165	p<.05
No. of days	10	21	p<.05
Phase II			
No. of patients	1	3	
Total dose (mg)	5	92.5	p<.05
No. of days	1	10	p<.05

and it was found that patients scored lower during clonazepam treatment on both these factors. The total score for all extrapyramidal symptoms also showed a significant ($p<.01$) difference favoring clonazepam over lithium.

In addition, patients tended to manifest more tardive dyskinesia during lithium treatment than during clonazepam treatment, although the difference did not achieve statistical significance (Table 6). The effect of clonazepam in tardive dyskinesia has been investigated, and it has been suggested that the drug may have a nonspecific beneficial effect related to sedation.[37,38] However, tardive dyskinesia is a difficult disorder to study, and long-term clinical trials are needed to determine whether clonazepam is of any value in this indication.

Lithium plasma levels averaged 0.90 mEq/l on day four and 0.98 mEq/l after 10 days of treatment—levels which are considered to be therapeutic in acute treatment. Some residual lithium concentrations appeared in the second phase clonazepam-treated group, but at the end of 20 days, the plasma concentrations averaged only 0.02 mEq/l.

The results of this study suggest that clonazepam's rapid onset of action and lack of serious side effects may make it an effective and safe agent for the control of acute mania. In addition, treatment with clonazepam may reduce the incidence and severity of extrapyramidal symptoms associated with the use of neuroleptics often given with lithium in these patients.

Clonazepam vs Haloperidol

After gaining extensive experience in using clonazepam in acute mania, we initiated a second study which is currently underway. This is a randomized double-blind

TABLE 5. Extrapyramidal symptom rating scale: clonazepam vs lithium (adapted from reference 5)

Symptom	Initial mean score	Final mean score Clonazepam	Final mean score Lithium	Difference between treatments[a]
Parkinsonism: physician's examination				
Expressive automatic movements	0	0	0.3	NS
Bradykinesia	0	0	0.1	NS
Rigidity	0.5	0.1	0.8	NS
Gait and posture	0.8	0.3	1.0	p<.05
Tremor[b]	5.4	2.8	6.3	p<.01
Akathisia	0.2	0	0.3	p<.10
Sialorrhea	0	0	0	NS
Acute dystonia	0	0	0	NS
Nonacute dystonia	0.3	0.8	0.5	NS
Factors				
Hypokinetic movements	1.3	0.3	2.2	p<.10
Hyperkinetic movements[b]	5.6	2.8	6.7	p<.05
Total score (nonacute dystonia excluded)	6.8	3.1	8.8	p<.01

[a] *Analysis of variance appropriate to crossover design.*
[b] *Mean scores at Day 10 significantly (p<.05) higher than those at Day 20.*
NS—not significant

TABLE 6. Tardive dyskinesia: clonazepam vs lithium (adapted from reference 5)

	Initial mean score	Final mean score Clonazepam	Final mean score Lithium	Difference between treatments[a]
Tardive dyskinesia				
Bucco-labial	0.2	0.2	1.0	p<.10
Factors				
Bucco-lingual-masticatory	1.0	1.9	3.7	NS
Extremities	0.8	1.7	1.5	NS
Total Score[b]	1.8	3.7	5.5	NS

[a] *Analysis of variance appropriate to cross-over design.*
[b] *Total score of all the items on the tardive dyskinesia scale.*
NS—not significant

controlled trial comparing the antimanic effect of clonazepam with that of haloperidol. The study will include a total of 48 newly admitted manic patients from emergency rooms, who will be administered either clonazepam or haloperidol for the first seven days of treatment (Phase I). Lithium carbonate will then

TABLE 7. Clonazepam vs haloperidol in acute mania

Study design

Randomized

Haloperidol	Week 1	Clonazepam
Haloperidol + lithium	Weeks 2-3	Clonazepam + lithium
Lithium + haloperidol PRN	Weeks 4-5	Lithium + clonazepam PRN

be given to both treatment groups, and clonazepam or haloperidol gradually decreased over a period of 14 days (Phase II). During Phase III, clonazepam or haloperidol will be available on a PRN basis for an additional 14 days (Table 7).

The following drug schedule is followed:

Phase I		**Clonazepam**	**Haloperidol**
	Level I (initial dose)	2 mg TID or QID	5 mg TID or QID
	Level II (maximum dose, not including PRN's)	4 mg QID	10 mg QID
Phase 2		+ lithium 300 mg TID	+ lithium 300 mg TID
		(Li dosage adjusted according to therapeutic effect and side effects)	
Phase 3		lithium + clonazepam 1-2 mg PRN	lithium + haloperidol 5-10 mg PRN

The study has not yet been completed. However, of 16 patients enrolled to date, only one terminated the trial prematurely, suggesting that clonazepam may be useful as a single therapeutic agent in the first week of treatment of acute mania and that the equivalency of 1 mg of clonazepam to 2.5 mg of haloperidol used in this trial is appropriate.

In cases where bipolar patients have been treated chronically with neuroleptics, it is the author's practice to initiate treatment for acute mania during the first week with either clonazepam plus haloperidol PRN or haloperidol plus clonazepam PRN. The author's preference is to initiate treatment with clonazepam 2 mg QID. Dosage can then be adjusted to achieve maximum therapeutic effect up to a maximum of 16 mg/day (excluding clonazepam PRN), given QID in equal doses. If the patient is treated with liquid haloperidol, the initial dose is 5 mg TID or QID unless significant side effects such as parkinsonism or hypotension develop. A maximum dose of 40 mg per day can be given. Treatment of these patients during the subsequent weeks is similar to that described above, with lithium added during the second week, while clonazepam or haloperidol are gradually tapered and administered only on a PRN basis.

We are also currently investigating a treatment protocol comparing intramuscular clonazepam versus intramuscular haloperidol for acutely manic patients in the emergency room. Treatment involves a rapid tranquilization method carried out over a three-hour period, each drug being administered every half-hour, then every hour for a total of four doses (hours 0, 0.5, 1, 2). Haloperidol is supplied in a 1 cc intramuscular injectable solution containing 5 mg of haloperidol. Clonazepam is supplied in a 2 cc intramuscular injectable solution containing 1 mg of clonazepam. (In the United States, however, clonazepam is not available for intramuscular injection.) In cases of side effects such as extreme sedation occurring in either treatment group, one dose of medication is omitted.

MAINTENANCE TREATMENT OF BIPOLAR PATIENTS

The need to use neuroleptics and tricyclic antidepressants in bipolar patients can be minimized by using a combination of other pharmacological agents with potentiating effects or different mechanisms of action. The drugs used in the treatment of bipolar patients can be divided into two categories: mood stabilizers and antimanic agents (Table 8). Lithium is the classic mood stabilizer. It has a weak effect when used alone for acute symptoms, a potentiating effect when given with another mood stabilizer or antimanic agent, and is especially effective in preventing mood swings. Neuroleptics, in addition to their anti-Tourette and antipsychotic effects, have definite antimanic properties and can be classified with the antimanic agents. Anticonvulsants like carbamazepine, clonazepam, and valproate appear to be efficacious in acute mania but there is also evidence that they may have mood stabilizing effects when given as monotherapy, although this aspect needs further investigation. They may also have potentiating effects when given with other mood stabilizing or antimanic agents (see Chapters 1 and 2 in this volume).

The author's stepwise approach to the pharmacological treatment of bipolar patients is outlined in Table 9. Because of its well documented efficacy, lithium is the first step in the maintenance treatment of bipolar illness. As a second step L-tryptophan, an amino acid with 5-HT potentiating properties, may be added up to doses of 12 g/day. Tryptophan appears to increase lithium concen-

TABLE 8. Two categories of drugs for bipolar patients

Mood-stabilizing drugs	Antimanic agents
Lithium, tryptophan	Neuroleptics, anticonvulsants (clonazepam, carbamazepine, valproate)
• Weak effect alone in acute symptoms	• Most efficacious for acute symptoms
• Potentiating effect when given in combination with antimanic drugs or mood-stabilizing drugs	• Variable mood stabilizing effect
	• Potentiating effect when given with mood stabilizer
• Mainly mood swing prevention	• Potentiating effect when two are combined

TABLE 9. Stepwise approach to pharmacotherapy for bipolar disorder

Step 1: Lithium

Step 2: Lithium + L-tryptophan

Step 3: Lithium + L-tryptophan + clonazepam (and/or carbamazepine)

Step 4: Lithium + L-tryptophan + clonazepam + atypical neuroleptic

Step 5: Lithium + L-tryptophan + clonazepam + atypical neuroleptic + classical neuroleptic

Step 6: Lithium + L-tryptophan + clonazepam + atypical neuroleptic + classical neuroleptic + tricyclic antidepressant (use with caution for short periods only)

trations in plasma quite significantly, perhaps by making lithium more bioavailable (thus, lithium dosage will often need to be reduced). If suitable control of manic symptoms is not achieved, in order to defer the use of neuroleptics, clonazepam can be added to the treatment regimen as a third step.

Clonazepam,[39-41] as compared with carbamazepine,[42-44] may produce fewer adverse effects when given in combination with lithium and neuroleptics. Furthermore, unlike clonazepam, carbamazepine may interact with a number of other drugs, such as erythromycin,[45] dextropropoxyphene,[46] phenytoin,[47] and the calcium antagonists diltiazem[48] and verapamil.[49]

The dose of clonazepam may vary from 0.5 mg/day to 16 mg/day, depending upon the patient's condition and phase of illness. It is the author's experience that clonazepam dosage can be adjusted and even significantly decreased in bipolar patients without adverse effects, because these patients, in contrast to some schizophrenic patients, do not appear to develop psychological dependency while taking the drug.

If patients have been treated with neuroleptics for at least one year prior to the manic episode, it may be necessary to add a neuroleptic as a further step, as these patients may have developed supersensitivity psychosis.[50] Possible choices include pimozide or other diphenylbutylpiperidines which have a higher affinity for D_2-dopamine receptors (ratio of D_2:D_1 blockade $\geqslant$ 1000).[51] Compared with typical neuroleptics, this class of antipsychotic drugs is easier to withdraw and induces less receptor supersensitivity. The daily dose of pimozide should not exceed 10 mg when given with lithium.

As a fifth step, haloperidol or other classical neuroleptics may occasionally be required. Fortunately, in the author's experience, only a small percentage of bipolar patients require continuation of haloperidol if the previous four steps are followed. Even in these few instances, the drug can usually be given in very small doses.

The use of tricyclic antidepressants in bipolar patients is generally avoided at our center because of the risk that they may perpetuate the illness by exacerbating cycling or triggering the switch process.[52,53] However, if necessary, a tricyclic can be administered as a sixth step, but for as short a period of time as possible. The dose should be quickly reduced as soon as a therapeutic effect is achieved.

It is unfortunate that, in many cases, polypharmacy cannot be avoided. However, by adjusting combinations and dosages among the three classes of drugs (mood stabilizers, anticonvulsants, and neuroleptics) maximum efficacy can be achieved with minimal adverse effects. Neuroleptic drugs provide the least flexibility and induce the most serious adverse side effects; therefore their use is discouraged. Tricyclic antidepressants, for the reasons mentioned above, should probably not be used on a long-term basis.

Clonazepam, therefore, may be a good adjunctive medication in the long-term treatment of bipolar patients.[39] Although sedation is often encountered during initiation of treatment, it generally subsides over time. In the author's experience approximately 66% of patients treated with lithium and tryptophan will require the addition of clonazepam, and about two-thirds of this group appears to benefit from clonazepam.

Of the patients who require clonazepam, approximately 10% will generally require further treatment with neuroleptics. Prospective controlled studies are necessary to delineate further the usefulness of clonazepam in the long-term maintenance treatment of bipolar disorder. Pending the results of such studies, it appears that in those patients for whom L-tryptophan is contraindicated or not available, clonazepam would be a logical adjunctive medication to lithium.

TREATMENT OF MANIC SPECTRUM DISORDERS AND OTHER PSYCHIATRIC DISORDERS

To our knowledge, a total of 84 patients treated with clonazepam for mania or manic spectrum behaviors has been reported in the English scientific literature. These reports include one controlled study[5] (n = 12 patients) and 11 case reports[39-41, 54-60] (n = 72 patients). Success rates varied between 44%[40] and 66%.[39] These reports demonstrate that clonazepam may be beneficial in patients presenting with manic spectrum behavioral disorders in which the target symptoms are agitation, pressure of speech, and increased motor activity. These symptoms are associated with a variety of psychiatric conditions, primarily mania, schizoaffective disorder, and schizophrenia.

Clonazepam is now being used for a variety of other psychiatric disorders — for example, in agitated adolescents in whom neuroleptics may be appropriate but where avoidance of tardive dyskinesia is important; in cases of agitation, such as that seen in steroid-induced psychosis[56] and mental retardation;[12] and in elderly patients with organic brain syndromes.[61] The drug has also been reported to be efficacious in antidepressant-induced mania.[57] Recently, Kishimoto and colleagues reported the successful treatment of 21 (84%) of 25 patients with depression (18 with major depression and nine with bipolar depression, including eight who had failed to respond to previous treatment with two or more antidepressants) with open-label clonazepam (maximum daily doses of 1.5 mg to 6.0 mg).[13] The onset of clonazepam's apparent antidepressant effect was rapid, with significant improvement attained within one week of commencement of treatment. There is no evidence, however, that clonazepam has antipsychotic effects in schizophrenia. Although there have been reports describing benzodiazepine use in schizophrenia,[62] the only placebo-controlled monotherapy study available shows that the drug is not superior to placebo.[63]

There have also been reports of the usefulness of clonazepam in various neuropsychiatric syndromes. For instance, clonazepam was shown to correct drug-induced EEG abnormalities in a case of neuroleptic-induced somnambulism and temporal epileptiform activity.[64] In addition, the successful treatment of one case of schizophrenia-like psychosis with epilepsy and three cases of atypical psychosis with clonazepam has been reported.[58] In animal studies, clonazepam appears to be one of the most efficacious drugs for correcting drug-induced seizures. In humans, clonazepam may prove to be useful in the detoxification of patients dependent on high doses of alprazolam.[65]

TREATMENT OF ANXIETY DISORDERS

Major advances have been made in the use of benzodiazepines in the treatment of psychiatric disorders. Up until 1982 the main indication for the use of benzodiazepines was generalized anxiety, manifested by insomnia or anxiety. That year, we reported the results of a double-blind placebo-controlled study demonstrating that alprazolam could effectively block panic attacks.[8] In 1983 we published the results of a study of clonazepam in severely ill patients with panic disorder.[9] The antipanic effect of clonazepam was significant and appeared more pronounced than the effect we observed with alprazolam; in addition, clonazepam did not appear to induce rebound anxiety.

These preliminary findings have now been confirmed in both open and controlled studies carried out in the United States.[10,11] The Boston group treated 50 patients with clonazepam; 78% were considered to demonstrate a good response.[10] Forty-one of these 50 patients were considered to have been poor responders to standard treatment. These same investigators published a one-year follow-up of these patients, and found that 18 of the 20 patients who were still being treated with clonazepam continued to show a positive response.[66] Of note, once their symptoms were controlled, fewer than half of the patients underwent subsequent dosage increases. Those needing increases had a mean dosage increase of 1.7 mg/day, leading the authors to conclude that the development of tolerance to therapeutic efficacy was not a problem. In a review of open clinical trials of clonazepam in patients with panic attacks, Pollack again concluded that the development of tolerance or abuse was not a problem.[67] Finally, these investigators have also reported successful treatment of seven of 10 panic patients not responsive to standard drug treatment.[68]

The amount of clonazepam necessary to treat panic disorder appears to be much less than that required to treat acute mania. In a recent investigation of 10 patients with diagnoses of panic disorder or agoraphobia with panic attacks at our center, successful doses began with 0.5 mg at dinner and bedtime and were increased by 0.5 mg every three days until the next visit or to a maximum of 2 mg.[69] Treatment was continued for three months, with dosage adjusted upward as needed to a maximum of 3 mg to 6 mg daily for most patients. The results of this investigation are shown in Table 10. Of note, there was statistically significant improvement in the three types of symptoms (anxiety, phobic anxiety, and panic attacks) predominant in these patients. In the majority of patients, panic attacks stopped after a few days of treatment with clonazepam—even in patients who had been unable to leave their homes for several years.

As mentioned above, phobic anxiety was significantly reduced with clonazepam treatment. In the author's experience, if the abrupt, acute panic attacks are blocked, patients eventually begin to approach previously feared situations, often without the supportive or instructive behavior therapy previously thought to be necessary. We concluded that, with clonazepam treatment, such ad-

TABLE 10. SCL-90 self-ratings: baseline and after clonazepam treatment (adapted from reference 69)

	Baseline evaluation mean (SD)	After clonazepam treatment	p
Anxiety (0-4)	2.5 (0.7)	0.8 (0.8)	<.001
Phobic anxiety (0-4)	2.9 (1.0)	0.9 (1.3)	<.01
Panic attacks (0-4)	3.6 (0.5)	1.0 (0.9)	<.001

junctive therapy is often not required, and patients quickly show ability face situations that were avoided previously.

Clonazepam vs alprazolam

Clonazepam and alprazolam are both potent benzodiazepines, but clonazepam's long half-life (80 hours) decreases the likelihood of withdrawal symptoms, including the rebound phenomena upon drug discontinuation, interdose rebound, clock-watching syndrome, and early morning rebound often associated with alprazolam.[69] In addition, the longer half-life allows dosage flexibility, so that clonazepam can be administered BID or in a single daily dose, whereas alprazolam most often requires a TID regimen.

In a placebo-controlled study comparing alprazolam and clonazepam, the two drugs were found to have similar antipanic efficacy, and both active treatments were found to be superior to placebo.[10] A procedure to switch patients from alprazolam to clonazepam has been suggested by Herman and colleagues, who sucessfully switched 48 consecutive patients, treated for panic disorder, from alprazolam to clonazepam.[70] Clonazepam is approximately twice as potent as alprazolam (0.5 mg of clonazepam equals 1 mg of alprazolam). As mentioned earlier, in one case clonazepam was also used successfully for detoxification from high doses of alprazolam.[65]

CONCLUSIONS

Preliminary evidence suggests that clonazepam, an antiepileptic agent given for myoclonic and absence seizures, may be effective in the treatment of patients with mania and panic disorder and may have an improved side-effect profile over standard treatments. Clonazepam provides a safe alternative to the use of neuroleptics in the acute and maintenance treatment of manic patients. In the management of patients with panic disorder, clonazepam may be an effective treatment alternative to alprazolam and imipramine. Clonazepam may also be used for a variety of psychiatric disorders which could be classified under the "manic spectrum" disorders concept.

REFERENCES

1. Browne TR. Clonazepam. N Engl J Med 1978; 299:812-6.
2. Sato S, Penry JK, Dreifuss FE, et al. Clonazepam in the treatment of absence seizures: a double-blind clinical trial. Neurology (Minneapolis) 1977; 27:371. Abstract.
3. Chandra B. Clonazepam in the treatment of petit mal. Asian J Med 1973; 9:433-5.
4. Dreifuss, FE. Treatment of seizure disorders and myoclonus. Psychosomatics 1985; 26:30S-5S.
5. Chouinard G, Young SN, Annable L. Antimanic effect of clonazepam. Biol Psychiatry 1983; 18:451-66.
6. Prange AJ, Wilson IC, Lynn CW, et al. L-tryptophan in mania. Arch Gen Psychiatry 1974; 30:56-62.
7. Chouinard G, Young SN, Annable L. A controlled clinical trial of L-tryptophan in acute mania. Biol Psychiatry 1985; 20:546-57.
8. Chouinard G, Annable L, Fontaine R, et al. Alprazolam in the treatment of generalized anxiety and panic disorders: a double-blind, placebo-controlled study. Psychopharmacology 1982; 77: 229-33.
9. Chouinard G, Labonte A, Fontaine R, et al. New concepts in benzodiazepine therapy: rebound anxiety and new indications for the more potent benzodiazepines. Prog Neuropsychopharmacol Biol Psychiatry 1983; 7:669-73.

10. Spier SA, Tesar GE, Rosenbaum JF, et al. Treatment of panic disorder and agoraphobia with clonazepam. J Clin Psychiatry 1986; 47:238-42.
11. Tesar GE, Rosenbaum JF, Pollack MH, et al. Clonazepam versus alprazolam in the treatment of panic disorder: interim analysis of data from a prospective, double-blind, placebo-controlled clinical trial. J Clin Psychiatry 1987; 48:16S-9S.
12. Freinhar JP. Clonazepam treatment of a mentally retarded woman (letter). Am J Psychiatry 1985; 142:1513.
13. Kishimoto A, Kamata K, Sugihara T. Treatment of depression with clonazepam. Acta Psychiatr Scand 1988; 77:81-6.
14. Greenblatt DJ, Miller LG, Shader RI. Clonazepam pharmacokinetics, brain uptake, and receptor interactions. J Clin Psychiatry 1987; 48:4S-10S.
15. Naito A, Wachi M, Nishida M. Clinical effects of plasma concentrations on long-term clonazepam monotherapy in previously untreated epileptics. Acta Neurol Scand 1987; 76:58-63.
16. Dreifuss FE, Penry JK, Rose SW, et al. Serum clonazepam concentrations in children with absence seizures. Neurology (Minneapolis) 1975; 25:255-8.
17. Miller LG, Greenblatt DJ, Paul SM, et al. Benzodiazepine receptor occupancy in vivo: correlation with brain concentrations and pharmacodynamic actions. J Pharmacol Exp Ther 1987; 240: 516-22.
18. Lai AA, Levy RH. Pharmacokinetic description of drug interactions by enzyme induction: carbamazepine-clonazepam in monkeys. J Pharmaceut Sci 1979; 68:416-21.
19. Miller ME, Garland WA, Min BH, et al. Clonazepam acetylation in fast and slow acetylators. Clin Pharmacol Ther 1981; 30:343-7.
20. Cohen LS, Rosenbaum JF. Clonazepam: new uses and potential problems. J Clin Psychiatry 1987; 48:50-5.
21. Sullivan FM, McElhatton PR. A comparison of the teratogenic activity of the antiepileptic drugs carbamazepine, clonazepam, ethosuximide, phenobarbital, phenytoin, and primidone in mice. Toxicol Appl Pharmacol 1977; 40:365-78.
22. Randall LO, Kappell B. Pharmacological activity in some benzodiazepines and their metabolites. In: Garattini S, Mussini E, Randall LO, eds. The benzodiazepines. New York: Raven Press, 1973:27-51.
23. Honer WG, Rosenberg RG, Turey M, et al. Respiratory failure after clonazepam and amobarbital (letter). Am J Psychiatry 1986; 143:1495.
24. Ghadirian AM, Gauthier S, Wong T. Convulsions in patients abruptly withdrawn from clonazepam while receiving neuroleptic medication (letter). Am J Psychiatry 1987; 144:686.
25. Jaffe R, Gibson E. Clonazepam withdrawal psychosis (letter). J Clin Psychopharmacol 1986; 6:193.
26. Richards JG, Mohler H, Haefely W. Benzodiazepine binding sites: receptors or acceptors? Trends Pharmacol Sci 1982; 3:233-5.
27. Jenner P, Chadwick D, Reynolds EH, et al. Altered 5-HT metabolism with clonazepam, diazepam and diphenylhydantoin. J Pharm Pharmacol 1975; 27:707-10.
28. Chadwick D, Hallett M, Harris R, et al. Clinical, biochemical, and physiological features distinguishing myoclonus responsive to 5-hydroxytryptophan, tryptophan with a monoamine oxidase inhibitor, and clonazepam. Brain 1977; 100:455-87.
29. Wagner HR, Reches A, Fahn S. Clonazepam-induced up-regulation of serotonin$_1$ binding sites in frontal cortex of rat. Neuropharmacology 1985; 24:953-6.
30. Okuma T, Inanaga K, Otsuki S, et al. A preliminary double-blind study on the efficacy of carbamazepine in prophylaxis of manic-depressive illness. Psychopharmacology 1981; 73:95-6.
31. Ballenger JC, Post RM. Carbamazepine in manic-depressive illness. A new treatment. Am J Psychiatry 1980; 137:782-90.
32. Folks DG, King LD, Dowdy SB, et al. Carbamazepine treatment of selected affectively disordered inpatients. Am J Psychiatry 1982; 139:115-7.
33. Emrich HM, von Zerssen D, Kissling W, et al. Therapeutic effect of valproate in mania (letter). Am J Psychiatry 1981; 138:256.
34. Miller F, Menninger J. Lithium-neuroleptic neurotoxicity is dose dependent. J Clin Psychopharmacol 1987; 7:89-91.

35. Chouinard G, Annable L, Ross-Chouinard A, et al. Ethopropazine and benztropine in neuroleptic-induced parkinsonism. J Clin Psychiatry 1979; 40:147-52.
36. Chouinard G, Ross-Chouinard A, Annable L, et al. Extrapyramidal symptom rating scale. Can J Neurol Sci 1980; 7:233.
37. Sedman G. Clonazepam in treatment of tardive oral dyskinesia (letter). Br Med J 1976; 2:583.
38. Bobruff A, Gardos G, Tarsy D, et al. Clonazepam and phenobarbital in tardive dyskinesia. Am J Psychiatry 1981; 138:183-9.
39. Chouniard G. Use of clonazepam in the maintenance treatment of manic depressive illness. In: Shagass C, Josiassen RC, Bridger WH, et al., eds. Biological psychiatry 1985. New York: Elsevier Science Publishing Co., 1986:723-5.
40. Harms L. Clonazepam and mania (letter). Pharmabulletin (Health Department of Victoria, Australia) 1985; 104:117-9.
41. Freinhar JP, Alvarez WA. Clonazepam: a novel therapeutic adjunct. Int J Psychiatry Med 1985-86; 15:321-8.
42. Shukla S, Godwin CD, Long LEB, et al. Lithium- carbamazepine neurotoxicity and risk factors. Am J Psychiatry 1984; 141:1604-6.
43. Kanter GL, Yerevanian BI, Ciccone JRF. Case report of a possible interaction between neuroleptics and carbamazepine. Am J Psychiatry 1984; 141:1101-2.
44. Arana GW, Goff DC, Friedman H, et al. Does carbamazepine-induced reduction of plasma haloperidol levels worsen psychotic symptoms? Am J Psychiatry 1986; 143:650-1.
45. Wroblewski BA, Singer WD, Whyte J. Carbamazepine-erythromycin interaction. JAMA 1986; 255:1165-7.
46. Yu YL, Huang CY, Chin D, et al. Carbamazepine interaction. Postgrad Med J 1986; 62:231-3.
47. Mutani DL, Sechi GP, Monaco F, et al. Carbamazepine/phenytoin cardiotoxicity: 3 case reports. Arch Neurol 1985; 42:1067-8.
48. Brodi MJ, MacPhee GJA. Carbamazepine neurotoxicity precipitated by diltiazem. Br Med J 1986; 292:1170-1.
49. MacPhee GJA, McInnes GT, Thompson GG, et al. Verapamil potentiates carbamazepine neurotoxicity: a clinically important inhibitory interaction. Lancet 1986; 1:700-3.
50. Chouinard G, Jones BD, Annable L. Neuroleptic-induced supersensitivity psychosis. Am J Psychiatry 1978; 135:1409-10.
51. Chouinard G, Steiner W. Remoxipride in the treatment of acute mania. Biol Psychiatry 1986; 21:1429-33.
52. Wehr TA, Goodwin FK. Rapid cycling in manic-depressives induced by tricyclic antidepressants. Arch Gen Psychiatry 1979; 36:555-9.
53. Wehr TA, Goodwin FK. Can antidepressants cause mania and worsen the course of affective illness? Am J Psychiatry 1987; 144:1403-11.
54. Zetin M, Freedman MJ. Clonazepam in bipolar affective disorder (letter). Am J Psychiatry 1986; 143:1055.
55. Victor BS, Link NA, Binder RL, et al. Use of clonazepam in mania and schizoaffective disorders. Am J Psychiatry 1984; 141:1111-2.
56. Jones BD, Chouinard G. Clonazepam in the treatment of recurrent symptoms of depression and anxiety in a patient with systemic lupus erythematosis. Am J Psychiatry 1985; 142:354-5.
57. Laporta M, Chouinard G, Goldbloom D, et al. Hypomania induced by sertraline, a new serotonin reuptake inhibitor (letter). Am J Psychiatry 1987; 144:1513-4.
58. Frykholm B. Clonazepam—antipsychotic effect in a case of schizophrenia-like psychosis with epilepsy and in three cases of atypical psychosis. Acta Psychiatr Scand 1985; 71:539-42.
59. Freinhar JP, Alvarez WH. Use of clonazepam in two cases of acute mania. J Clin Psychiatry 1985; 46:29-30.
60. Greenspan D, Levin D. Use of clonazepam in a patient with schizoaffective disorder (letter). Am J Psychiatry 1985; 142:774.
61. Freinhar JP, Alvarez WA. Clonazepam treatment of organic brain syndromes in three elderly patients. J Clin Psychiatry 1986; 47:525-6.
62. Nesteros JN, Nair NPV, Pulman JR, et al. High doses of diazepam improve neuroleptic-resistant chronic schizophrenic patients. Psychopharmacology 1983; 81:42-7.

63. Karson CN, Weinberger DR, Bigelow L, et al. Clonazepam treatment of chronic schizophrenia: negative results in a double-blind, placebo-controlled trial. Am J Psychiatry 1982; 139:1627-8.
64. Goldbloom D, Chouinard G. Clonazepam in the treatment of neuroleptic-induced somnambulism (letter). Am J Psychiatry 1984; 141:1486.
65. Albeck JH. Withdrawal and detoxification from benzodiazepine dependence: a potential role for clonazepam. J Clin Psychiatry 1987; 48:43S-8S.
66. Pollack MH, Tesar GE, Rosenbaum JF, et al. Clonazepam in the treatment of panic disorder and agoraphobia: a one-year follow-up. J Clin Psychopharmacol 1986; 6:302-4.
67. Pollack MH. Clonazepam: a review of open clinical trials. J Clin Psychiatry 1987; 48:12S-4S.
68. Tesar GE, Rosenbaum JF. Successful use of clonazepam in patients with treatment-resistant panic disorder. J Nerv Ment Dis 1986; 174:477-82.
69. Beaudry P, Fontaine R, Chouinard G, et al. Clonazepam in the treatment of patients with recurrent panic attacks. J Clin Psychiatry 1986; 47:83-5.
70. Herman JB, Rosenbaum JF, Brotman AW. The alprazolam to clonazepam switch for the treatment of panic disorder. J Clin Psychopharmacol 1987; 7:175-8.

CHAPTER 4

Psychiatric Effects of Phenytoin and Ethosuximide

Rolando Gutierrez-Esteinou, M.D. *Jonathan O. Cole, M.D.*
Belmont, Massachusetts

This chapter examines the psychiatric effects of two of the older anticonvulsants, phenytoin and ethosuximide. For each of these agents, we will present a brief synopsis of basic pharmacological data, followed by a detailed presentation of the available literature regarding their psychiatric effects.

PHENYTOIN

Synthesis and structure

The synthesis of phenytoin was the result of a careful search for a nonsedating anticonvulsant. Hydantoin was synthesized in 1908. Its derivative 5,5-phenylethylhydantoin has been available since the early 1900's as a sedative.[1] Phenytoin is the sodium salt of the 5,5-diphenyl derivative of hydantoin. The first clinical trials with phenytoin took place in 1937, when Putnam and Merritt found it to be an effective agent for grand mal seizures, without the sedative side effects of barbiturates and bromides.[2] Subsequent experience with phenytoin and related compounds suggests that a 5-phenyl or other aromatic substituent is essential for activity against generalized tonic-clonic seizures and abolition of maximal electroshock seizures (MES) in laboratory animals. Alkyl substituents in the 5 position contribute to sedation.[3]

Mechanism of action

At a cellular level, phenytoin has been shown to stabilize excitable membranes and possibly nonexcitable membranes as well. It appears to decrease resting fluxes of sodium ions and sodium currents during action potentials or chemically induced depolarizations, as well as the influx of calcium ions during depolarization. Phenytoin can also delay the activation of outward potassium current during the action potential, leading to an increased refractory period.[4] It increases the rate of serotonin (5-HT) synthesis from tryptophan, which may increase the seizure threshold.[5] In addition, it has been found to have neuroleptic-like[6] and antidepressant-like[7] effects in rat striatum and to reduce haloperidol-induced dopamine receptor supersensitivity.[8] It has been speculated that some of the psychotic reactions and movement disorders associated with phenytoin may be mediated by this mechanism.

Two properties of phenytoin thought to be relevant to its clinical usefulness are its ability to limit the development of maximal seizure activity and its ability to reduce the spread of the seizure process from an active focus (particularly in the cerebral cortex), possibly through its capacity to reduce post-tetanic potentiation.[9] Phenytoin does not elevate the threshold for seizures induced by injection of pentylenetetrazol or picrotoxin and has only limited ability to elevate the threshold for electroshock seizures. In fact, psychiatric patients undergoing electroshock therapy easily develop seizures despite treatment with phenytoin, although the drug blocks the initial tonic phase of the seizure and may prolong the clonic phase. The electroencephalogram (EEG) during such modified seizures shows reduction in both voltage and frequency of convulsive discharges.[10]

Phenytoin does not consistently retard the development of kindling in various animal species.[11] Also, it has little central nervous system (CNS) depressant action at therapeutic doses. In fact, toxic doses cause signs of excitation. An excitatory effect on the cerebellum, activating inhibitory pathways that extend to the cerebral cortex, has been thought to contribute to its anticonvulsant effect.[11]

Phenytoin is effective in the treatment of generalized tonic-clonic seizures and certain partial seizures but does not completely eliminate the sensory aura or other prodromal signs. It is not effective against absence seizures and can actually worsen them.

Pharmacokinetics

Absorption of phenytoin after oral ingestion is slow and sometimes variable. Peak concentrations after a single dose may occur in plasma as early as three hours or as late as 12 hours. It is rapidly distributed into all tissues, and concentrations in plasma and brain are equal within minutes of intravenous injection. Phenytoin is extensively bound to protein (90%). Less than 5% of phenytoin is excreted unchanged in the urine. It is metabolized primarily by hepatic microsomal enzymes, susceptible to alteration by other drugs. The major metabolite (60% of the dose), the parahydroxyphenyl derivative, is inactive and is excreted in the urine as a glucuronide. At plasma concentrations below 10 μg/ml, elimination follows first-order kinetics. The plasma half-life ranges between six and 24 hours. At higher concentrations, a dose-dependent elimination is apparent, so that the plasma half-life increases with concentration, possibly because of the saturability of the hydroxylation reaction. This characteristic explains the small margin between therapeutic and toxic doses at high plasma levels.[12] The therapeutic plasma level lies between 10 μg/ml and 20 μg/ml.

Toxicity

Acute toxicity is mostly related to CNS and cardiac effects. There are some claims that toxicity occurs as a predictable sequence in a dose-related manner, beginning with nystagmus at 15 μg/ml to 25 μg/ml, then ataxia at about 30 μg/ml, followed by lethargy and confusion at about 60 μg/ml.[12] Several cases of encephalopathy related to toxic serum levels have been reported.[13-15] This encephalopathy is manifested by worsening of seizures, slowing of the basic electroencephalographic rhythm, altered mood states, development of visual and haptic hallucinations, hyperactivity, confusion, dullness, schizophreniform reactions, and the appearance of focal neurologic signs.[15] Whether phenytoin-induced "forced normalization" of the EEG may contribute to psychotic symptoms has not been well studied.[16] Phenytoin seems to have an intermediate incidence of psychotic reactions, with ethosuximide more frequently and carbamazepine less frequently implicated.

Phenytoin has been incriminated in the irreversible cerebellar damage that occurs in some epileptic patients.[17] A frontal lobe syndrome with normal vitamin B_{12} serum levels has also been described in chronic phenytoin users.[17] In 30% of patients on phenytoin maintainence, a peripheral neuropathy may be documented by electrophysiologic studies, although it rarely has clinical significance. This neuropathy is related to the drug's effects on folate metabolism, which may also explain some of the psychiatric manifestations and the megaloblastic anemia of chronic phenytoin use.[17]

In addition to the ataxia associated with toxic levels, movement disorders such as athetosis and dystonia have been observed. Also of concern are the multiple reports of phenytoin-induced orofacial dyskinetic movements, clinically identical to those produced by neuroleptics.[18] Fortunately, these dyskinesias appear reversible with discontinuation of the medication. Other toxic effects include gingival hyperplasia, osteomalacia, hyperglycemia, hirsutism, and hypersensitivity reactions.

Dosage and administration

The initial daily dosage by the oral route for adults is 3 mg/kg to 5 mg/kg. Divided doses are recommended to avoid gastric intolerance or toxic peak concentrations. Intravenous administration should not exceed 50 mg per minute. Loading doses, if considered necessary, range from 600 mg to 1000 mg in divided portions over eight to 12 hours. Maintenance daily doses are highly variable but are generally approximately 300 mg. Weekly increases above 300 mg may be made until therapeutic results are achieved or toxicity ensues. Plasma level monitoring is desirable.

Some significant drug interactions include displacement of phenytoin from plasma protein by valproate, accelerated metabolism of phenytoin induced by carbamazepine and phenobarbital, and decreased metabolism induced by ethanol.

Use in psychiatry

Interest in the psychotropic effects of phenytoin was aroused by: (1) the initial observations of behavioral improvement in some epileptics treated with the drug; (2) the discovery of EEG abnormalities in particular psychiatric populations; (3) advances in the understanding of the function of the limbic system; and (4) the lack of effective pharmacologic treatments for most psychiatric disorders in the pre-neuroleptic era.[19] However, interest in phenytoin as an antipsychotic dwindled after the advent of the therapeutically superior phenothiazines in 1952.

With the advent of the theory that cerebral dysrhythmias and "sub-ictal neuronal discharges" could manifest as aggressiveness, impulsivity, anxiety, and agitation, the use of phenytoin under such circumstances seemed logical. In the late 1940's and early 1950's, initial open studies of phenytoin in the treatment of psychiatric patients yielded encouraging results.[20-24] Unfortunately, as will be seen in the following review, these results generally have not been replicated by more recent and rigorous studies, either with phenytoin alone or with phenytoin in combination with other major psychopharmacologic agents.[25-29]

Despite continuing occasional reports of successful treatment of diverse psychiatric disorders with phenytoin, it is still impossible to predict which patients will respond to the drug on the basis of diagnosis, EEG findings, symptomatology, or other characteristics.

Studies with chronically psychotic patients

The initial studies of phenytoin in psychiatric populations were based on chronically psychotic, agitated, hospitalized patients who often had not responded adequately to electroconvulsive therapy (ECT) or other non-neuroleptic treatments. Even under these adverse circumstances, a few studies yielded positive results in about half of the patients treated.

In 1943, Kalinowsky and Putnam performed the pioneering work on the use of phenytoin for psychiatric disorders.[22] They reported their experience in 60 psychiatric patients at a state hospital. Patients showing poor compliance with medication were excluded. The doses of phenytoin were increased to nearly toxic levels in order to elicit the maximum effect: patients were started on 300 mg or 400 mg a day, increasing by 100 mg/day until 600 mg/day was reached. The duration of the trial was between two and five weeks for each patient. None of the patients received any other treatment during this period. The diagnoses were distributed among the following categories: schizophrenia with symptoms of excitement, 22 patients; schizophrenia with catatonic stupor, six patients; other forms of schizophrenia, 13 patients; manic-depressive psychosis, manic type, nine patients; depressed type, five patients; involutional psychosis, four patients; mental deficiency with excitement, one patient. The improvement obtained with phenytoin was then compared to that of ECT, measured on a scale based on clinical judgment, as unimproved, moderately improved, and greatly improved. The best results were obtained in the "excited" group, whether schizophrenic (18% greatly improved, 55% moderately improved, 27% unimproved) or manic (56% greatly improved, 33% moderately improved, 11% unimproved). Only one depressed patient showed a marked improvement. The authors concluded that phenytoin had a purely symptomatic action on states of excitement, independent of diagnosis, not attributable to a sedative action. The improvement disappeared shortly after the medication was stopped and recurred when medication was resumed. Interestingly, subsequent ECT in several instances led to a remission after only one treatment, although the number of cases in which this occurred is not reported.

Two years later, Freyhan reported his experience with 45 chronic patients with varying diagnoses: manic-depressive psychosis, manic type; schizophrenia, catatonic, hebephrenic, and paranoid types; mental deficiency with excitement; dementia paralytica; and postencephalitic excitement.[23] The duration of the trial (two to five weeks) and the doses employed (300 mg to 500 mg/day) were similar to those used by Kalinowsky and Putnam. The patients' behavior was recorded daily before, during, and after the trial to minimize the confounding effect of spontaneous remissions. Only one manic patient, a 54-year-old female resistant to ECT, showed clear-cut improvement. In the schizophrenia group, only catatonic patients responded favorably, with a decrease in frequency of their sudden outbursts of assaultive and destructive behavior. The paranoid and hebephrenic groups showed no response. Little improvement was seen in the other patients. The patients who responded initially to phenytoin continued to respond during subsequent exacerbations of their illness. The author concluded that phenytoin was effective only in the treatment of excitement caused by the primary disease process, and not the secondary excitement due, for example, to the persecutory delusions of paranoid schizophrenia. Electroencephalograms were not performed in any of the cases. The patients who underwent ECT after the phenytoin trial did not show a decrease in the number of treatments required—in contrast to the findings of Kalinowsky and Putnam.

In 1946, Kubanek and Rowell reported the results of an open trial of phenytoin in 73 psychotic patients.[24] Fourteen had been symptomatic for less than a year; the mean duration of symptoms of the rest of the group was close to four and one-half years. Of the schizophrenics, one-third were described as greatly improved with phenytoin, as were two of 21 patients with general paresis. Among the manic depressives, five of nine in the manic phase and one of two in the depressive phase improved. The results were poor in patients with senile psychosis, paranoid condition, mental deficiency, and involutional melancholia. This was the first study to mention behavioral worsening in some of the patients, although no details are given. In congruence with the two previous studies, roughly half of the excited patients showed some response, while only one of nine depressed or retarded patients showed improvement. The authors concluded that phenytoin is useful in the treatment of excited chronic psychoses, especially those that are only partially responsive to other treatments such as barbiturates and ECT.

In 1967, Klein and Greenberg obtained less promising results in an open trial with hospitalized psychiatric patients.[26] Of the 28 patients studied, 13 received phenytoin alone and 15 received phenytoin in addition to other major psychotropic agents. The criteria for phenytoin administration were agitated depression, impulsive actions regardless of diagnosis, and episodic rage in response to trivial stimuli, especially if the patients had an EEG dysrhythmia.

All patients received phenytoin 100 mg TID for at least two weeks. Those who were treated with phenytoin alone had a minimum of four weeks of therapy. The response was measured through weekly interviews with the patient, the patient's psychiatrist, and ward staff, using an ordinal scale ranging from +3 for maximal improvement to -3 for maximal worsening of symptoms.

In the phenytoin-only group, seven patients were diagnosed as having character disorder; six of these had abnormal EEGs characterized by slow wave bursts; two of the six also had 14 Hz and 6 Hz positive spiking. Only one patient had a global improvement rating of +1, four received 0, and two received -1. Three other patients, two of whom had abnormal slow wave EEG activity, had depressive disorders. Their improvement ratings were +2, 0, and -1. Two patients had schizophrenia and one of these also had a diagnosis of psychomotor epilepsy with olfactory and haptic hallucinations and rage attacks. Two EEGs obtained in this patient during the study period showed only 14 Hz and 6 Hz positive spiking. This patient improved maximally with phenytoin, with an apparent complete remission of symptoms, and received a rating of +3.

Nevertheless, for the entire sample of 13 patients, the mean global improvement was 0. There was no relationship between the presence or type of EEG abnormality and the degree of clinical response in the 13 patients treated with phenytoin alone.

The other group comprised 15 patients partially responsive to other psychotropic agents (11 with phenothiazines and four with imipramine). Most of the patients in this group had symptomatology suggestive of psychomotor epilepsy, often in conjunction with an abnormal EEG (found in 11 patients). The predominant EEG abnormality was slow wave activity, either scattered or in bursts. Seven of these 11 patients had, in addition, 14 Hz and 6 Hz positive spiking. Ten of the 15 patients in this group were diagnosed as schizophrenic, of whom seven had abnormal EEGs. Their responses were distributed as follows: one patient was rated +1, eight were rated 0, and one was rated -1. The other five patients were diagnosed as having character disorders of hysterical or "emotionally unstable" type, with four of them showing abnormal EEGs. Of these patients, four received a clinical rating of -1, and one received a 0 rating. The authors concluded that no generally beneficial effect of phenytoin was apparent, whether alone or in combination with phenothiazines or imipramine. Indeed, the only patient with a good response had a previous diagnosis of psychomotor epilepsy.

In 1974, Simopoulos and colleagues published a report of a double-blind placebo-controlled study of the effects of phenytoin in 76 chronic schizophrenic patients in whom phenothiazine treatment had been discontinued.[29] To be included in the study, the patients had to have a primary clinical diagnosis of schizophrenia, continuous hospital treatment with phenothiazine medication for at least six months, no previous history of epilepsy, and at least one of the following behaviors: hostility, irritability, uncooperativeness, withdrawal, anxiety, tension, restlessness, or agitation. Patients were randomly assigned to phenytoin and placebo groups, with 38 in each group. The mean age for both groups was 42 ± 9 years, and the mean duration of current hospitalization was about 12 years, with a range of six months to 35 years. Patients were receiving daily chlorpromazine equivalent doses of 200 mg in 18 cases, 200 mg to 500 mg in 37 cases, 600 mg to 900 mg in 20 cases, and 1600 mg in one case.

On the first day of the study, all phenothiazines were discontinued and the patients randomly assigned to either placebo or phenytoin. Phenytoin was started at a daily dose of 375 mg, increasing weekly or biweekly by 125 mg to a maximum of 625 mg a day, for a total of eight weeks. The patients' responses were measured with the Brief Psychiatric Rating Scale (BPRS), administered before treatment and at the end of two, four, six, and eight weeks. The Crownsville Psychiatric Scale (CPS), part I, was also completed before treatment and at the end of the fourth and eighth weeks. This latter scale measures thinking disturbances (including items such as being worried, agitated, restless, angry, uncooperative, afraid, or withdrawn) and severity of illness (a composite of thinking and emotional disturbance). Other instruments used were the Nurses' Observation Scale for Inpatient Evaluation (NOSIE-30), administered before treatment and at the end of weeks two, four, six, and eight; and the CPS, part II, which measures habits (self-care and work), agitation, and sociability (quantity and type of verbal communications). Both groups of patients had CPS I and II scores above five, with no significant differences between groups, indicating that the entire group contained "hard-core" schizophrenic patients considered to have reached a plateau in their clinical progress with neuroleptic drugs. The initial BPRS scores were consistent with this impression.

There were 13 dropouts in the phenytoin group, seven because of increased assaultiveness, and 11 dropouts in the placebo group, eight because of increased assaultiveness. Although never reaching statistical significance, the adjusted mean scores for both groups tended to show deterioration over the course of the trial. Patients receiving phenytoin as compared to those receiving placebo showed less hostility and unusual thought content on the BPRS at the fourth week. At the eighth week, on the full dose of phenytoin, the patients on active medication showed worsened motor retardation and blunted affect when compared to the placebo group. There were no significant differences in the NOSIE or the CPS-II ratings. The authors concluded that the therapeutic effects of phenytoin, when they did occur, appeared early in the course of treatment when the daily doses were approximately 300 mg, and that improvement was not observed in the latter part of the study period because higher doses were employed.

Although all patients deteriorated off neuroleptics, the authors suggested that phenytoin might be useful in carefully adjusted doses, especially in schizophrenics showing high levels of hostility.

Uses in psychiatric populations with a high prevalence of EEG abnormalities

Phenytoin has been used in some psychiatric groups with a high prevalence of abnormal EEGs. These have included children with behavioral distrubances with or without concurrent mental retardation, patients with bulimia nervosa, and impulsive, explosive, or aggressive patients. As mentioned previously, there are several early, open reports of behavioral improvement with phenytoin in both adult and pediatric patients with epilepsy.[30-32] The improvements described include decreases in irritability,[33] hyperactivity,[34] and destructiveness and acting out.[35] Improvements in concentration,[31] cooperativeness, and general attitude[36] have also been observed. A double-blind controlled study in 47 "cultural retardates" showed trends toward decreased temper outbursts, lowered impulsivity, and lowered aggression.[37]

By contrast, more recent studies on the use of phenytoin in the pediatric population have focused on the deleterious effects of high blood levels or chronic exposure to the drug. Several well-designed studies with both retarded and nonretarded patients have shown a direct correlation between blood levels of phenytoin and cognitive deterioration. This process reversed upon discontinuation of the drug.[17,38] It has been estimated that 40% of the mentally retarded receive phenytoin, either alone or in combination with other psychotropic agents, making these findings of great importance for educational and rehabilitative efforts. Poor results with phenytoin have been observed more recently in the treatment of attention deficit disorder, conduct disorder, and autism.[39-42]

Patients with eating disorders have been reported to show 14 Hz and 6 Hz positive spikes over the temporal and occipital regions on their EEGs.[43] These spikes, also called ctenoids, might represent normal variants, but they have also been associated with episodic, aggressive impulse dyscontrol and somatic symptoms such as headache, nausea, dizziness, paresthesias, micropsias, and abdominal pain.[44] It has been argued that these spikes arise from deep structures such as the hypothalamus,[45] which is known to have a major role in the regulation of food intake. This evidence of a possible role of EEG abnormalities in eating disorders led Green and Rau to assess phenytoin in a series of patients with "compulsive eating disorders".[43,46,47] Subsequently, Wermuth and colleagues assessed phenytoin in 20 patients who would almost certainly have met modern diagnostic criteria for bulimia nervosa.[48] Briefly, although some patients with bulimic symptoms appeared to improve with phenytoin, the drug produced at best a modest effect and has not survived as a modern treatment for bulimia nervosa. Similarly, more recent studies have generally failed to show an elevated prevalence of EEG abnormalities in bulimic patients. The findings of these studies are discussed in detail in Chapter 9 in this volume.

The complexities in the study and treatment of aggression and implusivity have been widely acknowledged.[49-53] For example, Bach-y-Rita and colleagues have described a population with episodic loss of control resulting in violence.[54] In their experience evaluating and treating 130 such patients, they noted widely variable responses to psychotherapeutic and pharmacologic interventions. The authors used phenytoin in all patients with a history of seizure-like outbursts or an abnormal EEG. Although they do not describe the results of their medication trials, they emphasize that all patients benefited from any reduction in the level of anxiety and required close attention from clinicians.

Maletzky and Klotter reported a double-blind placebo-controlled study of phenytoin in the treatment of male patients with episodic dyscontrol.[55] Their population consisted of men with a mean age of 27 years, who had a history of episodic violence upon minimal or no provocation. Some patients reported apparent auras and post-ictal phenomena. The neurologic exam usually disclosed soft signs, and most of the EEGs showed nonspecific temporal lobe changes. Twelve pairs of subjects were formed, matched for age, military and marital status, the presence of alcoholism, and the frequency and severity of violent outbursts for the month prior to the trial. The study period lasted a maximum of 90 days, with average daily phenytoin doses of approximately 300 mg. One subject in each pair was assigned at random to the phenytoin group; the other was assigned to the placebo group. Improvement was measured in terms of: (1) severity of outbursts, using a scale from 1+ to 4+; (2) the frequency of outbursts; and (3) the latency between the initiation of the study and the first outburst rating 2+ or above. Only two phenytoin subjects had more outbursts than their respective placebo controls. One of these patients also had more severe outbursts than his control. This same patient and another one on phenytoin met the 2+ or above criterion sooner than their controls. However, aside from these unfavorable cases, when the patients were considered as a group, improvement with phenytoin appeared both statistically and clinically significant. The authors concluded that patients exhibiting the syndrome of legal difficulties, soft neurological signs, and outbursts of violence should undergo a trial of phenytoin.

Boelhouwer and colleagues, in 1968, published a study designed to examine the diagnostic and therapeutic significance of 14 Hz and 6 Hz positive spiking in the EEG.[56] They studied a total of 78 hospitalized adolescents and young adults, of mean age 18.8 years. To be included in the study, all subjects had to have uncontrollable, impulsive, self-destructive or aggressive behavior, antisocial behavior (stealing, acting out, truancy), and dissociative states during which the preceeding symptoms might have occurred. Patients with documented epilepsy, mental deficiency, or liver damage were excluded. Two groups were formed, one comprised of 47 patients with 14 Hz and 6 Hz positive spiking and a control group of 31 patients without EEG abnormalities. The research team remained blind to the EEG results during the study. All patients received a Minnesota-Hartford Personality Assay (MHPA) and a series of tests sensitive to the presence of mental deterioration as a result of organic brain damage. The subjects were then treated in a double-blind crossover design with either thioridazine 300 mg to 600 mg daily, phenytoin 300 mg daily, or both drugs in combination. Thus, patients who completed the study received three separate trials (two with individual drugs and one with the combination), each lasting eight weeks. Upon entry into the study, the group with the 14 Hz and 6 Hz positive spiking showed more anxiety, guilty self-concept, and poorer control mechanisms and judgement than the control group. Twelve patients from this group and 14 from the control group dropped out because of an increase in their disturbed behavior. Completers in both groups tended to show improvement on three MHPA items: lack of social conformity, lack of insight, and hostile aggessive behavior. These positive changes were more consistent in the group without positive spiking, although, surprisingly, the combination of drugs had significantly more influence on the positive spike group. This effect may be explained by the presence of a subgroup of patients with posterior quadrant slow activity within the positive spike group, who tended to have the poorest responses overall on any of the treatment combinations, although comparisons between the group without posterior slowing and the control group were not reported. The authors concluded that the issue of posterior slowing needed to be examined more closely.

Studies with nonpsychotic patients without an increased frequency of EEG abnormalities

There are several anecdotal reports on the use of phenytoin in anxiety neurosis, reactive depression, obsessive thinking, pseudoneurotic schizophrenia, and other conditions thought to be related to subictal discharges or "minimal epilepsy".[57,58] Jonas, in 1967, published his experiences with 211 patients from his private practice in which he used phenytoin at doses averaging 300 mg per day.[59] He reported some improvement in at least 50% of patients with only three patients having significant problems with the drug, namely, sedation. In his view, phenytoin improved many neurotic manifestations and cognitive disturbances. Turner also found good results with phenytoin in the treatment of several forms of nonpsychotic symptomatology.[60]

He treated 72 subjects in his personal practice with usual doses of phenytoin and found that 86% showed some improvement. In his hands, the target symptoms most amenable to relief by phenytoin were overthinking (i.e. brooding, ruminating), insomnia, depression (particularly when associated with irritability and hostility), anger, impatience and impulsiveness, fear, tension, tension headache, and paralysis in the ability to work because of a combination of the above symptoms.

Stephens and Shaffer studied the effects of phenytoin on neurotic patients in an open protocol.[61] They determined that the patients with "irritability, explosive temper, or anxiety" were the most likely to respond to phenytoin. Subsequently, they enrolled thirty outpatients with one or more of these characteristics in a double-blind placebo-controlled crossover study with phenytoin. They compared a standard oral dose of phenytoin (100 mg TID) to a dose thought to be equivalent to placebo (5 mg TID). The responses were recorded through self-evaluation and clinician-evaluation instruments. Five patients showed no response and 12 showed some response to both doses. The remainder tended to improve in symptoms related to irritability and anger while on full doses of medication and worsen while on the placebo-equivalent dose. These investigators replicated their findings in a subsequent study with a similar population and protocol.[62] However, other double-blind controlled crossover studies with somewhat different populations[28,63] did not show a benefit of phenytoin over placebo.

Conclusions

In conclusion, it appears that a phenytoin trial could be justified in some chronically psychotic, agitated patients, especially those with localized EEG abnormalities who have failed to respond to standard pharmacologic treatments. The drug could also be considered as a possible option in "resistant" patients with intermittent explosive disorder, impulse control disorder, bulimia nervosa, organic personality syndrome, organic affective syndrome, and selected patients with impulsivity and nonspecific EEG abnormalities.

The dearth of studies on the effects of phenytoin in patients with anxiety, irritability, and dysphoria prevents clear conclusions. However, it appears that phenytoin deserves further study in this population, given the current paucity of nonaddicting, nondisinhibiting therapeutic agents.

Conversely, it should be noted that a rare epileptic patient may experience protracted episodes of psychosis or encephalopathy secondary to the use of phenytoin. In such cases, another anticonvulsant may be substituted for phenytoin, sometimes with beneficial effects.

ETHOSUXIMIDE

Structure and mechanism of action

The succinimide derivatives, of which ethosuximide is a dialkyl derivative, were first synthesized and tested in 1951.[64] Little is known about their mechanism of action, although they are valuable resources in the treatment of absence seizures.

Succinimide itself is devoid of anticonvulsant activity, but three derivatives have been introduced for clinical use: ethosuximide, methsuximide, and phensuximide. They have been reported to suppress or prevent experimental seizures produced by pentylenetetrazol or MES.[65]

Antiepileptic effects

In animals ethosumixide has an anticonvulsant spectrum similar to that of trimethadione. Since ethosuximide is a succinimide with a dialkyl substitution in the 2 position, it has only anti-pentylenetetrazol and not anti-MES activity.[66] Specifically, ethosuximide completely prevents pentylenetetrazol seizures in rodents at doses that do not cause neurotoxic effects, unlike methsuximide and phensuximide, which require doses that produce ataxia to completely prevent seizures. Ethosuximide is practically devoid of anti-MES activity except at anesthetic doses exceeding 2 gm/kg, in contrast with methsuximide and phensuximide, which are effective against MES at nontoxic doses.[67] Ethosuximide suppresses other experimental seizures such as those produced by local application of conjugated estrogens to cat cerebral cortex,[68] application of frontal aluminum hydroxide implants in monkeys,[69] and seizures induced by gamma-hydroxybutyrate,[70] leu-enkephalin,[71] and penicillin[72]—characteristics that anti-absence agents share and that phenytoin possesses to a lesser degree. It is thought that absence seizures may involve paroxysmal activity of the inhibitory corticofugal pathways, which are inhibited by ethosuximide.[73] This effect may explain the emergence or increased frequency of generalized tonic-clonic seizures in some patients taking ethosuximide, while their absence seizures improve.

Ethosuximide is highly effective in the treatment of absence seizures but has little or no action against generalized tonic-clonic or partial seizures. Methsuximide and phensuximide are effective against generalized tonic-clonic, partial, and absence seizures, although they are not frequently used because of their high incidence of neurotoxicity at therapeutic doses.[74]

Usual doses of ethosuximide range from 20 mg/kg/day to 40 mg/kg/day in divided doses, although doses up to 60 mg/kg/day are tolerated by some patients.[75]

Pharmacokinetics

After oral ingestion of ethosuximide, absorption appears to be complete, with serum concentrations peaking approximately three hours after a single dose. The drug is not significantly bound to plasma proteins and the steady state concentration in CSF is similar to that of plasma. The volume of distribution is close to 0.7 liter per kilogram. The drug is relatively evenly distributed in all tissues and does not accumulate in fat.

Approximately 20% of an ingested dose of ethosuximide is excreted unchanged in the urine. The remainder is metabolized in the liver, where it undergoes hydroxylation and conjugation with glucuronic acid. The major metabolite is the hydroxyethyl derivative, which accounts for about 40% of the administered dose and is inactive.[76] The plasma half-life averages between 40 and 50 hours in adults and around 30 hours in children. Therapeutic plasma levels range from 40 to 100 μg/ml. Clinically significant drug interactions are rare, although an added neurotoxic effect can be expected when the drug is used in combination with other anticonvulsants.

Toxicity

The most common dose-related side effects are gastrointestinal (nausea, vomiting, and anorexia) and neurological (drowsiness, lethargy, euphoria, dizziness, headache, and hiccoughs). Parkinson-like symptoms have been reported, in congruence with evidence of a central dopamine blocking activity, observed both *in vitro* and in animal behavioral studies.[77]

Psychiatric uses

The only published study on the psychiatric use of ethosuximide is a 1980 preliminary report, by Andrulonis and colleagues, of a double-blind placebo-controlled crossover trial of ethosuximide in the treatment of episodic dyscontrol syndrome, as defined by DSM-III.[78] The study population was composed of patients with a history of violence, substance abuse, suicide attempts, and resistance to conventional psychiatric interventions. The subjects were likely to have had head trauma, learning disabilities, or hyperactivity as children. Their EEGs had nonspecific temporal and frontal abnormalities, 14 Hz and 6 Hz per second spiking in the temporal lobes, and sharp or slow wave activity in the posterior quadrant. Most had soft neurologic signs. The investigators hypothesized that the subjects' acts of violence were triggered by complex partial ictal events resulting from recurrent, excessive disorderly discharges from the temporal lobes. Ethosuximide was thought to be able to prevent such events. The instruments used to measure clinical change were the Minnesota Multiphasic Personality Inventory (MMPI), Minnesota-Hartford Personality Assay (MHPA), daily nursing notes, nursing special behavior reports, standard EEGs, and neurological examinations. At the time of publication, only seven patients had completed the protocol, so no statistical analyses were done.

However, the investigators describe the course of a 14-year-old girl with the diagnosis of episodic dyscontrol syndrome characterized by self-mutilation, assaultiveness, property damage, and multiple suicide attempts. Her admission EEG showed slow wave activity in the posterior quadrant and 6 Hz to 10 Hz positive spiking over the right temporal lobe during sleep. The patient underwent eight weeks of ethosuximide treatment, eight weeks of placebo, and then another eight weeks of ethosuximide. During the first period, the patient had four episodes of dyscontrol, including two of self-mutilation, before a therapeutic serum level was attained. At a therapeutic serum level (1250 mg/day, 73.6 μg/ml), she had two episodes of verbal threats without frank dyscontrol which did not require neuroleptic treatment. During the placebo period, she exhibitied 11 dyscontrol episodes requiring 34 doses of thioridazine (size of the dose not reported). When a therapeutic level of ethosuximide was restored, the patient did not suffer any further episodes of dyscontrol. Her MHPA results from both of the active medication periods showed less hostility, self-criticism, defective superego integration, and paranoid thinking than during the placebo period. However, baseline premedication testing was not performed. The MMPI showed lower scores during active medication periods on all scales except the masculine-feminine and ego strength scales. The daily nursing notes described less antisocial behavior during active treatment. The active treatment EEG showed a striking increase in alpha activity and a disappearance of the slow wave activity noted on the admission EEG. No change in the soft neurologic signs or medication side effects were noted. The authors concluded that this observation, under blind and controlled conditions, was consistent with their experience in treating 70 patients with open label ethosuximide for episodic dyscontrol disorders over a two-year period. Unfortunately, the controlled study was never finished (Glueck BC, personal communication, January, 1988), and a detailed presentation of the authors' experience was never published. To our knowledge, there are no other reports of psychiatric use of ethosuximide. Given these encouraging preliminary results, further research would seem warranted.

Adverse neuropsychiatric effects

The literature on the adverse neuropsychiatric effects of ethosuximide is scanty and inconclusive. This is partly due to the adverse consequences that absence seizures themselves may have on intellectual functions. Older studies, such as that of Guey and co-workers, showed global intellectual impairment with prominent disturbances in memory and speech following the addition of ethosuximide to phenobarbital in 25 children treated for absence seizures.[79] These observations were replicated by Soulayrol and Roger in 100 children receiving ethosuximide, the majority of whom showed similar intellectual deterioration.[80] More recent studies have not showed evidence of intellectual deterioration or behavior disturbances with ethosuximide. In fact, there was some evidence of improvement in psychological function in a controlled multicenter trial.[81] Similarly, Browne and colleagues were unable to detect detrimental effects of the drug on psychometric performance over a period of eight weeks in 37 epileptic children.[82] Indeed, 17 of the patients had improved performance, but this might have been due to good seizure control.

Several case reports of psychotic episodes associated with ethosuximide have appeared since 1961. Lairy described three cases of psychosis in a series of 32 patients treated with the drug,[83] and Lorentz de Haas and Stoel observed psychotic episodes in three cases among 60 ethosuximide-treated patients.[84] All patients had absence seizures and abnormalities in the pre-ethosuximide EEG that disappeared with treatment. Their psychoses remitted after stopping the anticonvulsant and recurred following resumption of treatment. Whether they became psychotic on other anticonvulsants is not specified. The psychosis was thought to be due to "forced normalization" of the EEG as described by Landolt.[16]

Fischer and associates reported three cases of psychosis in a series of 105 patients treated with ethosuximide for absence seizures, or absence plus tonic-clonic seizures.[85] In the patients with more than one type of seizure, multiple drugs were employed. The dose of ethosuximide used was 30 mg/kg/day. Their success rate in the treatment of the seizures was comparable to that of other investigators (i.e. improvement in

70% of children and 40% of adults with absence seizures). The three cases of psychosis shared the following characteristics: absence seizures with abnormal EEGs (3 Hz spike-waves and diffusely increased delta activity); age greater than 27; no clear personal or family psychiatric history; some evidence of depression preceeding the exposure to ethosuximide; a prodromic phase with delirium and hallucinations; affective symptoms such as self-reproach, depressed mood, and agitation; and improved control of the seizures with normalization of the EEG during treatment with ethosuximide. The psychotic symptoms disappeared after stopping ethosuximide and recurred in the two patients who resumed the drug. One of the patients who was treated with other unspecified anticonvulsants did not experience a recurrence of the psychosis in spite of normalization of her EEG with the new treatment. Nonetheless, the authors speculated that the cause of these psychotic episodes was "forced normalization" of the EEG as had been proposed by Lorentz de Haas and Stoel.[84]

Roger and colleagues[86] reported 15 new cases of neuropsychiatric complications related to ethosuximide and pooled these with 20 cases previously reported in the literature. They determined the incidence of psychotic reactions to be about 4% on doses usually considered therapeutic (mean 1250 mg/day). More than half of the patients were treated with combinations of anticonvulsants. No patients were reported to have had psychotic reactions on these drugs prior to the addition or substitution of ethosuximide, even in the presence of normalization of the EEG. Unfortunately, measurements of serum levels of anticonvulsants were not obtained in any of these patients, and there were no assessments of their metabolic status, including folate and B12 serum levels. Age was thought to be an important factor, given that only three of the 35 cases were younger than 15 years and the mean age at index episode was over 22 years. The mean duration of the seizure disorder was 14 years; half of the cases presented a mixed form of grand mal plus absence seizures and 71% of the cases had a positive family history of seizures. Six had a history of psychosis, and several others had "neurotic traits of hysteric or obsessive type" or character pathology.

The clinical picture of the psychosis included a prodromic phase of variable length with half of the episodes appearing in the first three weeks following initiation of treatment or a major increase in the dose. The prodrome was characterized by anxiety, depression, and worsening of behavioral disorders, followed by depersonalization, oneiroid states, and confusion. Hallucinations, more frequently auditory than visual, were mood-congruent and often accompanied by persecutory delusions. Two-thirds of the cases ceased to have absence seizures and 75% of the cases showed normalization of the EEG. The total duration of the psychotic episodes was extremely variable, from days to several months, averaging three months. One exceptional case lasted for five years. All cases of psychosis resolved *ad integrum*. The management in most cases was limited to discontinuation of the drug, but some patients were prescribed neuroleptics and/or antidepressants, so that improvement in the psychosis may have been due to any of the measures taken. In only two cases was improvement of seizure control maintained after stopping ethosuximide.

In their discussion, the authors favor the hypothesis that psychotic episodes are a direct toxic effect of ethosuximide, and they argue that the role of "forced normalization" of the EEG remains unclear. They recommend lowering the dose or switching to a different anti-absence drug when prodromes of the psychotic episode (depression, asthenia, anxiety, behavorial worsening) appear or if a brisk normalization of the EEG occurs.

In summary, it is clear that the occurrence of "forced normalization" of the EEG is neither sufficient nor necessary for the development of psychosis, as evidenced by the 25% of cases that had persistently abnormal EEGs during ethosuximide-related psychoses. Conversely, anticonvulsants have been shown to produce forced normalization without precipitation of psychosis.[87,88]

CONCLUSIONS

Presently available data on the psychiatric actions of ethosuximide are extremely limited. On the one hand, the drug showed an apparent beneficial effect in a single study of patients with episodic dyscontrol syndromes. On the other hand, the drug has been reported to cause occasional psychotic episodes in epileptic patients, possibly related to "forced normalization" of the EEG. Although these episodes eventually resolve following withdrawal of ethosuximide, psychotic symptoms have persisted for months in many cases. Clearly, further studies of ethosuximide in special psychiatric populations and studies of the mechanism of ethosuximide-induced psychosis are warranted.

REFERENCES

1. Blitz H. Uber die Konstitution der Einwekungsprodukte von substituierte Harnstoffen auf Benzil über einige neue Methoden zur Darstellung der 5,5 diphenylhydantoine. Berl Dtsch Chem Ges 1908; 41:45-55.
2. Putnam TJ, Merritt HH. Experimental determination of anticonvulsant properties of some phenyl derivatives. Science 1938; 85:525-6.
3. Toman JEP, Goodman LS. Anticonvulsants. Physiol Rev 1948; 28:409-32.
4. Woodbury DM, Fingl E. Drugs effective in the treatment of the epilepsies. In: Goodman LS, Gilman A, eds. The pharmacologic basis of therapeutics. 5th ed. New York: MacMillan, 1975:201-26.
5. Chadwick D, Jenner P, Reynolds EH. Serotonin metabolism in human epilepsy: the influence of anticonvulsant drugs. Ann Neurol 1977; 1:218-24.
6. Elliot PN, Janner P, Chadwick D, et al. The effect of diphenylhydantoin on central catecholamine-containing neuronal systems. J Pharm Pharmacol 1988; 29:41-3.
7. Poncelet M, Hakkou F, Simon P. Psychopharmacological profile of diphenylhydantoin in mice. Prog Neuropsychopharmacol Biol Psychiatry 1984; 8:373-8.
8. Lepore V, Di Reda N, Defazio G, et al. Dopaminomimetic action of diphenylhydantoin in rat striatum: effect on homovanillic acid and cyclic AMP levels. Psychopharmacolgy 1985; 86:27-30.
9. Woodbury DM, Kemp JW. Pharmacology and mechanisms of action of diphenylhydantoin. Psychiatry Neurol Neurochir 1971; 74:91-115.
10. Toman JEP, Swinyard EA, Goodman LS. Properties of maximal seizures and their alterations by anticonvulsant drugs and other agents. J Neurophysiol 1946; 9:231-40.
11. Julien RM, Halpern LM. Effects of diphenylhydantoin and other antiepileptic drugs on epileptiform activity and Purkinje cell discharge rates. Epilepsia 1972; 13:387-400.
12. Kutt H, Winters W, Kokenge R, et al. Diphenylhydantoin metabolism, blood levels, and toxicity. Arch Neurol 1964; 2:642-8.

13. McLellan DL, Swash M. Choreoathethosis and encephalophathy induced by phenytoin. Br Med J 1984; 2:204-5.
14. Vallarta JM, Bell DB, Reichert A. Progressive encephalopathy due to chronic hydantoin intoxication (letter). Am J Dis Child 1974; 128:2734.
15. Hoaken PCS, Kane FJ. Unusual brain syndrome with diphenylhydantoin and phenobarbital (letter). Am J Psychiatry 1963; 120:282.
16. Landolt H. Serial EEG investigation during psychotic episodes in epileptic patients during schizophrenic attacks. In: Lorenz de Haas A, ed. Lectures in epilepsy. Amsterdam: Elsevier, 1958:91-102.
17. Oxley J, Janz D, Meinardi H, eds. Chronic toxicity of antiepileptic drugs. New York: Raven Press, 1983.
18. Chadwick D, Reynolds EH, Marsden CD. Anticonvulsant-induced dyskinesias: a comparison with dyskinesias induced by neuroleptics. J Neurol Neurosurg Psychiatry 1976; 39:1210-8.
19. Elkes J. American College of Neuropsychopharmacology session on diphenylhydantoin. Introductory remarks. Int J Neuropsychiatry 1967; 2:6S-7S.
20. Silverman D. The electroencephalograph and therapy of criminal psychopaths. Criminal Psychopathology 1944; 5:439-57.
21. Brill NQ, Walker EF. Psychopathic behavior with latent epilepsy. J Nerv Ment Dis 1945; 101:545-9.
22. Kalinowsky LB, Putnam TJ. Attempts at treatment of schizophrenia and other non-epileptic psychoses with Dilantin. Arch Neurol Psychiatry 1943; 49:414-20.
23. Freyhan FA. Effectiveness of diphenylhydantoin in management of non-epileptic psychomotor excitement states. Arch Neurol Psychiatry 1945; 53:370-4.
24. Kubanek JL, Rowell RC. The use of Dilantin in the treatment of psychotic patients unresponsive to other treatments. Dis Nerv Syst 1946; 7:47-50.
25. Pasamanick B. Anticonvulsant drug therapy of behavior problem children with abnormal electroencephalograms. Arch Intern Med 1951; 104:752-66.
26. Klein DF, Greenberg IM. Behavioral effects of diphenylhydantoin in severe psychiatric disorders. Am J Psychiatry 1967; 124:847-9.
27. Kanzler M, Malitz S, Higgins JC. How effective are antidepressants (letter)? JAMA 1968; 204:34.
28. Lefkowitz MM. Effects of diphenylhydantoin on disruptive behavior: study of male delinquents. Arch Gen Psychiatry 1969; 20:643-5.
29. Simopoulos AM, Pinto A, Uhlenhuth EH, et al. Diphenylhydantoin: effectiveness in the treatment of chronic schizophrenics. Arch Gen Psychiatry 1974; 30:106-11.
30. Merritt HH, Putnam TJ. A new series of anticonvulsant drugs tested by experiments on animals. Arch Neurol Psychiatry 1938; 39:1003-15.
31. Kimball OP, Horan TN. The use of Dilantin in the treatment of epilepsy. Ann Intern Med 1939; 13:787-93.
32. Frankel SI. Dilantin sodium in the treatment of epilepsy. JAMA 1940; 114:1320-1.
33. McCartan W, Carson J. The use of sodium diphenylhydantoinate. J Ment Sci 1939; 85:965-71.
34. Rossi AO. Psychoneurologically impaired child: community mental health clinic approach. NY Med 1967; 67:902-12.
35. Itil TM, Rizzo AE, Shapiro DM. Study of behavior and EEG correlation during treatment of disturbed children. Dis Nerv Syst 1967; 28:731-6.
36. Ross AT, Jackson V. Dilantin sodium: its influence on conduct and on psychometric ratings of institutionalized epileptics. Ann Intern Med 1940; 14:770-3.
37. Goldberg JB, Kurland AA. Dilantin treatment of cultural-familial retardates. J Nerv Ment Dis 1970; 150:133-7.
38. Glaser GH. Diphenylhydantoin toxicity. In: Woodbury DM, Penry JK, Schmidt RP, eds. Antiepileptic drugs. New York: Raven Press, 1972:219-41.
39. Luhdorf K, Lund M. Phenytoin-induced hyperkinesia. Epilepsia 1977; 18:409-15.
40. Stores G. Behavioural effects of anti-epileptic drugs. Dev Med Child Neurol 1975; 17:647-58.
41. Saccar CL. Drug therapy in the treatment of minimal brain dysfunction. Am J Hosp Pharm 1978; 35:544-52.

42. Aman MG, Paxton JW, Field CJ, et al. Prevalence of toxic anticonvulsant drug concentrations in mentally retarded persons with epilepsy. Am J Ment Defic 1986; 90:643-50.
43. Rau JH, Struve FA, Green RS. Electroencephalographic correlates of compulsive eating. Clin Electroencephalogr 1979; 10:180-9.
44. Refsum S, Presthus J, Skulstad AA, et al. Clinical correlates of the 14 and 6 per second positive spikes: an electroencephalographic and clinical study. Acta Psychiatr Scand 1960; 35:330-44.
45. Berilaqua AR, Little SC. Fourteen and six per second dysrhythmia with proven hypothalamic disease. Electroencephalogr Clin Neurophysiol 1961; 13:314-5.
46. Green RS, Rau JH. Treatment of compulsive eating disturbances with anticonvulsant medication. Am J Psychiatry 1974; 131:428-32.
47. Green RS, Rau JH. The use of diphenylhydantoin in compulsive eating disorders: further studies. In: Vigersky RA, ed. Anorexia nervosa. New York: Raven Press, 1977:377-83.
48. Wermuth BM, Davis KL, Hollister LE, et al. Phenytoin treatment of the binge eating syndrome. Am J Psychiatry 1977; 134:1249-53.
49. Monroe RR. Anticonvulsants in the treatment of aggression. J Nerv Ment Dis 1975; 160: 119-26.
50. Smith WL, Kling A, eds. Issues in brain behavior control. New York: Spectrum, 1976.
51. Sandler M, ed. Psychopharmacology of aggression. New York: Raven Press, 1979.
52. Lion JR. Conceptual issues in the use of drugs for the treatment of aggression in man. J Nerv Ment Dis 1975; 160:76-82.
53. Woodcock JH. A neuropsychiatric approach to impulse disorder. Psychiatr Clin N Am 1986; 9:341-52.
54. Bach-y-Rita G, Lion JR, Climent CE, et al. Episodic dyscontrol: a study of 130 violent patients. Am J Psychiatry 1971; 127:1473-8.
55. Maletzky BM, Klotter J. Episodic dyscontrol: a controlled replication. Dis Nerv Syst 1974; 35:175-8.
56. Boelhouwer C, Henry CE, Glueck BC. Positive spiking: a double-blind control study on its significance in behavior disorders, both diagnostically and therapeutically. Am J Psychiatry 1968; 125:473-81.
57. Haward LR. The use of phenytoin in neurotic disorders treated in general practice. Curr Med Res Opin 1982; 8:134-8.
58. Dreyfus J. A remarkable medicine has been overlooked. New York: Simon and Schuster, 1970.
59. Jonas AD. The diagnostic and therapeutic use of diphenylhydantoin in the subictal state and non-epileptic dysphoria. Int J Neuropsychiatry 1967; 2:21S-9S.
60. Turner WJ. The usefulness of diphenylhydantoin in the treatment of non-epileptic emotional disorder. Int J Neuropsychiatry 1967; 2:8S-20S.
61. Stephens JH, Shaffer JW. A controlled study of the effects of diphenylhydantoin on anxiety, irritability and anger in neurotic patients. Psychopharmacologia (Berlin) 1970; 17:169-81.
62. Stephens JH, Shaffer JW. A controlled replication of the effectiveness of diphenylhydantoin on anxiety, irritability and anger in neurotic patients. J Clin Pharmacol 1973; 13:351-6.
63. Case WG, Rickels K, Bazilian S. Diphenylhydantoin in neurotic anxiety. Am J Psychiatry 1969; 126:254-5.
64. Chen G, Portman R, Ensor CR, et al. The anticonvulsant activity of alpha-phenylsuccinimides. J Pharmacol Exp Ther 1951; 103:54-61.
65. Chen G, Weston JK, Bratton AC. Anticonvulsant activity and toxicity of phensuximide, methsuximide and ethosuximide. Epilepsia 1963; 4:66-76.
66. Vida JA, ed. Medicinal chemistry, a series of monographs. Vol. 15. Anticonvulsants. New York: Academic Press, 1977.
67. Ferrendelli JA, Kupferberg HJ. Antiepileptic drugs: succinimides. In: Glaser GH, Penry JK, Woodbury DM, eds. Antiepileptic drugs: mechanisms of action. New York: Raven Press, 1980:587-96.
68. Julien RM, Fowler GW, Danielson MG. The effects of antiepileptic drugs on estrogen-induced electroencephalographic spike-wave discharge. J Pharmacol Exp Ther 1975; 193:647-56.

69. David J, Marathe SB, Patil SD, et al. Behavioral and electrical correlates of absence seizures induced by thalamic stimulation in juvenile rhesus monkeys with frontal aluminum hydroxide implants: a pharmacologic evaluation. J Pharmacol Methods 1982; 7:219-29.
70. Snead OC. Gamma-hydroxybutyrate in the monkey. III. Effect of intravenous anticonvulsant drugs. Neurology (Minneapolis) 1978; 28:1173-8.
71. Snead OC, Bearden LJ. Anticonvulsants specific to petit mal antagonize epileptogenic effect of leucine enkephalin. Science 1980; 21:1031-3.
72. Guberman A, Gloor P, Sherwin AL. Response of generalized pencillin epilepsy in the cat to ethosuximide and diphenylhydantoin. Neurology (Minneapolis) 1975; 25:758-64.
73. Fromm GH, Kohli CM. The role of inhibitory pathways in petit mal epilepsy. Neurology (Minneapolis) 1972; 22:1012-20.
74. Millichap JG. General principles. Clinical efficacy and use. In: Woodbury DM, Penry JK, Schmidt RP, eds. Antilepileptic drugs. New York: Raven Press, 1972: 97-101.
75. Woodbury DM, Fingl E. Drugs effective in the treatment of the epilepsies. In: Goodman LS, Gilman A, eds. The pharmacologic basis of therapeutics. 5th ed. New York: MacMillan, 1975:459-61.
76. Horning MG, Butler CM, Lertratanangkoon K, et al. Gas chromatography-mass spectrometry-computer studies of the metabolism of anticonvulsant drugs. In: Kellaway P, Petersen I, eds. Quantitative analytic studies in epilepsy. New York: Raven Press, 1976:95-114.
77. Jodhav JH, Balsara JJ, Jeurkar AJ, et al. Effect of ethosuximide on dopaminergically mediated behaviours. Indian J Physiol Pharmacology 1981; 25:274-8.
78. Andrulonis PA, Donnelly J, Glueck BC, et al. Preliminary data on ethosuximide and the episodic dyscontrol syndromes. Am J Psychiatry 1980; 137:1455-6.
79. Guey J, Charles C, Conquery C, et al. Study of psychological effects of ethosuximide (Zarontin) on 25 children suffering from petit mal epilepsy. Epilepsia 1967; 8:129-41.
80. Soulayrol R, Roger J. Effets psychiatriques défavorables des médications anti-épileptiques. Revue Neuropsychiatr Infant 1970; 18:591-8.
81. Buchanan RA. Ethosuximide toxicity. In: Woodbury DM, Penry JK, Schmidt RP, eds. Antiepileptic drugs. New York: Raven Press, 1972:377-86.
82. Browne TR, Dreifuss FE, Dyken PR, et al. Ethosuximide (Zarontin) in the treatment of absence (petit mal) seizures. Neurology (Minneapolis) 1975; 25:515-25.
83. Lairy CG. Signes psychotiques survenant chez des épileptiques au cour d'un traitement par éthosuccimide. Rev Neurol 1964; 110:225-6.
84. Lorentz de Haas A, Stoel LMK. Experiences with alpha-ethyl, alpha-methyl-succinimide in the treatment of epilepsy. Epilepsia 1960; 1:501-11.
85. Fischer M, Korskjaer, Pederson E. Psychotic episodes in Zarontin treatment, effects and side-effects in 105 patients. Epilepsia 1965; 6:325-34.
86. Roger J, Grangeon H, Guey J, et al. Incidences psychiatriques et psychologiques du traitement par l'éthosuximide chez les épileptiques. Encephale 1968; 57:146-52.
87. Chkhenkeil SA, Geladze TS. The forced normalization EEG phenomenon and several mechanisms of psychopathologic symptoms in epileptic patients. Zh Neuropatol Psykhiatr 1979; 79:680-5.
88. Pakalnis A, Drake M, Kuruvilla J, et al. Forced normalization. Acute psychosis after seizure control in seven patients. Arch Neurol 1987; 44:289-91.

CHAPTER 5

Combining Anticonvulsants with Conventional Psychopharmacologic Agents

Barry S. Fogel, M.D.
Providence, Rhode Island

INTRODUCTION

The combination of anticonvulsants with other psychotropic drugs is widespread, although it has been the focus of little systematic study. Both pharmacokinetic and pharmacodynamic interactions can affect clinical efficacy and toxicity. A judicious choice of the specific anticonvulsant and psychotropic used can reduce adverse interactions and promote additive or synergistic effects. This chapter will describe common clinical situations in which anticonvulsant-psychotropic combinations are rational. It will then discuss the most common and important drug interactions, and mention special considerations regarding the prevention of suicide and appropriate use of the electroencephalogram (EEG) to guide and monitor therapy.

OCCASIONS FOR COMBINATION THERAPY

Epilepsy with concurrent psychopathology

Patients with epilepsy, particularly those with complex partial seizures, are known to be at increased risk for both depression and psychosis.[1-3] In a typical outpatient epilepsy clinic, at least 10% of the patients receive drug treatment for depression,[4,5] and among patients with poorly controlled temporal lobe epilepsy, the prevalence of psychosis is between 10% and 15%.[6] The psychiatric concomitants of epilepsy frequently go beyond mere adjustment reactions and constitute major psychiatric syndromes requiring pharmacologic treatment. Depression and psychosis may contribute substantially to disability and may indirectly aggravate seizures because of their effect on sleep, medication compliance, and stress level.[7,8] State hospitals treating the chronically mentally ill encounter a high proportion of patients with associated seizure disorders, with a 10% estimate in one large state hospital in New York.[9] Both institutionalized and community-dwelling retarded populations also have a high prevalence of epilepsy as a secondary diagnosis, and many retarded patients concurrently receive neuroleptics for psychosis or agitation[10] (and see Chapter 11 in this volume). Making conservative assumptions about the prevalence of chronic mental disorder and of epilepsy, we can estimate that at least 250,000 patients in the United States are receiving concurrent anticonvulsant and psychotropic drug therapy because of epilepsy associated with a major mental disorder.

Bipolar disorder

While lithium is the mainstay of treatment for bipolar disorder, many patients do not respond to lithium or are intolerant of its side effects. Recent work has brought attention to the antimanic efficacy of three anticonvulsants—carbamazepine, valproate, and clonazepam[11-14] (and see Chapters 1-3 in this volume). Controlled studies provide the strongest evidence for the antimanic and prophylactic efficacy of carbamazepine,[15-17] and randomized studies show it to be as effective as lithium.[18,19] Anticonvulsants may be particularly valuable in rapid-cycling illness, because unlike antidepressants and even lithium, they have not been reported to aggravate this condition[20-22] (and see Chapter 7 in this volume). Many patients have been reported who have responded neither to lithium alone nor to an anticonvulsant alone, but have done well on a combination. Combination therapy has been reported using lithium and carbamazepine, lithium and valproate, and lithium and clonazepam.[14,23-27]

Patients with bipolar disorder may have successful control of manic episodes with an anticonvulsant, yet have less satisfactory control of depressive episodes. Depressive episodes in patients on antimanic anticonvulsants might be an occasion for the concurrent use of a tricyclic antidepressant or monoamine oxidase (MAO) inhibitor. There is scant literature on these combinations, although the safe concurrent use of carbamazepine and tranylcypromine has been reported.[28]

Violence and agitation in institutionalized patients

Carbamazepine has been used as an alternative or adjunct to neuroleptic therapy in violent or agitated patients with schizophrenia,[29] borderline personality,[30,31] dementia,[32] mental retardation,[33,34] other chronic psychoses,[35] and aggressive behavior.[36] In the treatment of aggressive behaviors combinations with neuroleptics and with lithium are most common. Beta blockers have been also used widely for agitation and violence in institutionalized patients,[37-39] so anticonvulsant-beta blocker combinations almost certainly have been employed. Details, however, have not been reported.

Atypical psychosis

Patients with atypical psychotic disorders may be suspected of having an epileptic psychosis, even if there is no abnormality on surface EEG. Case series have identified patients with psychotic symptoms aggravated by neuroleptics and helped by anticonvulsants, particularly carbamazepine.[40,41] Many of these patients have normal waking EEGs, with abnormalities evident only on sleep deprivation or on depth electrode studies. Some of these patients might require a combination of anticonvulsant and neuroleptic therapy.

Bulimia

The literature on bulimia has suggested that a subgroup of bulimic patients responds to anticonvulsants. This group includes some with abnormal EEGs[42,43] and others with rapid-cycling bipolar illness plus bulimia[44] (and see Chapter 9 of this volume). The latter group may be particularly responsive to valproate or carbamazepine.[44,45] Because there is a high prevalence of depression in bulimia, and because antidepressants may ameliorate bulimia,[46] antidepressant- anticonvulsant combinations could rationally be prescribed in this disorder.

Prophylaxis in psychiatric patients with risk factors for seizures

Both neuroleptics and tricyclic antidepressants lower the seizure threshold and provoke clinical seizures in a small but significant proportion of patients.[47-51] Patients with other risk factors for epilepsy are particularly at risk. These factors include paroxysmal EEG abnormalities, a family history of epilepsy, and a history of focal lesions with epileptic potential, such as those from head trauma, stroke, infection, multiple sclerosis, or congenital central nervous system (CNS) disease. In such patients, it may be rational to use anticonvulsants prophylactically, to prevent the emergence of seizures during treatment of a psychiatric disorder with an antidepressant or neuroleptic. There would be a particularly compelling reason to do so in the patient with neurologic risk factors but no history of epilepsy who had a seizure shortly after initiating therapy with an antidepressant or neuroleptic.

Chronic pain

Neuropathic pain with a lancinating or "shooting" quality may be responsive to anticonvulsants, including carbamazepine, phenytoin, clonazepam, and valproate. Anticonvulsant-responsive painful conditions include trigeminal neuralgia, glossopharyngeal neuralgia, paroxysmal pains of multiple sclerosis, and some cases of diabetic neuropathy, as well as lancinating pains following laminectomy, amputation, or an episode of herpes zoster.[52,53] In many of these situations antidepressants may also be indicated, either to treat a concurrent depression or to treat a steady, persistent, and nonlancinating aspect of the pain itself. For example, a patient with painful diabetic neuropathy might require a tricyclic-carbamazepine combination for optimal pain relief; a patient with multiple sclerosis, a mood disorder, and paroxysmal pain might be treated with a tricyclic plus clonazepam.

COMMON AND IMPORTANT DRUG INTERACTIONS

Drug interactions between anticonvulsants and other psychotropic drugs can be divided into two main groups—pharmacokinetic interactions, mediated through changes in drug absorption, metabolism, protein binding, or receptor binding; and pharmacodynamic interactions, mediated through additive, synergistic, or antagonistic effects of the two drugs on the CNS. In the first instance, the interaction would be associated with some change in a drug level or other measurable parameter such as percentage of protein binding. In the second instance, the toxicity would be reflected by neurologic or mental status changes in the presence of apparently appropriate drug levels.

The literature on the interaction between anticonvulsants and other psychotropics can be confusing for several reasons. First, pharmacokinetics of both anticonvulsants and psychotropics are subject to enormous interindividual variation. Because blood levels may be unusually low or high on a standard dose of a one-drug regimen, interactive effects with a second drug can be demonstrated conclusively only by challenge, removal, and rechallenge with the second drug.

Second, drug interactions may oppose one another, cancelling clinical effect. Two hypothetical examples will illustrate this: (1) If drug B displaces drug A from protein binding sites, drug A may be cleared more rapidly, leading to a lower blood level. On the other hand, the displacement of drug A from protein binding sites could raise the proportion of free drug, canceling out the effects of a lower total blood level. (2) Drug B may induce the hepatic cytochrome system, leading to more rapid metabolism of both drug B itself, and drug A. On the other hand, drug B may compete with drug A for sites on the metabolic enzymes, and the decrease in metabolism of drug A, due to competition, may exactly counterbalance the increased rate of metabolism due to enzyme induction, with no net effect on the level of drug A. Pharmacokinetic variability implies that cancelation may take place in one patient but not in another, depending on individual differences in factors such as enzyme activity, protein binding sites, and clearance rates.

Third, a drug interaction may become apparent only when one of the drugs is stopped. For example, in the case where enzyme induction is counterbalanced by competition for enzyme sites, removal of one drug may eliminate competition effects while the metabolizer enzyme remains induced. This could lead to a sudden drop in the blood level of the drug being continued.

Because of these considerations, a general principle of combining anticonvulsants with other psychotropic drugs is to regularly obtain blood levels of all drugs for which levels are therapeutically meaningful, and to recheck levels whenever there is a significant change in the patient's status—either a relapse of the mental disorder, a relapse of seizures, or the appearance of clinical toxicity. In situations where protein binding is thought to be an issue, free drug levels, when available, may settle the point. This is particularly helpful for phenytoin, which is highly protein bound and subject to displacement by numerous other drugs, and for which an assay of free drug level is widely available.

REPORTED PHARMACOKINETIC INTERACTIONS

With phenytoin

Addition of tricyclic antidepressants to the regimen of patients on phenytoin has been reported to increase serum phenytoin levels, but the effect is inconsistent.[54,55] Similarly, benzodiazepines have been reported to increase phenytoin levels[56,57] but on occasion have been associated with decreased levels.[58] Phenothiazines, including chlorpromazine and thioridazine, have been associated with increased phenytoin levels due to inhibited metabolism,[59] but some patients have decreased phenytoin levels,[60] and, in a recent retrospective series, most patients showed no change in phenytoin levels after thioridazine was started.[61] A recent case report suggests that trazodone may precipitate phenytoin intoxication, perhaps by competing for phenytoin's hepatic site of metabolism.[62]

With valproate

Valproate increases diazepam levels, with a disproportionate rise in the free (unbound) level of diazepam.[63] Lorazepam, however, is not displaced from binding protein by valproate.[64] The clinical relevance of the valproate/benzodiazepine pharmacokinetic interaction is unknown, but might be expected to be greater in elderly patients or malnourished patients with a low serum albumin.[65] Amitriptyline raises the plasma half-life of valproate, leading to increased blood levels, possibly by increasing the binding of valproate to tissue.[66] It is not known whether other antidepressant drugs have a similar effect.

With carbamazepine

When carbamazepine is added to the regimen of schizophrenic patients taking haloperidol, haloperidol levels are often reduced, and occasionally this reduction leads to clinical deterioration.[67-70] A similar effect may be seen with thioridazine.[70] Viloxazine, a second-generation antidepressant with relatively low epileptogenic effects, may produce a marked increase in carbamazepine levels in epileptics previously stable on carbamazepine.[71] Standard antidepressants currently available in the United States have not been not known to have this dramatic effect on carbamazepine blood levels.

With tricyclics

Considering the effect of anticonvulsants on psychotropic drug levels, several small case series suggest that phenytoin may lower tricyclic antidepressant blood levels on standard dosages, and that patients chronically treated with phenytoin may need larger than usual oral dosages of tricyclics to obtain an adequate therapeutic effect.[72,73] Nonetheless, there are certainly epileptic patients on chronic phenytoin therapy who respond to standard dosages of tricyclics. The effect of carbamazepine has been less well studied, although it is the author's impression that carbamazepine-treated patients also tend to require relatively large tricyclic dosages to obtain therapeutic blood levels.

NONPHARMACOKINETIC INTERACTIONS AT THE CNS LEVEL

As the above suggests, pharmacokinetic interactions between anticonvulsants and other psychotropic drugs are highly variable, and the literature can serve only to put one on guard to obtain more frequent levels in situations where interactions have previously been found. Interactions at the CNS level, not predictable by blood levels, pose greater difficulties, as therapeutic benefits and toxic interactions may be mediated by similar mechanisms.

Readers familiar with lithium-haloperidol combination treatment know that the combination of lithium and a neuroleptic may work better than either agent alone for treating severe psychotic mania, but that severe extrapyramidal reactions and even life-threatening CNS neurotoxicity have been reported from the combination.[74-76] Lithium and neuroleptics influence dopaminergic transmission by different and synergistic mechanisms; this fact may underlie both the rapid therapeutic effect and the occasional occurrence of profound toxicity.

Similar considerations apply to the combination of lithium and carbamazepine, lithium and phenytoin, neuroleptics and carbamazepine, and neuroleptics and valproate. The lithium and carbamazepine combination has been reported by several authors to be uniquely valuable in some patients with severe and refractory bipolar disorder[24,25] (and see Chapter 1 in this volume). Nonetheless, severe neurotoxic reactions have been reported from the combination of these two drugs, even when both are at therapeutic blood levels.[77,78] The precise mechanism of interactive toxicity at the CNS level is unknown, although risk factors have been identified, including a history of lithium neurotoxicity and preexisting neurologic compromise.[77] When employing lithium-carbamazepine therapy, the levels of both drugs should be kept at the lower end of the therapeutic range, and both cognitive mental state and extrapyramidal motor signs should be monitored closely.

Phenytoin has been reported to precipitate lithium toxicity without raising lithium levels.[79] Perhaps this pharmacodynamic interaction is related to the tendency of phenytoin to produce delirium, involuntary movements, and rarely, parkinsonism if given alone at toxic levels.

Delirium has also been reported from the combination of carbamazepine with haloperidol at a daily dosage of 16 mg of haloperidol and a carbamazepine blood level of 6.7 μg/ml.[80] In this case a higher level of carbamazepine was tolerated without side effects after haloperidol was discontinued. The mechanism of this interaction is also unknown, but one possibility is that carbamazepine inhibits the induction of cyclic AMP by dopamine in cells with dopamine receptors.[81,82] Perhaps this effect potentiates the clinical action of dopamine receptor blockers, whether for better or for worse.

Delirium and stupor have been reported from the combination of valproate with neuroleptics. The cases were associated with diffuse EEG slowing, down to the delta range.[83] Other investigators have reported an increased frequency of neuroleptic-induced parkinsonism and sedation during combined valproate-neuroleptic therapy, necessitating a 25% to 50% reduction in the usual daily doses of neuroleptic drugs.[84] Patients receiving combined neuroleptic and valproate therapy should receive relatively low doses of neuroleptics, and their mental status must be closely monitored. An EEG should be considered if new or increased cognitive impairment develops.

Because the anticonvulsants carbamazepine and valproate both may increase extrapyramidal side effects of neuroleptics, the author strongly favors prophylactic antiparkinson medication when these drugs are used in combination. Among the antiparkinson drugs, amantadine may be preferable because of its lesser cognitive side effects.[85]

MAO inhibitors potentiate the sedative effects of barbiturates and benzodiazepines.[86] The clinical relevance of this phenomenon varies greatly among individuals and may be partially offset by some reduction in anticonvulsant blood levels due to enzyme induction by the MAO inhibitor. This issue is discussed later in this chapter.

In the author's experience, there is an increased incidence of ataxia when anticonvulsants are combined with antidepressants or with benzodiazepine anxiolytics. A patient who tolerates either an anticonvulsant alone or a psychotropic alone at the usual therapeutic dosage may develop significant gait disturbance when the two drugs are combined. Patients with underlying neurologic disorders affecting gait, such as multiple sclerosis or congenital hemiparesis, are especially at risk. In the author's experience, secondary amine tricyclics may be less likely than tertiary amines or trazodone to precipitate this interaction with anticonvulsants. Among the benzodiazepines, clonazepam, whether used as a psychotropic or an anticonvulsant, appears to cause the most problems with ataxia at usual clinical dosages. Carbamazepine produces ataxia at rather low dosages if the dose is raised too rapidly. The need for small dosage increments is even greater when the drug is added to a tricyclic or a benzodiazepine.

Finally, another theoretically possible interaction is that valproate could aggravate the action tremor produced by lithium or tricyclic antidepressants. The possibility arises because a tremor with physiologic properties of essential tremor occurs in about 10% of patients who receive valproate alone.[87] Tricyclic and lithium tremors are physiologically similar, raising the possibility of an additive pharmacodynamic effect. However, the author has not seen any unusual problems with tremor in patients whom he has treated with antidepressant-valproate combinations.

CONFLICTING OR ADDITIVE EFFECTS ON BLOOD COUNT AND CHEMISTRIES

In addition to pharmacokinetic interactions and direct CNS effects, both anticonvulsant and psychotropic drugs may significantly affect blood counts, electrolytes, and hormone levels.

Lithium raises the white blood count, and carbamazepine lowers it; one case reports use of lithium to counteract carbamazepine-induced leukopenia.[88] It is doubtful, however, that lithium reduces the probability of agranulocytosis, which is a rare idiosyncratic reaction to carbamazepine.

Lithium induces hypothyroidism in susceptible patients.[89] Both carbamazepine and phenytoin lower thyroxine levels,[90] and carbamazepine lowers the TSH response to TRH.[91] These overlapping effects place patients on a lithium-carbamazepine or lithium-phenytoin combination at greater risk for hypothyroidism than patients receiving lithium alone.[92]

Lithium may raise serum calcium,[89] while carbamazepine may lower it.[93] Carbamazepine, either alone or with lithium, might thus be rational for the patient with bipolar disorder who has developed hypercalcemia on lithium.

Carbamazepine and phenytoin have been associated with inappropriate ADH secretion and consequent hyponatremia. Tricyclics, MAO inhibitors, and phenothiazines have also been associated with this effect.[94] It is not known whether anticonvulsant-psychotropic combinations lead to additive, sub-additive, or super-additive risk, but periodic electrolyte determinations are prudent after instituting any such combination, especially since blood must be drawn anyway to check drug levels.

SEIZURES FROM PSYCHOTROPICS

It is well known that both neuroleptics and antidepressants can induce seizures in susceptible patients. Particular drugs, such as maprotiline and chlorpromazine, have a special association with drug-induced seizures.[47-51] However, seizures occurring in patients on appropriately selected anticonvulsant-psychotropic drug combinations usually result from excessive levels of the psychotropic or nontherapeutic levels of the anticonvulsant. The only common exception occurs in patients with poorly controlled epilepsy. In these patients, particularly those with complex partial seizures, the effects of drug combinations are unpredictable and idiosyncratic, with the addition of antidepressants or neuroleptics improving seizure control in some patients and worsening it in others, seemingly without regard to measurable drug levels or surface EEG changes.

BEHAVIORAL TOXICITY FROM ANTICONVULSANTS

The psychotoxicity of anticonvulsants is usually quite predictable and manageable. Virtually any anticonvulsant can produce a confusional state at toxic levels, and phenytoin in particular can produce extraordinarily bizarre behavior as a symptom of intoxication.[95] The sedating anticonvulsants, including phenobarbital, primidone, and clonazepam, can disinhibit behavior, producing impulsiveness, violence, and a clinical impression of personality disorder or drug abuse. Alternatively, the sedating anticonvulsants can produce an apathetic picture easily mistaken for a retarded major depression. When psychiatric symptoms newly develop in any patient on anticonvulsant therapy, the first step is to ascertain that drug levels are therapeutic, and whenever possible, to remove sedating anticonvulsants and substitute nonsedating ones. Carbamazepine and valproate are generally regarded as the least psychotoxic of the commonly prescribed anticonvulsants.[96-98] If symptoms apparently due to a primary psychiatric disorder are in fact caused by anticonvulsant toxicity, the addition of psychotropic drugs may simply obscure the picture.

Anticonvulsants, including phenytoin and phenobarbital, interfere with folic acid metabolism, and substantial numbers of chronically treated epileptics may be folate deficient.[99] This folate deficiency may produce a behavioral picture of depression or may aggravate cognitive problems or abnormal behavior. Replacement therapy with folic acid at 1 mg per day can correct the folate deficiency without interfering with seizure control.

PRINCIPLES OF ANTICONVULSANT SELECTION

Experience in the drug therapy of epilepsy suggests that certain simple rules minimize the psychotoxicity of anticonvulsants. First, monotherapy should be employed whenever possible. Behavioral and neurologic toxicity from anticonvulsants are more likely when two or three drugs are used than when just one drug is used.[100-102] Second, the drugs of choice for primary generalized tonic-clonic epilepsy are carbamazepine, valproate, and phenytoin.[103] Of these three, phenytoin is most likely to produce cognitive or behavioral side effects. Phenobarbital and primidone have greater behavioral toxicity and may be less effective, so they should be used only if the former drugs are either ineffective or not tolerated. For patients with mixed seizure types that include absence, valproate is the drug of choice, because of its high efficacy and relatively low psychotoxicity. For partial seizures, including complex partial seizures and secondarily generalized seizures, carbamazepine has been regarded as the drug of choice with phenytoin the runner-up.[104] The proper role of valproate in partial seizures is not yet settled. Some studies have shown a good response of partial seizures to valproate, while others have been less positive.[105-109] To this author, it appears that valproate is a reasonable alternative therapy for partial seizures if carbamazepine and phenytoin are not tolerated; however, it is unlikely that valproate will abolish seizures if carbamazepine has failed at high doses. While ethosuximide is effective and well tolerated for classic absence seizures, it is less effective for patients with mixed seizure types,[110] and it can cause psychotic episodes (see Chapter 4 in this volume).

As noted previously, carbamazepine, valproate, and clonazepam have antimanic effects. Carbamazepine may also be an antidepressant,[111] although it is generally less effective than the tricyclics. Clonazepam is effective for anxiety and insomnia, as well as for panic attacks.[112] When a patient with epilepsy also has an affective or anxiety disorder, it may be possible to select an anticonvulsant with concurrent antimanic, antidepressant, or antianxiety effects. However, clonazepam is not as effective for partial epilepsy as carbamazepine or phenytoin. Valproate, on the other hand, may be as effective as phenytoin for complex partial seizures.[113] Thus, in the patient with partial epilepsy and a psychiatric disorder for which clonazepam might be appropriate, a two-drug regimen with carbamazepine or phenytoin might be necessary if seizures were not controlled on clonazepam alone. If valproate were used as a psychotropic/anticonvulsant, the need for multiple anticonvulsants would be less likely to arise, but remains possible.

The benzodiazepines and barbiturates tend to be depressing and disinhibiting, and to have negative effects on cognitive performance. Often, in patients on multiple drug therapy, the gradual discontinuation of these agents not only improves their mental state, but actually improves their seizure control and functional status as well.[114] Thus, there should be a compelling reason for choosing a sedating anticonvulsant for any patient. If impulsive or disinhibited behavior, such as suicide attempts or violence, is a major behavioral problem, every effort should be made to switch the patient to an agent such as carbamazepine that may actually have a positive effect on impulse control (see Chapter 8 of this volume).

PRINCIPLES OF PSYCHOTROPIC DRUG SELECTION

Because of the relatively frequent co-occurrence of psychosis and epilepsy, it is not uncommon to administer neuroleptics to patients on anticonvulsants. Also, patients receiving anticonvulsants for prophylaxis of bipolar disorder may require short-term treatment with neuroleptics if psychotic symptoms break through the prophylactic regimen. Since all neuroleptics are equally effective antipsychotics, the choice of neuroleptic in this situation should be based on minimizing side effects and risk of precipitating seizures.

Among neuroleptics, chlorpromazine probably has the worst epileptic potential. Surprisingly, thioridazine and mesoridazine, although also low-potency aliphatic phenothiazines, do not aggravate seizures as greatly.[115] Among the higher-potency agents, molindone and fluphenazine appear most benign *in vitro*,[116] and pimozide appears somewhat less likely than haloperidol to precipitate seizure activity in photosensitive baboons.[48] Thus, in two nonhuman models, haloperidol is slightly inferior to other agents. Based on these admittedly insufficient studies, this author uses primarily molindone or fluphenazine when a high-potency agent is needed, and thioridazine or mesoridazine when a low-potency, more sedating agent is desired. I am not enthusiastic about the use of haloperidol and on several occasions have seen apparent aggravation of seizures by haloperidol in "rapid neuroleptization" dosages of 5 mg to 10 mg per hour in agitated epileptic patients. In summary, aggravation of seizures can be prevented by keeping neuroleptic doses as low as possible and choosing those agents that appear least likely to provoke seizures.

When combining antimanic anticonvulsants and neuroleptics for the treatment of mania in the nonepileptic patient, precipitation of seizures is quite unlikely. Neuroleptic choice here should be based on minimizing unwanted anticholinergic effects, or excessive ataxia or sedation. If the antimanic anticonvulsant is carbamazepine, and the focus is avoiding anticholinergic effects, fluphenazine, haloperidol, or molindone are all good choices. If the antimanic anticonvulsant is clonazepam or valproate, and the focus is on minimizing ataxia and sedation, the same neuroleptics are useful. If, however, the patient is very excited and sleep-deprived, sedation may be appropriate. Thus, thioridazine or mesoridazine should be considered. However, with these neuroleptics, anticholinergic side effects of constipation and blurred vision are frequent, particularly if carbamazepine is the antimanic anticonvulsant agent.

Regarding choice of antidepressant, of those currently marketed in the United States, the tetracyclic antidepressant maprotiline is undoubtedly most likely to provoke seizures.[51] The more serotonergic antidepressants clomipramine, trazodone, and amitriptyline are perhaps a bit more likely to provoke seizures than doxepin, nortriptyline, trimipramine, or desipramine.[50] However, all antidepressants available in the United States have been associated with convulsions.

In patients with known epilepsy, well controlled on adequate doses of anticonvulsant drugs, it is unusual for any antidepressant to produce a lapse in seizure control, unless pharmacokinetic factors or poor compliance cause anticonvulsant blood levels to deviate from the therapeutic range. Thus, the selection of an antidepressant should be based primarily on the desirability or undesirability of sedation and the relative tolerance of the patient to the differential side effects of the various agents. A secondary consideration favoring nortriptyline or despiramine is the availability of meaningful blood levels,[117] which can be of great help when evaluating nonresponse to antidepressant therapy.

A common clinical problem is the epileptic patient with a troublesome dysthymia that does not respond to tricyclics or trazodone. Such patients often can be dramatically helped with MAO inhibitors. While phenelzine has been reported to raise carbamazepine levels, tranylcypromine has not been reported to affect carbamazepine levels,[28] and it is probably the simplest agent to use in treating dysthymic epileptics. There are, however, several caveats. First, carbamazepine raises plasma tryptophan levels.[82] Elevated tryptophan levels may lead to increased central serotonin in the presence of an MAO inhibitor, producing drowsiness and ataxia, particularly after meals. Patients may need to avoid large high-carbohydrate meals during the daytime or may need to increase caffeine consumption to compensate. Second, patients taking MAO inhibitors together with sedating anticonvulsants such as barbiturates or clonazepam may suffer from excessive daytime sleepiness or from paroxysmal sleep attacks. If the drug combination is otherwise satisfactory, a planned midday nap may help prevent sleep attacks. Third, although they are less provocative of seizures than tricyclics, MAO inhibitors can produce increased seizure frequency, particularly in epileptics who are not fully controlled prior to the initiation of the MAO inhibitor (McNamara E, personal communication, December, 1987). Sometimes, a few weeks' wait will reveal that seizure frequency then falls to baseline, or even below baseline, as the antidepressant benefits on sleep, stress level, and medication compliance are fully realized.

In using MAO inhibitors and carbamazepine together, the physician should be aware that the combination is listed by the manufacturers as contraindicated, in view of the chemical similarity between carbamazepine and tricyclic antidepressants. However, the combination of tricyclics and MAO inhibitors is relatively safe if administered carefully, with particular caution not to institute the tricyclic in a fully MAO-inhibited patient. Similarly, in the author's experience, there is no unusual problem with hypertension if the MAO inhibitor is added to carbamazepine and the dosage of the MAO inhibitor is increased slowly. Compared with phenelzine, tranylcypromine, with its short half-life and reversible MAO inhibition, would decrease the duration of a potential adverse reaction.

It is comforting to know that at the time of this writing litigation from adverse effects of MAO inhibitor-carbamazepine combinations has not been reported,[118] nor have problems been reported in the clinical literature. Nonetheless, because of the manufacturers' explicit statement of a contraindication, patients for whom the combination seems desirable should be fully informed of the manufacturers' recommendation, and the risk, benefits, and rationale for combination treatment should be explained. The conversation should be documented in the patient's medical record. There are no published contraindications to the combined use of valproate and MAO inhibitors, and the author has used the combination successfully in one case.

If a patient requires simultaneous treatment for epilepsy and anxiety, it is natural to consider using an anticonvulsant with anxiolytic effects as part of the patient's regimen. In this regard, there are two oral agents that are both potent anti-anxiety drugs and approved by the United States Food and Drug Administration for the treatment of epilepsy: clonazepam and clorazepate. Clonazepam is primarily indicated for myoclonic seizures—a seizure type rather uncommon in adults—but it is useful as a second-line adjunct drug in partial epilepsy. Clorazepate is approved by the Food and Drug Administration as an adjunctive anticonvulsant, but not as a primary anticonvulsant.

Clonazepam has a number of drawbacks, including the quite frequent occurrence of sedation, ataxia, disinhibition, and cognitive impairment. On the other hand, it not only is a potent drug for anxiety, but also may be effective for panic attacks, so that it warrants consideration in the epileptic patient with troublesome panic episodes. Clorazepate, however, is relatively free of side effects, and its pharmacokinetic profile is nearly ideal. Given twice a day, clorazepate leads to virtually unchanging levels of its active metabolite nordiazepam.[119] Thus, problems of sedation shortly after a dose, or rebound anxiety when a dose is due, are virtually eliminated. In most epileptic patients who require a benzodiazepine, clorazepate would appear to be the drug of choice. If the patient's seizure disorder appears to be uniquely responsive to clonazepam, or if panic attacks are highly prominent, clonazepam would be preferable. Long-acting drugs such as diazepam or chlordiazepoxide, which have rapid absorption and high peak levels, are less satisfactory because they can give the patient a euphoric effect shortly after taking the drug. The shorter-acting agents, such as lorazepam and alprazolam, may be troublesome in epileptic patients because they may produce rebound anxiety shortly before the next dose is due, and this rebound anxiety may be associated with an increased risk of seizures in patients whose seizure control is marginal.

Because of the tendency of benzodiazepines to impair cognition and memory, buspirone, if it proves to be equally effective, may be an attractive alternative to the benzodiazepines for anxious epileptic patients. However, seizures have been reported as a side effect of buspirone in the product literature supplied by the manuacturer, and potential interactions of buspirone with anticonvulsants are largely unexplored.

Some epileptic patients will develop intense anxiety states during the prodrome of seizures, or as post-ictal phenomena. In these situations, the patient often needs fast relief of anxiety and cannot wait for the absorption of an oral drug. Lorazepam is well absorbed sublingually,[120-123] and, anecdotally, so is clonazepam. A small dose of one of these benzodiazepines taken under the tongue at the first sign of anxiety can sometimes avert the seizure for which the anxiety is the prodrome. In patients with relatively poorly controlled seizures and substantial peri-ictal anxiety, such a strategy is worth trying.

SPECIAL CONSIDERATIONS

Suicidal risk

Patients with epilepsy are at substantially greater risk for death by suicide than the general population,[124] and the risk of suicide during depressive episodes is elevated when depressed epileptic patients are compared with other depressed patients.[4] Because multiple drug overdoses tend to be more lethal than single drug overdoses, the patient with epilepsy and affective disorder on a combination regimen requires particularly close monitoring of suicidal ideation. Further, because epilepsy is a chronic disease, epileptics often have a large stock of drugs, including anticonvulsants and psychotropics prescribed by previous physicians, so that the means for suicide are always at hand. Therefore, even if one personally prescribes relatively small, nonrefillable prescriptions, the patient may still be at risk.

Many epileptic patients are dysthymic and have intermittent or chronic suicidal thoughts. In such patients, assessment and record keeping should focus on cognitive, affective, and behavioral deviations from the patient's baseline, rather than simply whether morbid thinking is present or absent.

USING THE EEG

As psychiatrists become more involved in using anticonvulsants as psychotropics and in treating the psychopathology associated with epilepsy, they must become more familiar with the EEG. It is not enough to rely on the interpretation of EEG reports, because the EEG is a relatively nonspecific test, and EEG data are most useful if related to the clinical situation by the psychiatrist, rather than interpreted solely by an electroencephalographer who does not know the patient. For example, both an EEG with a background alpha rhythm of 11 Hz and an EEG with a background alpha rhythm of 8 Hz may be within normal limits, but if the same patient develops the second EEG one week after the first, it is presumptive evidence for an acute toxic or metabolic process affecting the brain.

If anticonvulsant drug therapy is contemplated, whether for epilepsy or for a psychiatric indication, it is valuable to obtain a baseline EEG. In the patient with epilepsy, the baseline EEG may confirm the diagnosis, but more importantly may offer information about the seizure type or seizure focus which may be helpful in selecting an optimal anticonvulsant. In the nonepileptic patient, a baseline EEG assists in the future evaluation of changes in mental status. EEG slowing from the baseline is an excellent marker of toxic-metabolic influences that might explain an apparent deterioration in mood or cognitive function when a patient is on an exotic multiple-drug therapy.

Patients with seizures and psychopathology are particularly problematic diagnostically, as they may exhibit paroxysmal behavior of both epileptic and nonepileptic origin. An EEG obtained at the time of, or immediately following a change in mental status or behavior can shed light on whether the phenomenon in question is ictal or post-ictal. If the behavior is sufficiently frequent, intensive monitoring, either by a portable cassette EEG recorder or by telemetry,[125] may settle the question. Such monitoring is important, since prescribing anticonvulsants for a nonepileptic problem may be counterproductive, producing a toxic encephalopathy or behavioral disinhibition. An EEG obtained at a time of behavioral change may also reveal an unexpected EEG pattern, such as generalized spike-and-wave, that would call for a different therapy, such as substituting valproate for carbamazepine.

CONCLUSIONS

The combination of anticonvulsants with other psychotropic drugs is essential in a large proportion of epileptic patients and may offer novel approaches to a number of nonepileptic neuropsychiatric disorders. The safe and effective application of combination therapy requires a solid working knowledge of the relevant clinical pharmacology, along with meticulous patient follow-up, including serial assessments of cognitive function, drug levels, and, where appropriate, repeated EEGs. When polypharmacy is approached with adequate theoretical knowledge and appropriate precautions, it can be as safe and rational as single-drug therapy, while substantially improving quality of life for patients unresponsive to simpler treatments.

REFERENCES

1. Trimble MR. Psychopathology and epilepsy—introduction. In: Trimble MR, ed. The psychopharmacology of epilepsy. Chichester: John Wiley & Sons, 1985:1-16.
2. Robertson MM, Trimble MR. Depressive illness in patients with epilepsy: a review. Epilepsia 1983; 24:109S-16S.
3. Trimble MR. The psychoses of epilepsy and their treatment. Clin Neuropharmacol 1985; 8: 211-20.
4. Mendez MF, Cummings JL, Benson DF. Depression in epilepsy. Arch Neurol 1986; 43: 766-70.
5. Curri ES, Heathfield KWG, Henson RA, et al. Clinical course and prognosis of temporal lobe epilepsy: a survey of 666 patients. Brain 1971; 94:173-90.
6. Sherwin I, Peron-Magnan P, Bancaud J, et al. Prevalance of psychosis in epilepsy as a function of the laterality of the epileptogenic lesion. Arch Neurol 1982; 39:621-5.
7. Trimble MR. Psychosomatic aspects of epilepsy. Adv Psychosom Med 1985; 13:133-50.
8. McNamara ME. Neurology. In: Stoudemire A, Fogel BS, eds. Principles of medical psychiatry. Orlando: Grune & Stratton, 1987:521-52.
9. Siris JH, Werner WL. Epilepsy control, neuroleptics, and mental state. JAMA 1978; 239: 402-3.
10. Martin JE, Agran M. Psychotropic and anticonvulsant drugs used by mentally retarded adults across community residential and vocational placements. Appl Res Ment Retard 1985; 6:33-49.
11. Emrich HM, Dose M, von Zerssen D. The use of sodium valproate, carbamazepine and oxcarbazepine in patients with affective disorders. J Affect Dis 1985; 8:243-50.
12. Lerer B. Alternative therapies for bipolar disorder. J Clin Psychiatry 1985; 46:309-16.
13. Victor BS, Link NA, Binder RL, et al. Use of clonazepam in mania and schizoaffective disorders. Am J Psychiatry 1984; 141:1111-2.
14. Chouinard G. Clonazepam in acute and maintenance treatment of bipolar affective disorder. J Clin Psychiatry 1987; 48:29S-36S.
15. Stromgren LS, Boller S. Carbamazepine in treatment and prophylaxis of manic-depressive disorder. Psychiatr Dev 1985; 4:349-67.
16. Nolen WA. Carbamazepine, a possible adjunct or alternative to lithium in bipolar disorder. Acta Psychiatr Scand 1983; 67:218-25.
17. Kishimoto A, Okura C, Hazama H, et al. Long-term prophylactic effects of carbamazepine in affective disorder. Br J Psychiatry 1983; 143:327-31.
18. Lerer B, Moore N, Meyendorff E, et al. Carbamazepine versus lithium in mania: a double-blind study. J Clin Psychiatry 1987; 48:89-93.
19. Placidi GF, Lenzi A, Lazzerini F, et al. The comparative efficacy and safety of carbamazepine versus lithium: a randomized, double-blind 3-year trial in 83 patients. J Clin Psychiatry 1986; 47:490-4.
20. Roy-Byrne PP, Joffe RT, Uhde TW, et al. Approaches to the evaluation and treatment of rapid-cycling affective illness. Br J Psychiatry 1984; 145:543-50.
21. Nurnberg HG, Finkel JA. Carbamazepine in bipolar-depressed disorder complicated by tricyclic antidepressant switching: case report. J Clin Psychiatry 1985; 46:487-8.
22. Dunner DL, Fieve RR. Clinical factors in lithium carbonate prophylaxis failure. Arch Gen Psychiatry 1974; 30:229-33.
23. Lovett L, Watkins SE, Shaw DM. The use of alternative drug therapy in nine patients with recurrent affective disorder resistant to conventional prophylaxis. Biol Psychiatry 1986; 21:1344-7.
24. Lipinski JF, Pope HG, Jr. Possible synergistic action between carbamazepine and lithium carbonate in the treatment of three acutely manic patients. Am J Psychiatry 1982; 139:948-9.
25. Inoue K, Arima S, Tanaka K, et al. A lithium and carbamazepine combination in the treatment of bipolar disorder—a preliminary report. Folia Psychiatr Neurol Japon 1981; 35:465-76.
26. Adler LW. Mixed bipolar disorder responsive to lithium and clonazepam. J Clin Psychiatry 1986; 47:49-50.

27. Kwamie Y, Persad E, Stancer H. The use of carbamazepine as an adjunctive medication in the treatment of affective disorders: a clinical report. Can J Psychiatry 1984; 29:605-8.
28. Joffe RT, Post RM, Uhde TW. Lack of pharmacokinetic interaction of carbamazepine with tranylcypromine (letter). Arch Gen Psychiatry 1985; 42:738.
29. Klein E, Bewlat E, Leven B, et al. Carbamazepine and haloperidol versus placebo and haloperidol in excited psychoses. Arch Gen Psychiatry 1984; 41:165-70.
30. Luchins DJ. Carbamazepine in psychiatric syndromes: clinical and neuropharmacological properties. Psychopharmacol Bull 1984; 20:569-71.
31. Mattes JA. Carbamazepine for uncontrolled rage outbursts. Lancet 1984; 2:1164-5.
32. Jenike MA. Handbook of geriatric psychopharmacology. Littleton: PSG Publishing Co., 1985.
33. Buck OD, Havey P. Combined carbamazepine and lithium therapy for violent behavior (letter). Am J Psychiatry 1986; 143:1487.
34. Greenberg WM. Sedative or antimanic effects of carbamazepine and treatment of behavioral dyscontrol (letter). Am J Psychiatry 1986; 143:1486.
35. Neppe VM. Carbamazepine as adjunctive treatment in non-epileptic chronic inpatients with EEG temporal lobe abnormalities. J Clin Psychiatry 1983; 44:326-31.
36. Luchins DJ. Carbamazepine for the violent psychiatric patient (letter). Lancet 1983; 1:766.
37. Greendyke RM, Kanter DR, Schuster DB, et al. Propranolol treatment of assaultive patients with organic brain disease. J Nerv Ment Dis 1986; 174:290-4.
38. Mattes JA, Rosenberg MA, Mays D. Carbamazepine versus propranolol in patients with uncontrolled rage outbursts: a random assignment study. Psychopharmacol Bull 1984; 20:98-100.
39. Ratey JJ, Mikkelsen EJ, Bushnel LS, et al. Beta blockers in the severely and profoundly mentally retarded. J Clin Psychopharmacol 1986; 6:103-7.
40. Brodsky L, Shah A, Casenas E. Two distinct "paradoxical" reactions to neuroleptics. Psychiatr J Univ Ottawa 1984; 9:61-4.
41. Monroe RR. Limbic ictus and atypical psychoses. J Nerv Ment Dis 1982; 170:711-5.
42. Rau JH, Green RS. Compulsive eating: a neuropsychologic approach to certain eating disorders. Compr Psychiatry 1975; 16:223-31.
43. Rau JH, Struve FA, Green RS. Electroencephalographic correlates of compulsive eating. Clin Electroencephalography 1979; 10:180-9.
44. Herridge PL, Pope HG, Jr. Treatment of bulimia and rapid-cycling bipolar disorder with sodium valproate: a case report. J Clin Psychopharmacol 1985; 5:229-30.
45. Kaplan AS, Garfinkel PE, Darby PL, et al. Carbamazepine in the treatment of bulimia. Am J Psychiatry 1983; 140:1225-6.
46. Pope HG, Jr, Hudson JI. Antidepressant drug therapy of bulimia: current status. J Clin Psychiatry 1986; 47:339-45.
47. Edwards JG, Long SK, Sedgwick EM, et al. Antidepressants and convulsive seizures: clinical, electroencephalographic, and pharmacological aspects. Clin Neuropharmacol 1986; 9:329-60.
48. Meldrum BS. The effect of psychotropic drugs on seizure threshold: animal studies. In: Trimble MR, ed. The psychopharmacology of epilepsy. Chichester: John Wiley & Sons, 1985:107-18.
49. Edwards JG. Antidepressants and seizures: epidemiological and clinical aspects. In: Trimble MR, ed. The psychopharmacology of epilepsy. Chichester: John Wiley & Sons, 1985:119-40.
50. Itil TM, Soldatos C. Epileptogenic side effects of psychotropic drugs: practical recommendations. JAMA 1980; 244:1460-3.
51. Dessain EC, Schatzberg AF, Woods BT, et al. Maprotiline treatment in depression. A perspective on seizures. Arch Gen Psychiatry 1986; 43:86-90.
52. Fields HL. Anticonvulsants, psychotropics, and antihistaminergic drugs in pain management. In: Fields HL, ed. Pain. New York: McGraw-Hill, 1987:285-306.
53. Swerdlow M. The treatment of shooting pain. Postgraduate Med J 1980; 56:159-61.
54. Perucca E, Richens A. Interaction between phenytoin and imipramine. Br J Clin Pharmacol 1977; 4:485-6.
55. Richens A, Houghton GW. Effect of drug therapy on the metabolism of phenytoin. In: Schneider H, Janz D, Gardner-Thorpe C, et al., eds. Clinical pharmacology of anti-epileptic drugs. Berlin: Springer Verlag, 1975:87-95.

56. Huang CY, McLeod JG, Sampson D, et al. Clonazepam in the treatment of epilepsy. Med J Australia 1974; 2:5-8.
57. Vajda FJE, Prineas RJ, Lovell RRH. Interaction between phenytoin and the benzodiazepines (letter). Br Med J 1971; 1:346.
58. Houghton GW, Richens A. The effect of benzodiazepines and pheneturide on phenytoin metabolism in man. Br J Clin Pharmacol 1974; 1:344-5.
59. Vincent FM. Phenothiazine-induced phenytoin intoxication. Ann Int Med 1980; 93:56-7.
60. Siris JH, Pippenger CE, Werner WL, et al. Anticonvulsant drug serum levels in psychiatric patients with seizure disorders. NY State J Med 1974; 74:1554-6.
61. Sands CD, Robinson JD, Salem RB, et al. Effect of thioridazine on phenytoin serum concentration: a retrospective study. Drug Intell Clin Pharm 1987; 21:267-72.
62. Dorn JM. A case of phenytoin toxicity possibly precipitated by trazodone. J Clin Psychiatry 1986; 47:89-90.
63. Dhillon S, Richens A. Valproic acid and diazepam interaction *in vivo* (letter). Br J Clin Pharmacol 1982; 13:553.
64. Calvo R, Carlos R, Erill S. Differential effects of valproic acid on the serum protein binding of lorazepam and diazepam. Int Clin Pharmacol Res 1986; 6:213-5.
65. Greenblatt DJ, Koch-Weser J. Clinical toxicity of chlordiazepoxide and diazepam in relation to serum albumin concentration: a report from the Boston Collaborative Drug Surveillance Program (letter). Eur J Clin Pharmacol 1975; 7:259.
66. Pisani F, Primerano G, D'Agostino A, et al. Valproic acid-amitriptyline interaction in man. Therap Drug Monit 1986; 8:382-4.
67. Jann MW, Ereschefsky L, Saklad SR, et al. Effects of carbamazepine on plasma haloperidol levels. J Clin Psychopharmacol 1985; 5:106-9.
68. Kidron R, Averbuch I, Klein E, et al. Carbamazepine-induced reduction of blood levels of haloperidol in chronic schizophrenia. Biol Psychiatry 1985; 20:219-22.
69. Arana GW, Goff DC, Friedman H, et al. Does carbamazepine-induced reduction of plasma haloperidol levels worsen psychotic symptoms? Am J Psychiatry 1986; 143:650-1.
70. Linnoila M, Viukari M, Valsanen K, et al. Effect of anticonvulsants on plasma haloperidol and thioridazine levels. Am J Psychiatry 1980; 137:819-21.
71. Pisani F, Fazio A, Oteri G. Carbamazepine-viloxazine interaction in patients with epilepsy. J Neurol Neurosurg Psychiatry 1986; 49:1142-5.
72. Fogel BS, Haltzman S. Desipramine and phenytoin: a potential drug interaction of therapeutic relevance. J Clin Psychiatry 1987; 48:387-8.
73. Braithwaite RA, Flanagan RA, Richens A. Steady-state plasma nortriptyline concentrations in epileptic patients. Br J Clin Pharmacol 1975; 2:469-71.
74. Spring G, Frankel M. New data on lithium and haloperidol incompatibility. Am J Psychiatry 1981; 138:818-21.
75. Cohen WJ, Cohen NH. Lithium carbonate, haloperidol, and irreversible brain damage. JAMA 1974; 230:1283-7.
76. Pope HG, Jr, Keck PE, Jr, McElroy SL. Frequency and presentation of neuroleptic malignant syndrome in a large psychiatric hospital. Am J Psychiatry 1986; 143:1227-33.
77. Ghose K. Interaction between lithium and carbamazepine (letter). Br Med J 1980; 280:1122.
78. Price WA, Zimmer B. Lithium-carbamazepine neurotoxicity in the elderly. J Am Geriatr Soc 1985; 33:876-7.
79. MacCallum W. Interaction of lithium and phenytoin. Br Med J 1980; 280:610-1.
80. Yerevanian BL, Hodgman CH. Haloperidol-carbamazepine interaction in a patient with rapid-cycling bipolar disorder (letter). Am J Psychiatry 1985; 142:785-6.
81. Shukla S, Godwin LD, Long LEB, et al. Lithium-carbamazepine neurotoxicity and risk factors (letter). Am J Psychiatry 1984; 141:1604.
82. Post RM, Uhde TW, Rubinow DR, et al. Biochemical effects of carbamazepine: relationship to its mechanisms of action in affective illness. Prog Neuropharmacol Biol Psychiatry 1983; 7:263-71.
83. van Sweden B, van Moffaert M. Valproate as psychotropic agent. Acta Psychiatr Scand 1985; 72:315-7.

84. Puzynski S, Klosiewicz L. Valproic acid amide in the treatment of affective and schizoaffective disorders. J Affect Dis 1984; 6:115-21.
85. McEvoy JP. A double-blind crossover comparison of antiparkinson drug therapy: amantadine versus anticholinergics in 90 normal volunteers, with an emphasis on differential effects on memory function. J Clin Psychiatry 1987; 48:20S-23S.
86. Sjoqvist F. Psychotropic drugs (2). Interaction between monoamine oxidase (MAO) inhibitors and other substances. Proc Roy Soc Med 1965; 58:967S-78S.
87. Karas BJ, Wilder BJ, Hammond EJ, et al. Treatment of valproate tremors. Neurology 1983: 33:1380-2.
88. Brewerton TD. Lithium counteracts carbamazepine-induced leukopenia while increasing its therapeutic effect. Biol Psychiatry 1986; 21:677-85.
89. Lazarus JH. Endocrine and metabolic effects of lithium. New York: Plenum Medical Book Co., 1986.
90. Rootwelt K, Ganes T, Johannessen SI. Effect of carbamazepine, phenytoin, and phenobarbitone on serum levels of thyroid hormones and thyrotropin in humans. Scand J Clin Lab Invest 1978; 38:731-6.
91. Joffe RT, Gold PW, Uhde TW, et al. The effects of carbamazepine on thyrotropin response to thyrotropin-releasing hormone. Psychiatry Res 1984; 12:161-6.
92. Vieweg WVR, Yank GR, Stekler TL, et al. Grades 1 and 2 hypothyroidism in a state mental hospital: risk factors and clincial findings. Psychiatr Q 1986; 58:135-43.
93. Joffe RT, Post RM, Uhde TW. Effects of carbamazepine on serum electrolytes in affectively ill patients. Psychol Med 1986; 16:331-5.
94. Caird FI, Scott PJW. Drug-induced diseases in the elderly. Amsterdam: Elsevier, 1986.
95. Franks RD, Richter AJ. Schizophrenia-like psychosis associated with anticonvulsant toxicity. Am J Psychiatry 1979; 136:973-4.
96. Vining EPG, Mellits ED, Dorsen MM, et al. Psychologic and behavioral effects of antiepileptic drugs in children: a double-blind comparison between phenobarbital and valproic acid. Pediatrics 1987; 80:165-74.
97. Vining EPG. Cognitive dysfunction associated with antiepileptic drug therapy. Epilepsia 1987; 28:18S-22S.
98. Beghi E, DiMascio R, Sasanelli F, et al. Adverse reactions to antiepileptic drugs: a multicenter survey of clinical practice. Epilepsia 1986; 27:323-30.
99. Trimble MR, Corbett JA, Donaldson D. Folic acid and mental symptoms in children with epilepsy. J Neurol Neurosurg Psychiatry 1980; 43:1030-4.
100. Schmidt D. Reduction of two-drug therapy in intractable epilepsy. Epilepsia 1983; 24:368-76.
101. Shorvan SD, Reynolds EH. Reduction in polypharmacy for epilepsy. In: Johnannessen SI, Morselli PL, Pippenger CE, et al., eds. Antiepileptic therapy: advances in drug monitoring. New York: Raven Press, 1980:203-9.
102. Reynolds EH, Shorvan D. Monotherapy or polytherapy for epilepsy? Epilepsia 1981; 22:1-10.
103. Drugs for epilepsy. Med Lett Drugs Ther 1986; 28:91-4.
104. Mattson RH, Cramer JH, Collins JF, et al. Comparison of carbamazepine, phenobarbital, phenytoin and primidone in partial and secondarily generalized tonic-clonic seizures. N Engl J Med 1985; 313:145-51.
105. Covanis A, Gupta AK, Jeavons PM. Sodium valproate: monotherapy and polytherapy. Epilepsia 1982; 23:693-720.
106. Turnbull DM, Rawlins M.D., Weightman D, et al. Comparison of phenytoin and valproate in previously untreated adult epileptic patients. J Neurol Neurosurg Psychiatry 1982; 45:55-9.
107. Browne TR. Valproic acid. N Engl J Med 1980; 302:661-6.
108. Dasheiff RM, McNamara D, Dickinson L. Efficacy of second line antiepileptic drugs in the treatment of patients with medically refractive complex partial seizures. Epilespia 1986; 27: 124-7.
109. Callaghan N, Kenny RA, O'Neill B, et al. A prospective study between carbamazepine, phenytoin and sodium valproate as monotherapy in previously untreated and recently diagnosed patients with epilepsy. J Neurol Neurosurg Psychiatry 1985; 48:639-44.
110. Porter RJ. Epilepsy: 100 elementary principles. London: W.B. Saunders Co., 1984.

111. Post RM, Uhde TW, Roy-Byrne PP, et al. Antidepressant effects of carbamazepine. Am J Psychiatry 1986; 143:29-34.
112. Tesar GE, Rosenbaum JF, Pollack MH, et al. Clonazepam versus alprazolam in the treatment of panic disorder: interim analysis of data from a prospective, double-blind, placebo-controlled trial. J Clin Psychiatry 1987; 48:16S-9S.
113. Turnbull DM, Rawlins M.D., Weightman D, et al. Long-term comparative study of phenytoin and valproate in adult onset epilepsy. Br J Clin Pract 1983; 27:3S-5S.
114. Theodore WH, Porter RJ. Removal of sedative-hypnotic antiepileptic drugs from the regimens of patients with intractable epilepsy. Ann Neurol 1983; 13:320-4.
115. Trimble MR. The psychoses of epilepsy and their treatment. In: Trimble MR, ed. The psychopharmacology of epilepsy. Chichester: John Wiley & Sons, 1985:83-94.
116. Oliver AP, Luchins DJ, Wyatt RJ. Seizures with neuroleptics; an *in vitro* technique for assessing relative risk. Arch Gen Psychiatry 1982; 39:206-9.
117. American Psychiatric Association. Task force report on antidepressant drug levels. Am J Psychiatry 1985; 142:155-62.
118. Patterson RM, ed. Drugs in litigation: damage awards involving prescription and nonprescription drugs. Charlottesville, Virginia: Michie Co., 1987.
119. Griffith JL, Murray GB. Clorazepate in the treatment of complex partial seizures with psychic symptomatology. J Nerv Ment Dis 1985; 73:185-6.
120. Gale GD, Galloon S, Porter WR. Sublingual lorazepam: a better premedication? Br J Anaesth 1983; 55:761-5.
121. Greenblatt DJ, Divoll M, Harmatz JS, et al. Pharmacokinetic comparison of sublingual lorazepam with intravenous, intramuscular, and oral lorazepam. J Pharm Sci 1982; 71:248-52.
122. Caille G, Spenard J, Lacasse Y, et al. Pharmacokinetics of two lorazepam formulations, oral and sublingual, after multiple doses. Biopharm Drug Dispos 1983; 4:31-42.
123. Singh AN, Saxena B, Marshall AM. A dose-finding study of sublingual lorazepam in anxiety. Cur Ther Res 1983; 34:227-38.
124. Matthews WS, Barabas G. Suicide and epilepsy: a review of the literature. Psychosomatics 1981; 22:515-24.
125. Ramani V. Intensive monitoring of psychogenic seizures, aggression, and dyscontrol syndromes. In: Gummit RJ, ed. Intensive neurodiagnostic monitoring. New York: Raven Press, 1987.

CHAPTER 6

Effect of Anticonvulsants on Circadian Rhythms: Implications for Major Affective Disorder and Primary Sleep Disorders

David Borsook, M.D.
Boston, Massachusetts

INTRODUCTION

Understanding the physiological basis of circadian systems may be useful for the development of effective treatments of putative circadian-based diseases such as bipolar disorder. Conversely, an understanding of the mechanism of action of drugs used in the treatment of such disorders may offer insight into the underlying pathophysiology of the disease.

The first portion of this chapter provides a brief overview of the anatomy and neurochemistry of the suprachiasmatic nucleus (SCN), the putative central pacemaker of the central nervous system (CNS). Although numerous neuromodulators and neurotransmitters are present in the SCN, few agents, including agonists and antagonists of these neurotransmitters, have been shown to alter the circadian system by producing phase shifts or changes in periodicity of rhythms in animal models. The majority of these agents are not clinically useful.

However, the benzodiazepines and several anticonvulsants, including valproate, which are thought to exert their effects via GABAergic systems, have effects on the circadian system and may be used therapeutically, i.e. valproate in bipolar disorder and benzodiazepines in certain sleep disorders. Gamma-aminobutyric acid (GABA) is present in those structures important in the modulation and control of the central clock: the suprachiasmatic nucleus itself, the afferent pathways to this nucleus, the retinohypothalamic tract, and a pathway via the lateral geniculate body.

The second portion of this chapter provides an overview of the circadian basis of bipolar disorder, agents used in the treatment of this disorder, the effect of these agents on the circadian system, and experimental evidence for the effects of valproate on circadian rhythms in a primate model.

The final portion of this chapter discusses the role of benzodiazepines, used clinically for the treatment of sleep disorders, in circadian-based disorders.

THE CIRCADIAN SYSTEM IN MAMMALS

The suprachiasmatic nucleus

The earliest evidence indicating that the suprachiasmatic nucleus (SCN) of the ventromedial hypothalamus plays a significant role in the generation of circadian rhythms was provided by Moore and Eichler[1] and by Stephan and Zucker.[2] Lesions of this area of the hypothalamus significantly disrupted free-running rhythms of various physiological parameters. Since this seminal observation, extensive research has been undertaken to characterize the anatomy, physiology, and chemistry of the endogenous clocks.[3,4]

Normally, animals entrain to the 24-hour period of their environment. However, when animals, including man, are placed in isolation, free of environmental time cues, their rhythms only approximate 24 hours. Thus, some animals such as the mouse (Mus musculus) and the pigtail monkey (Macaca nemestrina) have endogenous rhythms shorter than 24 hours.[5,6] Other animals, like man, have endogenous or free-running rhythms longer than 24 hours.[7,8]

Endogenous pacemakers are responsive to environmental stimuli, particularly the daily alteration between light and dark. Through such alterations, the internal milieu of an animal is ordered in an appropriate temporal sequence to allow for adaptation to the environment. It has been postulated that abnormalities of this timing system may result in or result from various psychiatric disorders such as bipolar disorder or certain sleep disorders.

The SCN consists of two small groups of cells located in the anterior hypothalamus, dorsal to the optic chiasm. There is abundant evidence that the SCN constitutes the major pacemaker in mammals.[9-17] The function and anatomy of the SCN have been thoroughly reviewed by Moore,[18] Rusak and Zucker,[19] and Van Den Pol and Tsujimoto.[3] Specialized photoreceptors located in the retina are responsible for mediating the effects of light on the SCN.[20-22] Light information is transmitted to the SCN via two specialized pathways: the retinohypothalamic tract and a pathway via the ventrolateral geniculate nuclei.[23,24] GABA is located in all of these structures: the retina, the lateral geniculate body, and the SCN itself.

Numerous neurotransmitters and neuropeptides in addition to GABA have been shown to be located in the cell bodies and axon terminals in the SCN. Acetylcholine, norepinephrine, serotonin, and the neuropeptides somatostatin, vasopressin, vasoactive intestinal peptide, avian pancreatic peptide, substance P, cholecystokinin, leu-enkephalin, molluscan cardioexcitatory peptide, and bombesin have all been demonstrated in the SCN through the use of various staining techniques.[3,18]

Despite the existence and presumed functional importance of these neuroactive substances in the SCN, relatively few pharmacological agents, when administered exogenously, produce any significant effects on the two fundamental parameters used in assessing perturbations of the circadian system: circadian phase (relative position in time) and period (cycle length). Those pharmacological agents shown to affect the period in various mammalian species are listed in Table 1.[25-53]

Few of these agents mimic or block the effects of light, the most important zeitgeber affecting the central pacemaker, and until very recently, only two substances found in the SCN or its afferent pathways were known to affect circadian output: acetylcholine and neuropeptide Y.[54-57]

GABA serves as an important neurotransmitter in the central nervous system.[58,59] Neurons containing GABA are found throughout the brain, with high concentrations in the hypothalamus of rats,[60] monkeys,[61] and man.[62] Significantly, Van Den Pol and Tsujimoto noted that of all the classes of immunoreactive neurons stained within the SCN, the most numerous were those immunoreactive for glutamic acid decarboxylase (GAD), the synthetic enzyme for GABA.[3] In a more recent study, Van Den Pol showed that GABA and GAD immunoreactivity was found in the presynaptic boutons

TABLE 1. Pharmacological agents which alter the circadian period in vertebrates

Agent	Species	Period change: decrease	Period change: increase	Rhythm	Reference
Deuterium oxide	Mouse		+	Act.	25-27
	Hamster		+	Act.	28-30
Propylthiouracil	Hamster		+	Act.	31
Thiourea	Hamster		+	Act.	32
Imipramine	Rat		+	Recept.	33
Estradiol	Rat	–		Act.	34
	Hamster	–		Act.	35
Lithium	Man		+	Temp.	36-38
			+	Act.	36-38
		–		Act.	39
			+	S/W	40,41
	Rat		+	Act.	42-44
	Hamster		+	Act.	45
		–	+	Act.	46
	Goldfish		+	Act.	47
	Bat	–		Act.	48
Testosterone	Hamster	no change		Act.	49
	Mouse[a]		+	Act.	50
Clorgyline	Hamster		+	Act.	51
Valproate	Monkey	–	+	Act.	52
	Rat	–		Act.	53

Act.–Activity; Temp.–temperature; Recept.–receptors; S/W–sleep/wake; [a] castrated mice

as well as the perikarya of the SCN, suggesting that GABA may be involved in local circuit interactions between neurons within the SCN.[63] Furthermore, Makara and colleagues, using autoradiographic techniques, have shown high uptake of tritiated GABA in the neuropil of the SCN.[64] The identification of GABAergic neurons within the SCN, the retina,[65,66] and the ventral lateral geniculate body[67] therefore suggests that its presence may have some significance in the neurochemical modulation of circadian timekeeping.

Gaba and circadian timekeeping

In 1984, a putative role for GABAergic agents in circadian timekeeping was presented.[52] Other reports followed showing that GABA, GABA agonists, and GABA antagonists could produce changes in the circadian system of animals. Bicuculline, a specific $GABA_A$ receptor antagonist, was found to block phase delays normally induced by light pulses without affecting phase advances produced by light pulses given during the late subjective night.[68] The authors concluded that GABA could be involved in mediating the response to light in the SCN. Bicuculline was shown to inhibit the phase delaying effect of light pulses in a dose dependent manner (about 70% at maximal doses administered [4mg/kg] and approximately 40% at 2.5mg/kg). The authors further concluded that GABA could be involved in mediating some of the light input to the SCN, either in the input pathway or in the SCN itself.

Shibata and colleagues investigated the influence of GABA on single unit discharges of the SCN using hypothalamic slice preparations.[69] Iontophoresis of GABA onto these slices inhibited 90% of SCN neurons examined. These authors concluded that GABA modulated neuronal activity of the SCN via direct action as an inhibitory neurotransmitter. Our own preliminary data indicate that there is a diurnal variation of inhibition of neuronal firing within the SCN produced by application of GABA to brain slices, suggesting a phase-dependent effect.[52] Interestingly, in the frontal lobe of rats there is a diurnal variation of GABA receptors that is abolished by lesions of the SCN (Borsook D, Boulos Z, Brennan MJW, unpublished observations). No evidence for a diurnal variation of GABA or GABA receptors within the SCN itself is presently available.

Valproate, thought to act via GABAergic mechanisms, has been shown to alter the period length of free-running circadian rhythmicity in a primate model[52,70,71] as well as a rat model.[53] The effects of pineal N-acetyl-transferase activity in rats can be mimicked by diazepam, an agent that acts on the GABA benzodiazepine-chloride ionophore macromolecular complex. Diazepam can also alter the rate of reentrainment in rats to a shift in light cycle.[72] Alcohol, thought to mediate some of its actions via GABAergic pathways, has been reported to lengthen the free-running activity rhythms in hamsters or rats.[10]

More recent work has confirmed a role for the effects of benzodiazepines on the circadian system. Turek and Losee-Olsen have shown that benzodiazepines phase shift hamster rhythms.[73] Benzodiazepines potentiate the action of GABA by binding to the GABA benzodiazepine-chloride ionophore macromolecular complex. Acute administration of 2.5 mg of triazolam, a short-acting benzodiazepine, to golden hamsters (Mesocricetus auratus) under free-running conditions of either constant light or constant darkness caused phase shifts of the activity rhythm. The phase shifts were dependent on the circadian time of administration. The drug caused both advances and delays of approximately 90 minutes, with advances occurring during the subjective night (sleep/low activity) and delays occurring during the subjective day (awake/high activity). Thus, this agent is capable of inducing fundamental changes in an important parameter of the circadian system, i.e. the phase of the rhythm. The phase response curves determined for triazolam were opposite to those found for light. In some of the results presented by Turek and Losee-Olsen, there was, in addition to an abrupt phase shift, a substantial change in the period of the free-running rhythm for about a week following the phase shift.[73] Ralph and Menaker have shown that the benzodiazapine diazepam can block the effects of phase advances induced by light pulses given in the late subjective night in hamster locomotor activity rhythms.[74] No effects on phase delays induced by light pulses were shown when diazepam was given at the same doses that blocked the phase advance. The effects of blocking the phase advance due to light were dose dependent in the range 2.5 mg/kg to 12.5 mg/kg. Diazepam, when given without a light pulse, caused small phase delays of the free-running rhythm. The authors did not produce a full phase response curve for diazepam.

A PUTATIVE ROLE FOR VALPROATE, A GABAMIMETIC, IN THE TREATMENT OF BIPOLAR DISORDER

Circadian rhythms and bipolar disorder

Abnormalities in several neurotransmitter systems have been implicated in the pathogenesis of affective disorders. Data supporting the involvement of catecholamines derive largely from observations that a variety of antidepressant treatments have powerful effects on the metabolism, uptake, release, and receptor interaction of norepinephrine and serotonin. Although these findings are intriguing, they do not provide a neurophysiological basis for the understanding of affective symptoms. Recently, a variety of disturbances in the circadian rhythms of several behavioral and biological variables have been identified in patients with affective disorders. Since control of these rhythms is known to be dependent on central neural pacemakers (the SCN), it is possible that affective symptoms are associated with disordered pacemaker function. Whether abnormalities in circadian rhythms themselves cause affective symptoms or are merely further manifestations of the underlying neural pathology, however, is not known.

A number of authors have supported the hypothesis that alterations in the circadian timing system play a key role in the pathogenesis of bipolar disorder.[75] The plausibility of these circadian-based hypotheses has been strengthened by the demonstration that pharmacological agents effective in the treatment of certain psychiatric disorders have specific effects on circadian variables.[76] Of the neurotransmitters and neuromodulators known to be present in the SCN, only acetylcholine and neuropeptide Y have been shown to affect the circadian parameters of phase or period. Benzodiazepines, thought to be GABAmimetic in their action, have also been shown to affect this system (as discussed in the last portion of this chapter). However, none of these agents nor their analogues have provided a therapeutic basis for the treatment of presumed pathological disruptions of circadian function such as those thought to occur in bipolar disorder.

Bipolar patients exhibit several features suggestive of disruptions in the timing of phase control of the circadian system, including cyclic variations in mood, early morning awakening during depressive phases, reduction in the amplitude of circadian rhythms, and systematic advances and delays in phase.[75,77-85] In one chronobiological study of bipolar disorder, Kripke and colleagues identified two subpopulations of patients.[77] One group had abnormally rapid cycles (less than 24 hours) of their temperature, activity, urinary electrolyte, and cortisol rhythms. Another had abnormally slow cycles (greater than 25 hours).

Pharmacotherapy in bipolar disorder

Lithium is one of a few agents effective in the prophylaxis of affective episodes in a majority of bipolar patients.[86,87] Lithium is not used as an anticonvulsant, and although it may have anticonvulsant effects,[88] there is a general consensus that it is epileptogenic.[89] Significantly, this agent, by unknown mechanism(s), causes a lengthening in circadian parameters in man and most animals studied.[36-38,40-47] However, in two species, lithium has been shown to shorten the circadian period.[46,48] Clinically, there exists a subgroup of bipolar patients who do not respond to lithium and who are often called "lithium-resistant." Of note, the subgroup of bipolar patients identified by Kripke and associates with abnormally long circadian periods appeared to be "lithium-resistant", as they tended not to respond to lithium administration and in fact seemed to worsen.[77]

Figure 1 outlines a hypothetical model comprised of two groups of bipolar patients, one group with an abnormally shortened endogenous period in which lithium is clinically effective, and another group with an abnormally long endogenous period in which lithium is clinically ineffective.

FIGURE 1.

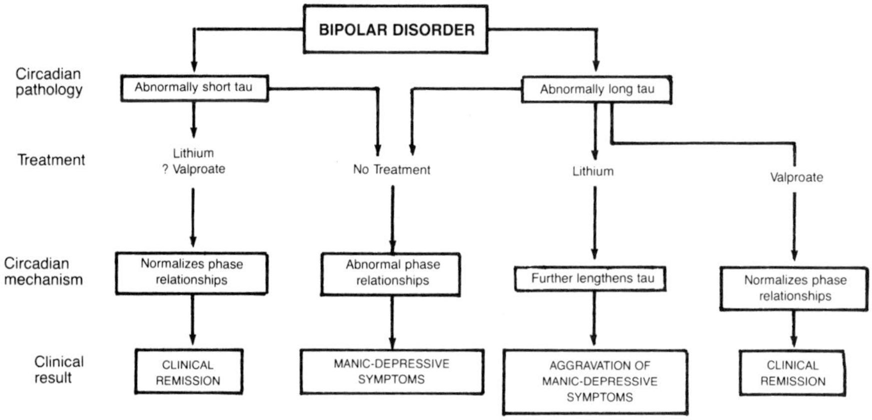

Hypothetical model outlining the possible circadian basis for pharmacotherapy of bipolar disorder. This diagram defines two groups of patients, one with an abnormally shortened endogenous period (or tau) and one with an abnormally lengthened period. Depending on this parameter, patients may respond to therapeutic agents which allow for resynchronization or normalization of phase relationships between the endogenous oscillator and the external environment.

Table 2 lists a number of agents, including valproate, valpromide, and carbamazepine, purportedly effective in both acute mania and the long-term prophylaxis of recurrent affective episodes.[90-115] Of significance is that these agents have been reported to be effective in bipolar patients who are lithium nonresponders.[96,99,109,112] It may be speculated

TABLE 2. Effectiveness of pharmacological agents used in the treatment of bipolar disorder

Agent	Acute mania	Depression	Prophylaxis Lithium responders	Prophylaxis Lithium resistant	Reference
Lithium	Yes	Yes (mild)	Yes	No	90-95
Valproate	Yes	? Yes	?	Yes	96-99
Valpromide	Yes	Yes (mild)	?	Yes	100-103
Carbamazepine	Yes	Yes	?	Yes	104-112
Tricyclics	No	Yes	No	No	113,114
Monoamine oxidase inhibitors	No	Yes	No	No	115

Yes–effective therapy; No–not effective therapy; ?–unknown therapeutic benefit

that GABAmimetics act to alter circadian cycles by shortening the period in patients with an endogenous long period. On the other hand, GABAmimetics may act to lengthen the period in patients with an endogenous short period, resynchronizing the patient's circadian system and allowing for clinical manifestations of the illness to be under control. In lithium nonresponders, it might be that agents such as valproate or carbamazepine shorten the endogenous cycles in certain patients (Figure 1), thereby allowing for therapeutic response.

PHARMACOLOGY OF CLINICALLY USEFUL "ANTICONVULSANTS"

Several lines of evidence now suggest that modulation of GABA levels may underlie the mechanisms of action of agents effective in the treatment of bipolar disorder. Valproate, a highly GABAergic compound, was first shown to possess anticonvulsant activity by Meunier and colleagues.[116] At high concentrations valproate elevates GABA levels through inhibition of GABA-transaminase (GABA-T) and succinic semi-aldehyde dehydrogenase (SSD) (two enzymes important in the catabolism of GABA)[117,118] and also through weak activation of glutamate decarboxylase (GAD), the enzyme which catalyzes the production of GABA from glutamate.[119] Furthermore, receptors on the presynaptic nerve terminals, which normally exert a negative feedback on GABA release, are inhibited by low concentrations of valproate.[120] Valproate also has been shown to induce a significant increase in the GABA content in the brain.[121,122] Iontophoretic application of valproate onto single neurons of rat cortex (containing high concentrations of GABA-mediated neurons per volume of brain) potentiates postsynaptic inhibitory responses.[123] The agent also increases GABA concentrations in synaptosomes of dogs *in vivo*.[124] Loscher and Nau have shown a possible regional selectivity of valproate in the dog and the rat brain,[125] and studies on the effects of valproate in various regions of the rat and the mouse brain have shown topographical differences in the degree of GABA increase after treatment with the drug.[126-128] Concentrations of valproate in the hypothalamus were the highest of thirteen regions of the dog brain. Valpromide, the amidation product of valproate, has similar actions, since it is converted to valproate *in vivo*. It has been suggested that carbamazepine may act on the GABA benzodiazepine-chloride ionophore macromolecular complex to prolong chloride channel opening time,[129] although opinion is divided on this point.

The mechanism of lithium's mood-stabilizing effect is unclear.[130] However, several observations suggest that the drug may alter GABA function. When chronically administered to rats, lithium induces a decrease in GABA receptor levels, specifically those in the striatum and the hypothalamus.[131] In man, lithium therapy has been shown to elevate GABA levels in cerebrospinal fluid (CSF).[132] Such an effect may be explained on the basis that lithium exerts a primary effect on receptor levels and that the increase in CSF GABA represents a compensatory response to decreased GABAergic transmission. This is supported by the observation that chronic administration of lithium to rats causes an increase in GABA levels in a number of regions of the rat brain, including the hypothalamus.[133,134]

THE EFFECT OF VALPROATE ON FREE-RUNNING RHYTHMS OF TEMPERATURE AND ACTIVITY IN THE SQUIRREL MONKEY

Circadian rhythms characteristically exhibit a very stable period. In mice, for example, circadian rhythms have a standard deviation of about nine minutes in estimating 24 hours,[135] and in man it has been estimated that the average day length over a period of a year in free-running temperature rhythms does not vary by more than about four minutes (Czeisler CA, personal communication, December, 1984). Richter recorded the activity rhythm of a blinded squirrel monkey (Saimiri sciureus) for over three years and showed that the rhythm remained very stable with a period of approximately 25 hours for the duration of the experiment.[136]

Pharmacological agents may alter timing of rest/activity cycles by affecting the temporal organization of sleep and wakefulness. Under conditions of constant light, the period change would reflect the drug effect on the output of the SCN. Table 1 lists agents that have been shown to alter the free-running period in mammals. A change of more than five to 10 minutes in the period is considered to be significant in most of these studies.

In our study, valproate was administered in drinking water to 10 male squirrel monkeys placed in conditions of constant light and humidity and in environmental

FIGURE 2.

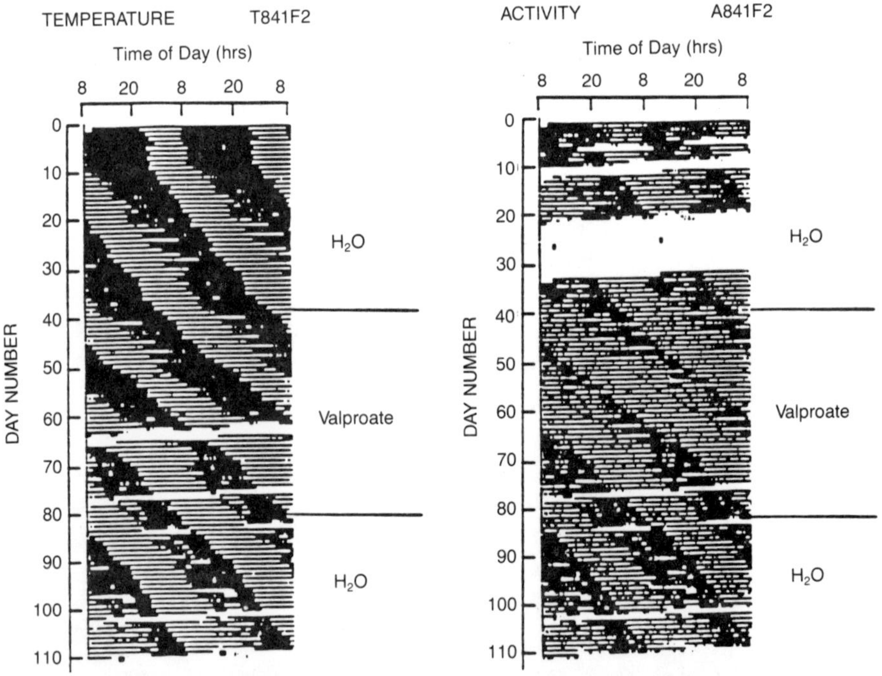

Actogram plots of the temperature and activity rhythms of monkey 841 showing a lengthening of the period on valproate (days 40 to 80) and a shortening when placed on water again (day 80). Note that the animal was entrained to a 12:12 light/dark schedule from days 1 to 10 and then released into a free-run. The missing data for the temperature and activity rhythms of monkey A841F2 occurred during data collection malfunctions.

chambers that shielded out other environmental stimuli. The daily doses of valproate consumed by the animals were between 80 mg/kg and 100 mg/kg. Plasma levels of valproate were shown to be within the "therapeutic" range for humans taking valproate for control of seizures, i.e. 50 μg/ml to 100 μg/ml. Temperature and activity data were recorded around the clock for the duration of the experiment.

Valproate was shown to increase the free-running period by 0.50 ± 0.11 hours in five animals (mean ± S.E.M.) and shorten the period by 0.61 ± 0.13 hours in five animals (mean ± S.E.M.). In some animals put through the experimental protocol for a second time, the administration of valproate caused the same change in the free-running period as initially demonstrated in the same monkey.

Figure 2 shows actogram plots of the activity and temperature rhythms of monkey 841, whose period lengthened from an initial period of 25 hours on water to a period of 25.25 hours on valproate. Note that the rhythms of activity and temperature revert to the initial period of 25.00 hours following withdrawal of the drug.

Figure 3 shows the effect of valproate on the free-running rhythms of monkey 902,

FIGURE 3.

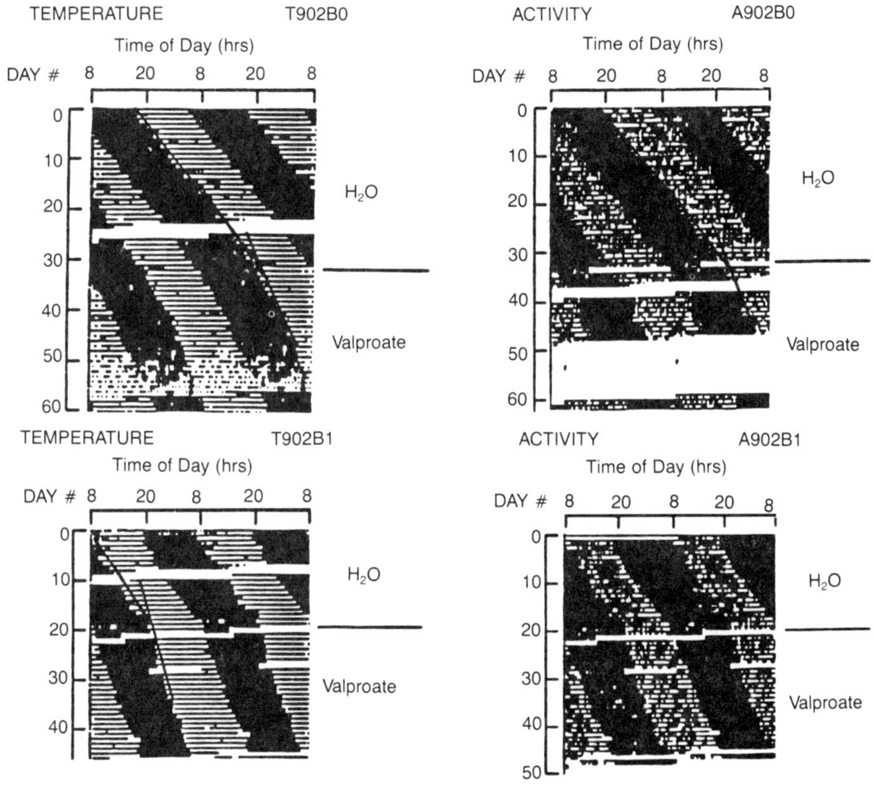

Actogram plots of the temperature and activity rhythms of monkey 902 showing data obtained when placing the animal in the protocol on two occasions four months apart. In both cases, both rhythms shortened on valproate. The missing data for the activity rhythm of monkey 902B0 occurred during a data collection malfunction. The animal was not interferred with during this period. Lines are drawn in to aid visual inspection of this data.

placed through the protocol on two occasions, four months apart. Administration of the drug at both times caused a shortening of the free-running period. Thus, as shown in Figure 3, the initial drug-free free-running periods of activity and temperature of 25.75 hours were shortened to 24.25 hours with addition of valproate (monkey 902B0). When the animal was placed through the protocol for the second time, the rhythms shortened from 25.00 hours to 24.25 hours.

FIGURE 4.

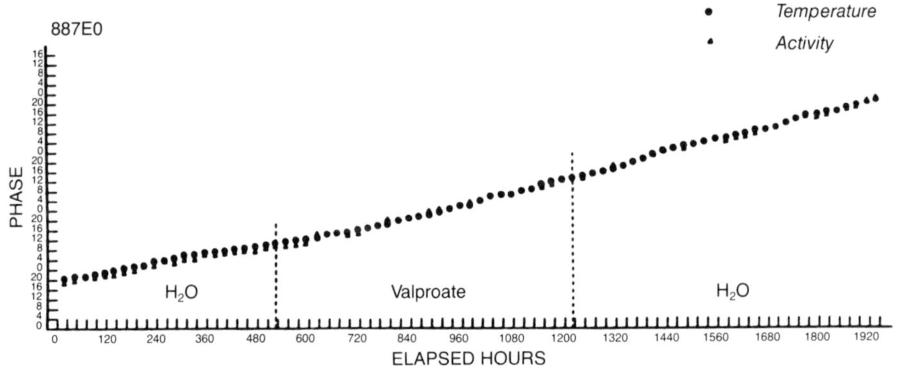

Phase plots of the free-running temperature and activity rhythms of monkey 887E0 on water (H_2O), on valproate, and then on water again. Each point on the graph represents the phase of the daily peak of temperature and activity. No significant difference between the temperature and activity phase positions was observed on water or on drug (paired Student's t-test for the inter-phase interval). Note that the slope of the curve increases on the drug compared with the initial water.

FIGURE 5.

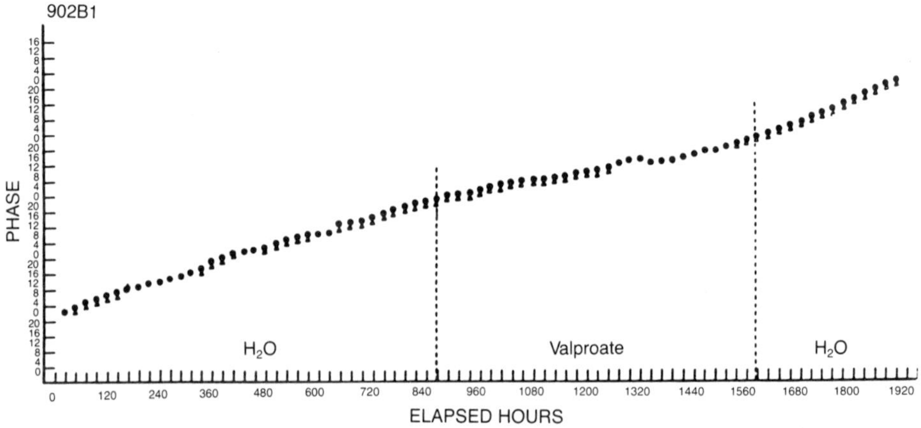

Phase plots of the free-running temperature and activity rhythms of monkey 902B1 on water (H_2O), on valproate, and then on water again. Each point on the graph represents the phase of the daily peak of temperature and activity. No significant difference between the temperature and activity phase positions was observed on water or on drug (paired Student's t-test for the inter-phase interval). Note that the slope of the curve decreases on the drug compared with the initial water and then increases again when the drug is discontinued.

There were no significant differences (paired Student's t-test) between the relative phases of the two rhythms (temperature and activity), suggesting that the rhythms are tightly coupled even during large period changes. Figures 4 and 5 show phase plots of the free-running temperature and activity rhythms in two monkeys, one of which displayed a shortened period on valproate (monkey 902). In all but one animal, when valproate was removed from the drinking water, the period reverted to or in the direction of the original free-running period.

FIGURE 6.

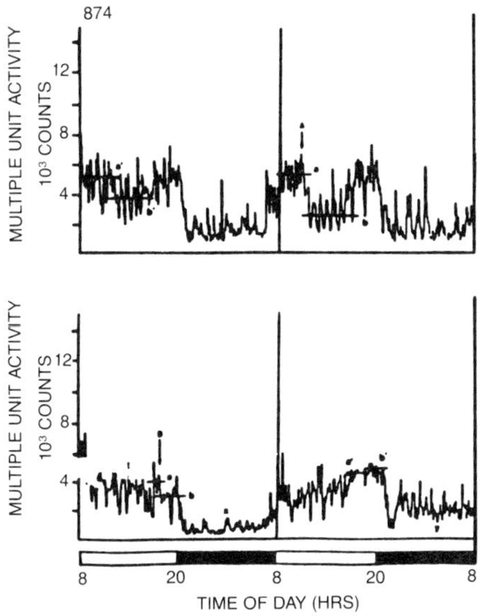

Multiple unit activity from the hypothalamus of monkey 874 recorded over 48 hours under a 12:12 light-dark cycle. The upper graph shows the effects of intraperitoneal injection of valproate during the subjective day (A), and the lower graph shows the drug effect following injection in the latter part of the subjective day (B). The lines a, b, a[1] and b[1] show the mean multiple unit activity for equivalent times during the two days. Note that following both injection times, multiple unit activity was shown to decrease within 30 minutes after the injection. Futhermore, following injection at B the mutliple unit activity during the subjective night (dark) decreased during the whole night when compared with the activity during the night of the following day.

Valproate was also administered intraperitoneally to monkeys with electrodes in the hypothalamus for multiple unit recording. When compared to the activity from previous days' recording, the drug caused a decrease in electrical activity when given either early in the day or late in the day just prior to lights off (Figure 6). This would suggest that valproate does have an effect on the electrical output of the hypothalamus.

While the above studies suggest that valproate may cause significant changes in the free-running period, the reason some animals shorten on the drug and others lengthen is unclear. Possible mechanisms may include a dose-dependent effect or a preferential drug effect on one portion of the SCN over another (the nucleus comprises a dorsomedial and a ventrolateral portion, each with different neuropeptides). Usually, partial lesions of the SCN cause a shortening of the period in species studies. However, there are reports of partial lesions causing a lengthening in about 20% of animals.[137-139] In a two-oscillator model as postulated by Kronauer and colleagues, differential coupling could produce either a lengthening or a shortening of the circadian output depending on which oscillator is preferentially affected.[140] Alternatively, changes in the hormonal milieu, which can be induced by valproate, could affect the circadian oscillator.[10,19] Examples of the latter point include the reciprocal relationship between growth hormone and cortisol secretion[141] and the effect of melatonin on synchronizing rhythms.[142] GABA enhances growth hormone secretion and inhibits ACTH/cortisol secretion.[143,144] When the Lotka[145] and Volterra[146] model is applied to the cyclic output of the SCN in a manner similar to Hobsen and McCarley's application of this model to the control of the REM/non-REM cycle, another possible explanation for the effects of valproate emerges.[147-150] In such a model, one agent or neurotransmitter could have an opposite effect on the cyclic output, thus either lengthening or shortening the circadian period. Lastly, valproate may have differential effects on two subpopulations of GABA receptors ($GABA_A$ and $GABA_B$) and hence produce opposite effects in individual animals. However, there is no experimental evidence to support this contention, since specific $GABA_B$ agents such as baclofen have not been used in experimental situations.

Although a clear mechanism of valproate's effect on free-running rhythms in a primate model has not been elucidated, valproate does cause significant changes in the free-running period of activity and temperature rhythms. The effect on the period in these animals placed under constant environmental conditions appears to be at the level of the SCN. It is relatively unusual for agents to cause a shortening of the circadian period in mammals. In the only other reported experiment of the effects of valproate on circadian rhythms, Rietveld and van Schravendijk showed that long-term application of valproate shortened the period length of the free-running rhythmicity of food intake of rats.[53] After withdrawal of the drug, the period length returned to pre-drug values.

These changes support a role for GABAergic agents in the treatment of affective disorder. While a group of lithium nonresponders has been well described, valproate nonresponders have not yet been systematically characterized. It is possible, therefore, if a circadian basis for affective illness holds, that valproate would be effective in lithium nonresponders, and lithium would be effective in valproate nonresponders. Although there is, in general, consensus in the literature that lithium lengthens the free-running period in mammals, including man, it should be pointed out that Welsh and associates reported the case of a patient whose rhythms shortened on lithium.[39] Similarly, in a report by Johnsson and colleagues the period of one or two subjects shortened on lithium.[37] The authors ascribe these effects to entrainment (the effects of outside cues). Lastly, it should be mentioned that lithium causes a shortening in the period of free-running rhythms in the bat.[48]

An understanding of the mechanism by which valproate alters the internal timing system could greatly enhance therapeutic intervention in bipolar disorder. For example, pulse therapy, rather than chronic therapy, may be a reasonable alternative if it is found that valproate alters the endogenous period in a well-defined manner. It would be essential to study normal volunteers under strict isolation conditions to determine whether valproate has any effect in human subjects. Many interventions such as light or drugs, when given at a particular phase of a circadian cycle, may have one effect, such as advancing the circadian phase, while when given at another point, could delay the system. Also, it may be of considerable importance to adjust a pharmacological approach for the above reasoning.

BENZODIAZEPINES, SLEEP AND CIRCADIAN RHYTHMS

Traditionally, benzodiazepines have been used as first-line drugs in treating sleep disorders, usually without a clear delineation of their specific pharmacology.[151] There are few controlled trials on the efficacy of benzodiazepines in specific circadian-based sleep disorders. Since benzodiazepines act to facilitate the action of GABA through a prolongation of the GABA-gated chloride channel opening time,[152] these agents should be capable of altering the phase relationships of rhythms such as the sleep-wake cycle relative to the light-dark cycle. Evidence for the effects of benzodiazepines on the circadian system in animal models has been discussed in the first portion of this chapter.

Although it is likely that many sleep disorders reflect an abnormality in circadian timing, the syndrome for which this has been most clearly demonstrated is delayed sleep phase insomnia.[153] This is a disorder characterized by a greatly increased nocturnal sleep latency and difficulty in awakening in the morning. This disorder reflects an inability of the circadian system to accomplish normal phase advances relative to environmental time cues. Nonpharmacological treatments which reschedule the phase of the sleep-wake cycle have been useful therapeutically,[153] although such treatment is time-consuming and costly.

Narcolepsy is another disorder of sleep that may reflect an abnormality of circadian timing. This sleep disorder presents with excessive daytime sleepiness manifested by automatic behaviours, lethargy, fatigue, hypersomnolence, and sleep attacks. The nighttime sleep of such individuals frequently is disrupted by awakenings.[154] This inability to maintain an alert state during the day and impaired maintenance of sleep at night implies that the disorder may involve the circadian ordering of the sleep-wake pattern.

The alterations of the sleep-wake cycle secondary to acute phase shifts are due to transient disruption of normal phase relationships between endogenous rhythms and exogenous or environmental cues such as the light-dark cycle. The "jet lag" syndrome is a consequence of abnormal phase relationships of endogenous rhythms relative to the environment, in which insomnia results from the inability to fall asleep at the wrong circadian phase.[155] Furthermore, daytime functioning such as alertness is diminished.[156]

The role of GABAergic agents, including benzodiazepines, in the treatment of these syndromes has not been well elucidated. The drug gamma-hydroxybutyrate (GHB) has been used in the treatment of narcolepsy.[157,158] Gamma-hydroxybutyrate is found in low concentrations in brain tissue, and is thought to be a derivative of GABA.[159] Although GHB has soporific effects, it seems to decrease daytime hypersomnolence as well as to improve nighttime sleep.

CONCLUSIONS

The pharmacological agents valproate and certain benzodiazepines have effects on the circadian system in animal models. It is presumed that these agents act via GABAergic systems known to be present in the anatomical pathways that mediate control of circadian rhythms. However, the effects of these agents on the circadian system in man have not been evaluated. Figure 7 is a summary of the effects that GABAmimetic agents have in circadian timekeeping.

FIGURE 7.

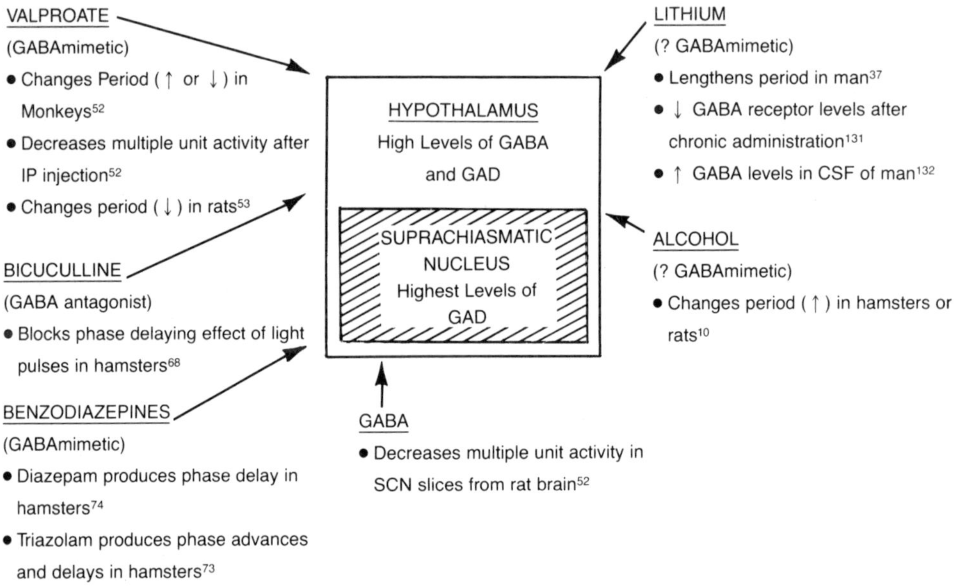

Also, there is a growing literature to support the clinical efficacy of valproate in the treatment of bipolar disorder (see Chapter 2 in this volume). Therefore, it is interesting to speculate that certain individuals who have hypernychthemeral rhythms (periods longer than 24 hours in a normal environment) may be effectively treated with valproate. However, in order to allow the comparison of biological rhythm data investigating either etiologic or therapeutic roles for the endogenous circadian oscillator in affective disease, it is essential that standardized experimental techniques are employed under controlled environmental conditions.

REFERENCES

1. Moore RY, Eichler VB. Loss of adrenal corticosterone rhythm following suprachiasmatic nucleus lesions. Brain Res 1972; 42:201-6.
2. Stephan FK, Zucker I. Circadian rhythms in drinking behavior locomotor activity of rats are eliminated by hypothalamic lesions. Proc Natl Acad Sci USA 1972; 69:1583-6.
3. Van Den Pol AN, Tsujimoto KL. Neurotransmitters of the hypothalamic suprachiasmatic nucleus: immunocytochemical analysis of 25 neuronal antigens. Neuroscience 1985; 15:1049-86.
4. Guldner FH. Synaptology of the rat suprachiasmatic nucleus. Cell Tissue Res 1976; 20:795-9.
5. Ebihara S, Tsuji K, Kondo K. Strain differences of the mouse's free-running circadian rhythm in continuous darkness. Physiol Behav 1978; 20:795-9.
6. Aschoff J. Circadian rhythms: general features and endocrinological aspects. In: Krieger DT, ed. Endocrine rhythms. New York: Raven Press, 1979:1-61.
7. Aschoff J, Wever R. Spontanperiodik des Menchen bei Ausschluss aller Zeitgeber. Naturwissenschaften 1962; 49:337-42.
8. Siffre M. Beyond time. New York: McGraw Hill, 1964.

9. Coindet J, Chouvet G, Mouret J. Effects of lesions of the suprachiasmatic nuclei on paradoxical sleep and slow wave sleep circadian rhythms in the rat. Neurosci Lett 1972; 1:243-7.
10. Zucker I. Hormones and hamster circadian organization. In: Suda M, Hayaishi O, Nakagawa H, eds. Biological rhythms and their central mechanisms. Amsterdam: Elsevier/North Holland Biomedical Press, 1979:369-81.
11. Rusak B, Groos G. Suprachiasmatic stimulation phase shifts rodent circadian rhythms. Science 1981; 215:1407-9.
12. Sawaki Y, Nihonmatsu I, Kawamura H. Transplantation of the neonatal suprachiasmatic nuclei into rats with complete bilateral suprachiasmatic lesions. Neurosci Res 1984; 1:67-72.
13. Lehman MN, Silver R, Gladstone WR, et al. Circadian rhythmicity restored by a neural transplant. Immunocytochemical characterization of the graft and its integration with the host brain. J Neurosci 1987; 7:1626-38.
14. Schwartz WJ, Gainer H. Suprachiasmatic nucleus: use of 14-C labelled deoxyglucose uptake as a functional marker. Science 1977; 197:1089-91.
15. Inouye ST, Kawamura H. Persistence of circadian rhythmicity in mammalian hypothalamic "island" containing the suprachiasmatic nucleus. Proc Natl Acad Sci USA 1979; 76:5961-6.
16. Green DJ, Gillette R. Circadian rhythm of firing rate recorded from single cells in the rat suprachiasmatic brain slice. Brain Res 1982; 245:198-200.
17. Groos G, Hendriks J. Circadian rhythms in electrical discharge of rat suprachiasmatic neurones recorded in vitro. Neurosci Lett 1982; 34:283-8.
18. Moore RY. Organization and function of a central nervous system oscillator: the suprachiasmatic hypothalamic nucleus. Fed Proc 1983; 42:2783-9.
19. Rusak B, Zucker I. Neural regulation of circadian rhythms. Physiol Rev 1979; 59:449-526.
20. Nelson RJ, Zucker I. Absence of extraocular photoreception in diurnal and nocturnal rodents exposed to direct sunlight. Comp Biochem Physiol 1981; 69:145-8.
21. Richter CP. Biological clocks in medicine and psychiatry. Springfield, IL: C. C. Thomas, 1965.
22. Takahashi JS, DeCoursey PJ, Bauman L, et al. Spectral sensitivity of a novel photoreceptive system mediating entrainment of mammalian circadian rhythms. Nature 1984; 308:186-8.
23. Moore RY. Retinohypothalamic projection in mammals: a comparative study. Brain Res 1973; 49:403-9.
24. Rusak B, Boulos Z. Pathways for photic entrainment of mammalian circadian rhythms. Photochem Photobiol 1981; 34:267-73.
25. Dowse HB, Palmer JD. The chronomutagenic effect of deuterium oxide on the period and entrainment of a biological rhythm. Biol Bull 1972; 143:513-24.
26. Daan S, Pittendrigh CS. A functional analysis of circadian pacemakers in nocturnal rodents. III. Heavy water and constant light: homeostasis of frequency? J Comp Physiol 1976; 106: 267-90.
27. Suter RB, Rawson KS. Circadian activity rhythm of the deer mouse, Peromyscus: effect of deuterium oxide. Science 1968; 160:1011-4.
28. Pickard GE, Zucker I. Influence of deuterium oxide on circadian rhythms of hamsters: role of the suprachiasmatic nucleus. Brain Res 1986; 376:149-54.
29. Fitzgerald KM, Zucker I. Circadian organization of the estrous cycle in the golden hamster. Proc Natl Acad Sci USA 1976; 73:2923-7.
30. Richter CP. Heavy water as a tool for study of the forces that control length of period of the 24-hour clock of the hamster. Proc Natl Acad Sci USA 1977; 74:1295-9.
31. Morin LP, Gavin ML, Ottenweller JE. Propylthiouracil causes phase delays and circadian period lengthening in male and female hamsters. Am J Physiol 1986; 250:151-60.
32. Beasley LJ, Nelson RJ. Thyroid gland influences the period of the hamster circadian oscillators. Experientia 1982; 38:870-1.
33. Wirz-Justice A, Kafka MS, Naber D, et al. Circadian rhythms in rat brain alpha- and beta-adrenergic receptors are modified by chronic imipramine. Life Sci 1980; 27:341-7.
34. Albers HE. Gonadal hormones organize and modulate the circadian system of the rat. Am J Physiol 1981; 241:62-6.
35. Morin LP, Fitzgerald KM, Zucker I. Estradiol shortens the period of hamster circadian rhythms. Science 1977; 196:305-7.

36. Johnsson A, Pflug B, Engelmann W, et al. Effect of lithium carbonate on circadian periodicity in humans. Pharmakopsychiatr Neuropsychopharmakol 1979; 12:423-5.
37. Johnsson A, Engelmann W. Influence of lithium ions on human circadian rhythms. Z Naturforsch 1980; 35:503-7.
38. Johnsson A, Engelmann W, Pflug B, et al. Period lengthening of human circadian rhythms by lithium carbonate, a prophylatic for depressive disorders. Int J Chronobiol 1983; 8:129-47.
39. Welsh DK, Nino-Murcia G, Gander PH, et al. Regular 48-hour cycling of sleep duration and mood in a 35-year-old woman: use of lithium in time isolation. Biol Psychiatry 1985; 21:527-37.
40. Kripke DF, Judd LL, Hubbard B, et al. The effect of lithium carbonate on the circadian rhythm of sleep in normal human subjects. Biol Psychiatry 1979; 14:545-8.
41. Sasaki M, Suzuki M, Onda M, et al. The effects of lithium on circadian rhythms. In: Langer S, Takahashi R, Segawa T, et al., eds. New vistas in depression. Oxford: Pergamon Press, 1982:303-8.
42. McEachron DL, Kripke DF, Hawkins R, et al. Lithium delays biochemical circadian rhythms in rats. Neuropsychobiol 1982; 8:12-29.
43. Hoffmann K, Gunderoth-Palmowski M, Wiedenmann G, et al. Further evidence for period lengthening effect of Li^+ ion on circadian rhythms. Z Naturforsch 1978; 33:231-4.
44. Kripke DF, Wyborney VG. Lithium slows rat circadian activity rhythms. Life Sci 1980; 26:1319-21.
45. Engelmann W. A slowing down of circadian rhythms by lithium ions. Z Naturforsch 1973; 28:733-6.
46. Delius K, Gunderoth-Palmowski M, Krause I, et al. Effects of lithium salts on the behaviour and circadian system of Mesocricetus auratus. J Interdiscipl Cycle Res 1984; 15:289-99.
47. Kavaliers M. Period lengthening and disruption of socially facilitated circadian activity rhythms of goldfish by lithium. Physiol Behav 1981; 27:725-8.
48. Subbaraj R. Effect of lithium chloride on the circadian rhythm in the flight activity rhythm of the microchiropteran bat, Taphozous melanopogan. Z Naturforsch 1981; 36:1068-71.
49. Morin LP, Cummings LA. Effect of surgical or photoperiodic castration, testosterone replacement or pinealectomy on male hamster running rhythmicity. Physiol Behav 1981; 26:825-38.
50. Daan, S, Damassa D, Pittendrigh CS, et al. An effect of castration and testosterone replacement on the circadian pacemaker in mice (Mus musculus). Proc Natl Acad Sci USA 1975; 72:3744-7.
51. Tamarkin L, Craig CJ, Garrich NA, et al. Effect on clorgyline (a MAO type A inhibitor) on locomotor activity in the Syrian hamster. Am J Physiol 1983; 245:215-21.
52. Borsook D, Moore-Ede MC, Richardson G, et al. Gamma-aminobutyric acid and the neural basis of circadian timekeeping: implications for pathophysiology and psychopharmacotherapy of circadian based disorders. In: Reinberg A, Smolensky M, Labrecque G, eds. Proceedings of the 1st International Montreux Conference of Chronopharmacology. Oxford: Pergamon Press, 1984:53-6.
53. Rietveld WJ, van Schravendijk K. Food intake and antiepileptic drugs: evidence for a role of GABA in circadian time-keeping. Prog Clin Biol Res 1987; 227:507-11.
54. Zatz M, Herkenham MA. Intraventricular carbachol mimics the phase-shifting effect of light on the circadian rhythms of wheel-running activity. Brain Res 1981; 212:234-8.
55. Earnest DJ, Turek FW. Phase shifting and entrainment of the hamster circadian system: role for acetylcholine in mediating the effects of light. Soc Neurosci Abstr 1983; 9:626.
56. Zatz M, Brownstein MJ. Intraventricular carbachol mimics the effects of light on the circadian rhythm in the rat pineal gland. Science 1979; 203:358-61.
57. Albers HE, Ferris CF, Leeman SE, et al. Avian pancreatic polypeptide phase shifts hamster circadian rhythms when micro-injected into the suprachiasmatic region. Science 1984; 223:833-6.
58. Roberts E, Chase TN, Tower DB, eds. GABA in nervous system function. New York: Raven Press, 1976.
59. Enna SJ, Gallagher JP. Biochemical and electrophysiological characteristics of mammalian GABA receptors. Int Rev Neurobiol 1983; 24:181-212.
60. Vincent SR, Hokfelt T, Wu J. GABA neuron systems in the hypothalamus and the pituitary gland. Neuroendocrinology 1983; 34:117-25.
61. Fahn S, Cote LJ. Regional distribution of gamma-aminobutyric acid (GABA) in brain of rhesus monkey. J Neurochem 1968; 15:209-13.

62. Perry TL, Berry K, Hansen S, et al. Regional distribution of amino acids in human brain obtained at autopsy. J Neurochem 1971; 18:513-9.
63. Van Den Pol AN. Gamma-aminobutyrate, gastrin releasing peptide, serotonin, somatostatin and vasopressin: ultrastructural immunocytochemical localization in presynaptic axons in the suprachiasmatic nucleus. Neuroscience 1986; 17:643-59.
64. Makara GB, Rappay G, Stark E. Autoradiographic localization of 3-H-gamma-aminobutyric acid in the medial hypothalamus. Exp Brain Res 1975; 22:449-55.
65. Enna SJ, Snyder SH. Properties of gamma-aminobutyric acid (GABA) receptor binding in rat brain synaptic membrane fractions. Brain Res 1975; 100:81-97.
66. Wu JY, Brandon C, Su YY, et al. Immunocytochemical and autoradiographic localization of GABA system in the vertebrate retina. Mol Cell Biochem 1981; 39:229-38.
67. Hendrickson AE, Ogren MP, Vaughn JE, et al. Light and electron microscope immunocytochemical localization of glutamic acid decarboxylase in monkey geniculate complex: evidence for GABA-ergic neurons and synapses. J Neurosci 1983; 3:1245-62.
68. Ralph MR, Menaker M. Bicuculline blocks circadian phase delays but not advances. Brain Res 1985; 325:362-5.
69. Shibata S, Oomura Y, Kita H, et al. Circadian rhythmic changes of neuronal activity in the suprachiasmatic nucleus of the rat hypothalamic slice. Brain Res 1982; 247:154-8.
70. Borsook D, Richardson GS, Moore-Ede MC, et al. GABA and circadian timekeeping: implications for manic-depression and sleep disorders. Med Hypotheses 1986; 19:185-98.
71. Borsook D. Gamma-aminobutyric acid and circadian timekeeping. Ph.D. Thesis, University of the Witwatersrand, Submitted.
72. Childs G, Redfern PH. A circadian rhythm in passive avoidance behavior: the effect of phase shift and benzodiazepines. Neuropharmacology 1981; 20:1365-6.
73. Turek FW, Losee-Olsen S. A benzodiazepine used in the treatment of insomnia phase-shifts the mammalian circadian clock. Nature 1986; 321:167-8.
74. Ralph MR, Menaker M. Effects of diazepam on circadian phase advances and delays. Brain Res 1986; 372:405-8.
75. Wehr TA, Sack D, Rosenthal N, et al. Circadian rhythm disturbances in manic-depressive illness. Fed Proc 1983; 42:2809-14.
76. Wirz-Justice A, Groos GA, Wehr TA. The neuropharmacology of circadian timekeeping in mammals. In: Aschoff J, Daan S, Groos GA, eds. Mammalian circadian rhythms. New York: Springer-Verlag, 1982:183-93.
77. Kripke DF, Mullaney DJ, Atkinson M, et al. Circadian rhythm disorders in manic-depressives. Biol Psychiatry 1978; 13:335-51.
78. Wehr TA, Goodwin FK. Biological rhythms and psychiatry. In: Arieti S, Brodie HK, eds. American handbook of psychiatry. New York: Basic Books, 1981:46-74.
79. Hall P, Spear MB, Stirland D. Diurnal variation of subjective mood in depressive states. Psychiatr Q 1974; 38:529-36.
80. Waldmann H. Die Tagesschwankung in der Depression als rhythmisches Phänomen. Fortschr Neurol Psychiatr 1972; 40:83-104.
81. Papousek M. Chronobiologische aspekte der Zyklothymie. Fortschr Neurol Psychiatr 1975; 43:381-440.
82. Sachar EJ, Hellman L, Roffwarg HP, et al. Disrupted 24-hour patterns of cortisol secretion in psychotic depression. Arch Gen Psychiatry 1973; 28:19-24.
83. Weeke A, Weeke J. The 24-hour pattern of serum TSH in patients with endogenous depression. Acta Psychiatr Scand 1980; 62:69-74.
84. Wehr TA, Goodwin FK, Wirz-Justice A, et al. Forty-eight-hour sleep-wake cycles in manic-depressive illness: naturalistic observations and sleep-deprivation experiments. Arch Gen Psychiatry 1980; 37:257-63.
85. Wehr TA, Muscettola G, Goodwin FK. Urinary 3-methoxy-4-hydroxyphenylglycol circadian rhythm: early timing phase advance in manic-depressives compared with normal subjects. Arch Gen Psychiatry 1980; 37:257-63.
86. Davis JM. Overview: maintenance therapy in psychiatry. II. Affective disorders. Am J Psychiatry 1976; 133:1-13.

87. Schou M. Pharmacology and toxicology of lithium. Ann Rev Pharmacol Toxicol 1976; 16:231-42.
88. Rao YV, Satischandran P, Kandlikar RP. Possible involvement of adrenergic nervous system in anticonvulsant effect of lithium carbonate in albino rats. Indian J Exp Biol 1986; 24:116-7.
89. Itil TM. Effects of psychotropic drugs on qualitatively and quantitativley analyzed human EEG. In: Clock WG, Guidice J, eds. Principles of psychopharmacology. New York: Academic Press, 1978:261-77.
90. Hartigan GP. The use of lithium salts in affective disorders. Br J Psychiatry 1963; 109:810-4.
91. Stallone F, Shelley E, Mendlewicz J, et al. The use of lithium in affective disorders. III. A double-blind study of prophylaxis in bipolar illness. Am J Psychiatry 1973; 130:1006-10.
92. Coppen A, Noguera R, Bailey J, et al. Prophylactic lithium in affective disorders. Lancet 1971; 2:275-9.
93. Baron M, Gershon ES, Rudy F, et al. Lithium carbonate response in depression. Arch Gen Psychiatry 1975; 32:1107-11.
94. Fieve RR, Platman SR, Plutchnik R. Use of lithium salts in affective disorders: II. Prophylaxis of depression in chronic recurrent affective disorder. Am J Psychiatry 1968; 125:492-8.
95. Goodwin FK, Murphy DL, Bunney WE. Lithium carbonate treatment in depression and mania: a longitudinal double-blind study. Arch Gen Psychiatry 1969; 21:486-95.
96. Brennan MJW, Sandyk R, Borsook D. Sodium valproate in the management of affective disorders: basic and clinical aspects. In: Emrich HM, Okuma T, Müller AA, eds. Anticonvulsants in affective disorders. Amsterdam: Excerpta Medica, 1984:56-65.
97. Emrich HM, von Zerssen DV, Kissling W, et al. Effect of sodium valproate in mania. The GABA-hypothesis of affective disorders. Arch Psychiatr Nervenkr 1980; 229:1-16.
98. Emrich HM, von Zerssen DV, Kissling W, et al. On a possible role of GABA in mania. Therapeutic efficacy of sodium valproate. In: Costa E, DiChiara G, Gessa GL, eds. GABA and benzodiazepine receptors. New York: Raven Press, 1981:287-96.
99. Emrich HM, Gunther R, Dose M. Current perspectives in pharmacopsychiatry of depression and mania. Neuropharmacology 1983; 22:385-8.
100. Lambert P-A, Carraz G, Borselli S, et al. Action neuropsychotrope d'un nouvel anti-épileptique: le Dépamide. Ann Méd Psychol 1966; 124:707-10.
101. Lambert P-A, Borselli S, Marcou G, et al. Action thymo-régulatrice à long terme du Dépamide dans la psychose maniaco-dépressive. Ann Méd Psychol 1971; 2:442-8.
102. Lambert P-A, Carraz G, Borselli S, et al. Le dipropylacétamide dans le traitement de la psychose maniaco-dépressive. Encephale 1975; 1:25-31.
103. Puzynski S, Klosiewicz L. Valproic acid amide in the treatment of affective and schizoaffective disorders. J Affect Dis 1984; 6:115-21.
104. Takezaki H, Hanaoka M. The use of carbamazepine (Tegretol) in the control of manic-depressive psychosis and other manic-depressive states [in Japanese]. Seishin Shinkeigaku Zasshi 1971; 13:173-83.
105. Okuma T, Kishimoto A, Inoue K, et al. Anti-manic and prophylactic effects of carbamazepine (Tegretol) on manic-depressive psychosis. Folia Psychiatr Neurol Japon 1973; 27:283-97.
106. Okuma T, Inanaga K, Otsuki S, et al. Comparison of the antimanic efficacy of carbamazepine and chlorpromazine: a double-blind controlled study. Psychopharmacology 1979; 66:211-7.
107. Okuma T, Inanaga K, Otsuki S, et al. A preliminary double-blind study of the efficacy of carbamazepine in prophylaxis of manic-depressive illness. Psychopharmacology 1981; 73: 95-6.
108. Ballenger JC, Post RM. Therapeutic effects of carbamazepine in affective illness: a preliminary report. Comm Psychopharmacol 1978; 2:159-78.
109. Ballenger JC, Post RM. Carbamazepine in manic-depressive illness: a new treatment. Am J Psychiatry 1980; 137:782-90.
110. Post RM, Uhde TW, Ballenger JC, et al. Prophylactic efficacy of carbamazepine in manic-depressive illness. Am J Psychiatry 1983; 140:1602-4.
111. Klein E, Belmaker RH. Carbamazepine in the treatment of affective disorders. Harefuah 1984; 107:176-80.
112. Post RM, Uhde TW. Carbamazepine in the treatment of affective illness. In: Doane BK, Livingston KE, eds. The limbic system: functional organization and clinical disorders. New York: Raven Press, 1986:267-84.

113. Kupfer DJ, Pickar D, Himmelhoch JM, et al. Are there two types of unipolar depression? Arch Gen Psychiatry 1975; 32:866-7.
114. Mandel MR, Klerman GL. Clinical use of antidepressants, stimulants, tricyclics and monoamine oxidase inhibitors. In: Clark WG, del Guidice J, eds. Principles of psychopharmacology. New York: Academic Press, 1978:537-51.
115. Lipper S, Murphy DL, Slater S, et al. Comparative behavioral effects of clorgyline and pargyline in man: a preliminary evaluation. Psychopharmacology 1979; 62:123-8.
116. Meunier H, Carraz G, Meunier Y, et al. Propriétés pharmacodynamiques de l'acide n-dipropylacétique. Thérapie 1963; 18:435-8.
117. Simler S, Ciesielski L, Maitre M, et al. Effect of sodium n-dipropylacetate on audiogenic seizures and brain gamma-aminobutyric acid level. Biochem Pharmacol 1973; 22:1701-8.
118. Harvey PKP, Bradford HF, Davison AN. The inhibitory effect of sodium n-dipropyl acetate on the degradative enzymes of the GABA shunt. FEBS Lett 1975; 52:251-4.
119. Loscher W, Frey HH. Zum Wirkungmechanismus von Valproinsaure. Arzneim-Forsch 1977; 27:1081-2.
120. Brennan MJW, Cantrill RC, Oldfield M, et al. Inhibition of gamma-aminobutyric acid release by gamma-aminobutyric acid agonist drugs: pharmacology of the gamma-aminobutyric acid autoreceptor. Mol Pharmacol 1981; 19:27-30.
121. Bernasconi R. The GABA hypothesis of affective illness: influence of clinically effective antimanic drugs on GABA turnover. In: Emrich HM, Aldenhof JB, Lux HD, eds. Basic mechanisms in the action of lithium. Amsterdam: Excerpta Medica, 1982:183-92.
122. Godin Y, Heiner L, Mark J, et al. Effects of di-n-propylacetate, an anticonvulsive compound, on GABA metabolism. J Neurochem 1969; 16:869-73.
123. Kerwin RW, Olpe H-R. The effect of sodium valproate on single unit activity in the rat brain. Br J Pharmacol 1980; 70:76P.
124. Loscher W. GABA in plasma, CSF and brain of dogs during acute and chronic treatment with gamma-acetylenic GABA and valproic acid. In: Okada Y, Roberts E, eds. Problems in GABA research. From brain to bacteria. Amsterdam: Excerpta Medica, 1982:102-9.
125. Loscher W, Nau H. Distribution of valproic acid and its metabolites in various brain areas of dogs and rats after acute and prolonged treatment. J Pharmacol Exp Ther 1983; 226:845-54.
126. Simler S, Gensburger C, Ciesielski L, et al. Time course of the increase in GABA level in different mice brain regions following n-dipropylacetate treatment. Comm Psychopharmacol 1978; 2:123-30.
127. Weissman D, Simler S, Ciesielski L, et al. Variations de la teneur en GABA de certaines zones du cerveau de la souris sous l'effet de l'acide propyl-2-pentene-2-oique. C R Soc Biol (Paris) 1978; 172:707-12.
128. Iadarola MJ, Raines A, Gale K. Differential effects of n-dipropylacetate and amino-oxyacetic acid on gamma-aminobutyric acid levels in discrete areas of rat brain. J Neurochem 1979; 33:1119-23.
129. Leeb-Lundberg F, Snowman A, Olsen RW. Some anticonvulsants interact with GABA receptor-ionophore complex at barbiturate/picrotoxin receptor sites. Fed Proc 1981; 40:309. abstract #432.
130. Hendler NH. Lithium pharmacology and physiology. In: Iversen LL, Iversen SD, Snyder SH, eds. Handbook of psychopharmacology. New York: Plenum Press, 1978:233-73.
131. Maggi A, Enna SJ. Regional alterations in rat brain neurotransmitter systems following chronic lithium treatment. J Neurochem 1980; 34:888-92.
132. Berrettini WH, Nurnberger JI, Hare TA, et al. Reduced plasma and CSF gamma-aminobutyric acid in affective illness: effect of lithium carbonate. Biochem Psychiatry 1983; 18:185-94.
133. Banay-Schwartz M, Wajda IJ, Manigault I, et al. Lithium effect on 3-H-spiperone binding, ionic content, and amino acid levels in the brain of rats. Neurochem Res 1982; 7: 179-89.
134. Wajda IJ, Banay-Schwartz M, Lajtha A. Lithium effects on neuronal membranes in rats of different ages. Neurosci Abstr 1983; 9:231. abstract.
135. Pittendrigh CS, Daan S. A functional analysis of circadian pacemakers in nocturnal rodents. IV. Entrainment: pacemaker as clock. J Comp Physiol 1976; 106:291-331.

136. Richter CP. Inherent twenty-four-hour and lunar clocks of a primate—the squirrel monkey. Comm Behav Biol 1968; 1:305-32.
137. Prosser RA, Satinoff E. Effects of partial SCN lesions on body temperature, drinking and activity rhythms in rats. Neurosci Abstr 1985; 11:817. abstract.
138. Pickard GE, Turek FW. The surpachiasmatic nucleus: two circadian clocks? Brain Res 1983; 268:201-10.
139. Ebihara S, Kawamura H. The role of the pineal organ and the suprachiasmatic nuclei in the control of circadian locomotor rhythms in the Java sparrow, Padda oryzivora. J Comp Physiol 1981; 141:207-14.
140. Kronauer RE, Czeisler CA, Pilato SF, et al. Mathematical model of the human circadian system with two interacting oscillators. Am J Physiol 1982; 242:R3-R17.
141. Czeisler CA. Internal organization of temperature, sleep-wake, and neuroendocrine rhythms monitored in an environment free of time cues. PhD Thesis, Stanford University, 1978.
142. Redman J, Armstrong S, Ng KT. Free-running rhythms in the rat: entrainment by melatonin. Science 1983; 219:1089-91.
143. Cavagnini F, Invitti C, Pinto M, et al. Effect of acute and repeated administration of gamma-aminobutyric acid (GABA) on growth hormone and prolactin secretion in man. Acta Endocrinol (Copenh) 1980; 91:149-54.
144. Grove J, Tell G, Schechter PJ, et al. Increased CSF gamma-aminobutyric acid after treatment with gamma-vinyl-GABA (letter). Lancet 1980; 2:647.
145. Lotka AJ. Elements of mathematical biology. New York: Dover, 1956:88-94.
146. Volterra V. Leçons sur la théorie mathématique de la lutte pour la vie. Paris: Gauthier-Villars, 1931.
147. Hobson JA, McCarley RW, Wyzinksi PW. Sleep cycle oscillation: reciprocal discharge by two brainstem neuronal groups. Science 1975; 189:55-8.
148. McCarley RW, Hobson JA. Neuronal excitibility modulation over the sleep cycle: a structural and mathematical model. Science 1975; 189:58-60.
149. McCarley RW, Massaquoi SG. A limit cycle mathematical model of the REM sleep oscillator system. Am J Physiol 1986; 251:1011-29.
150. Hobson JA, Lydic R, Baghdoyan HA. Evolving concepts of sleep cycle generation: from brain centers to neuronal populations. Behav Brain Sci 1986; 9:371-400.
151. Harvey SC. Hypnotics and sedatives. In: Gilman AG, Goodman LS, Gilman A, eds. The pharmacological basis of therapeutics. New York: Macmillan, 1980:339-49.
152. Costa E, Guidotti A. Molecular mechanism in the receptor action of benzodiazepines. Ann Rev Tox 1979; 18:531-45.
153. Czeisler CA, Richardson GS, Coleman RM, et al. Chronotherapy: resetting the circadian clocks of patients with delayed sleep phase insomnia. Sleep 1981; 4:1-21.
154. Rechtschaffen A, Wolpart EA, Dement WC, et al. Nocturnal sleep of narcoleptics. Electroencephalogr Clin Neurophysiol 1963; 15:599-609.
155. Weitzman ED, Kripke DF, Goldmader D, et al. Acute reversal of the sleep-waking cycle in man. Effect on sleep stage patterns. Arch Neurol 1970:483-9.
156. Klein KE, Wegmann HM. Circadian rhythms in air operations. In: Nicholson AN, ed. Sleep, wakefulness and circadian rhythms. Neuilly sur Seine, France: NATO Advisory Group for Aerospace Research and Development, 1979:105.
157. Broughton R, Mamelak M. The treatment of narcolepsy-cataplexy with nocturnal gamma-hydroxybutyrate. Can J Neurol Sci 1979; 6:1-6.
158. Mamelak M, Escrin JM, Stokan O. The effects of gamma-hydroxybutyrate on sleep. Biol Psychiatry 1977; 12:273-6.
159. Roth T, Hartze KM, Saab PG, et al. The effects of flurazepam, lorazepam, and triazolam on sleep and memory. Psychopharmacology 1980; 70:231-7.

I would like to thank Drs. Ziad Boulos, Martin Moore-Ede, and Michael Brennan who participated in the work on squirrel monkeys.

CHAPTER 7

Anticonvulsants in the Treatment of Rapid-Cycling Bipolar Disorder

Paul E. Keck, Jr., M.D. *Susan L. McElroy, M.D.*
Belmont, Massachusetts

INTRODUCTION

Emil Kraepelin[1] provided the nosologic foundation for manic-depressive illness, currently defined as bipolar disorder.[2] In his description of this illness, he emphasized its recurrent nature, marked by episodes of both mania and depression.[1] Decades of subsequent clinical experience and careful delineation of the natural history of bipolar disorder have borne out Kraepelin's observations.[3] However, the study of bipolar patients with frequent or continuous alternations between manic, depressed, and mixed affective states was not systematically approached until the early 1970's. In 1974, Dunner and Fieve introduced the term "rapid cycling" to describe a class of such patients who were disproportionately represented among patients poorly responsive to lithium prophylaxis.[4] Prior to this report, cases appeared only sporadically in the scientific literature. Kraepelin himself described only one such patient,[1] and two Scandanavian reports provided a smattering of cases.[5,6] Patients with "circular" and "chronic" variants of manic-depressive illness were described in early studies which may have included a portion with a rapid-cycling course.[7-10] In the 1960's, two patients with cyclical 48-hour alternations between mania and depression were reported.[11,12] Patients with more rapid alternations have not yet been described.

INCIDENCE

Dunner and Fieve defined rapid cycling as the occurrence of four or more affective episodes per year and found that 40 (13%) of 307 bipolar patients treated at the Lithium Clinic of the New York State Psychiatric Institute met this criterion.[4] In a recent report from another center, five (14%) of the 37 consecutive bipolar patients treated with valproate after proving intolerant or poorly responsive to lithium met Dunner and Fieve's criteria for rapid cycling.[13] A third survey, reported by Nurnburger and colleagues at the National Institute of Mental Health, again found that rapid cyclers constituted 13% of a cohort of bipolar and schizoaffective patients.[14] The actual prevalence of rapid cycling among bipolar patients, however, remains unknown and may well be less than the 13% proportion observed in these studies. Estimates of the prevalence of rapid cycling at these centers may be inflated, since each is a tertiary referral facility offering specialized evaluation and treatment of bipolar patients likely to be more treatment-resistant than a random cohort of such patients.

DISTINGUISHING CHARACTERISTICS

No consistent clinical or demographic factors, beyond the frequency of affective episodes themselves and general treatment resistance, have been found to distinguish rapid cyclers from other bipolar patients. In a follow-up analysis of their Lithium Clinic cohort, Dunner and colleagues could not distinguish rapid cyclers from the remainder of their bipolar patients by age, sex, age of onset, duration of illness, symptomatology, proportion of patients with bipolar I or bipolar II diagnosis, and family history of major affective disorder.[15] Subsequent studies have noted a greater proportion of females among the rapid cyclers.[14] Nurnberger and colleagues did not find evidence of increased genetic loading for major affective disorder in rapid cyclers (age-corrected morbid risk for major affective disorder was 23.5% in first-degree relatives of rapid cyclers and 31.0% in relatives of bipolar nonrapid cyclers).[14] In this study, rapid cycling did not "breed true" within families in which probands were afflicted with rapid-cycling bipolar disorder.[14] The Lithium Clinic cohort also failed to demonstrate differences between rapid cyclers and other bipolar patients with regard to the frequency of life events prior to onset of illness[16] and the presence of psychotic symptoms during manic episodes.[17] These findings support the concept that rapid cycling is a variant or extreme form of bipolar disorder, rather than a unique form of the illness that may arise from factors separable from the genetic susceptibility to bipolar disorder itself.[14]

ETIOLOGY

A variety of factors have been implicated as possible inducers or contributors to a rapid-cycling course in some patients. These factors have been thoroughly described in two recent reviews[18,19] and include treatment with or withdrawal from antidepressants,[20] treatment with lithium salts,[21,22] clinical or subclinical hypothyroidism,[20,21,23,24] and neurological disease or insult.[25-27] One intriguing and potentially unifying hypothesis of the pathophysiology of major affective disorder in general and rapid cycling in particular involves the desynchronization of circadian rhythms[28,29] and is supported by preliminary findings of an antidepressant effect of various sleep deprivation and sleep phase shift maneuvers.[30,31] Despite these interesting possibilities, the etiology of rapid-cycling bipolar disorder is unknown; a detailed analysis of the evidence supporting the various hypotheses listed in the preceeding discussion is beyond the scope of this chapter. For a more comprehensive discussion, the reader is referred to the reviews cited above.[18,19]

TREATMENT

Rapid-cycling bipolar disorder is notoriously difficult to treat and often refractory or only minimally responsive to lithium salts and neuroleptics.[18,19] Because rapid-cycling cases are uncommon, it is also difficult to assemble a cohort of sufficient size to conduct controlled trials of potentially useful treatments. To date, the findings regarding treatment results, briefly discussed earlier, have been based on case reports and small series of patients.

Although lithium is reputed to be of limited benefit in rapid cyclers, a small number of Dunner and Fieve's original cohort displayed a reduction in both the frequency and severity of episodes with ongoing lithium treatment, sometimes evident only upon prolonged follow-up.[15] Treatment with neuroleptics,[27] thyroid hormone,[32] electroconvulsive therapy (ECT),[18] clorgyline,[33] and repetitive sleep deprivation[34,35] have been suggested as alternative interventions in case reports and small series. However, for the reasons cited above, the efficacies of these treatments have not been systematically studied in larger patient samples.

A growing literature, reviewed below, suggests that the anticonvulsants carbamazepine, valproate, and possibly clonazepam may offer effective treatment for lithium-resistant patients in general and rapid-cycling bipolar patients in particular.[36-61] Of the available studies, 18 reports on 79 patients provide sufficient data for tabulation, as summarized in Table 1.

CARBAMAZEPINE

Ten reports examined carbamazepine, either alone or in combination with other psychotropic agents, in rapid-cycling bipolar disorder.[40-47,49,50] In these studies, 54 patients received the drug on an open basis and three under blind, controlled conditions (Table 1). Fifty-five (96%) of 57 patients studied had failed previous treatment with lithium salts, and the remaining two patients were noncompliant with lithium because of side effects.[47] Nevertheless, more than 70% of the total group showed sustained improvement with carbamazepine, maintained over follow-up periods of one month to three years. Twenty-nine patients received carbamazepine alone and 21 (72%) of these were described as responders (in this review, response was scored when a patient experienced a greater than 75% reduction in the frequency of affective episodes). The remaining 28 patients received carbamazepine in conjunction with lithium salts, neuroleptics, antidepressants, and various combinations of these agents.

In general, carbamazepine was well tolerated with a low incidence of adverse reactions. However, two patients experienced neurotoxic symptoms of lethargy, dysarthria, confusion, and ataxia when treated with carbamazepine in combination with haloperidol.[43,46] These patients subsequently responded to carbamazepine alone without adverse effects. During the trials in which carbamazepine was combined with haloperidol, carbamazepine levels were within the therapeutic range of 8.0 μg/ml to 12.0 μg/ml in both cases. The mechanism of this neurotoxicity is unknown and it has not been reported in larger series.[41,42,45,57]

Post and colleagues described a patient with rapid-cycling bipolar disorder responsive to carbamazepine who failed to respond to phenytoin and valproate administered in double-blind crossover trials.[44] Details of alternative anticonvulsant trials are not provided for the other 56 patients.

Post and his group have performed the only systematic assessment of possible predictors of antimanic response to carbamazepine to date. Their preliminary findings suggest that rapid cycling, as well as other factors associated with poor response to lithium in their bipolar patients (N = 19), including severity of mania, anxiety, dysphoria, and negative family history of major affective disorder, may predict response to carbamazepine[62] (and see Chapter 1 in this volume).

VALPROATE

While carbamazepine has been the anticonvulsant most extensively studied in the

TABLE 1. Studies and reports of anticonvulsants in rapid-cycling bipolar disorder

Study	Number of patients	Anticonvulsant	Concomitant medications	Outcome[a]	Comment
Kishimoto et al.[40]	24	Carbamazepine	Lithium added in 6/16 partial responders and 4/6 nonresponders	2 full remission; 16 partial remission 6 no response	Acute treatment and prophylaxis; up to 7-year follow-up
Nolen[41]	7	Carbamazepine	4 none; 1 lithium; 1 lithium + neuroleptic; 1 antidepressant	4/7 response	2/4 responders on carbamazepine alone
Post et al.[42]	6	Carbamazepine	3 none; 1 lithium; 1 neuroleptic; 1 antidepressant	5/6 response	
Kantner et al.[43]	1	Carbamazepine	Neuroleptic	Response	Neurotoxic side effects when added to haloperidol
Post et al.[44]	1	Carbamazepine	None	Response	No response to blind therapeutic trials of valproate and phenytoin
Greil et al.[45]	7	Carbamazepine	4 none; 2 lithium + neuroleptic + antidepressant; 1 neuroleptic + antidepressant	2/7 response	No responders among patients receiving carbamazepine alone
Yerevanian and Hodgman[46]	1	Carbamazepine	Neuroleptic after relapse	Response	Relapse after drop in blood level below therapeutic range; neurotoxic side effects when haloperidol added
Strömgren and Boller[47]	5	Carbamazepine	3 none; 1 neuroleptic; 1 neuroleptic + antidepressant	3/5 response	2/3 responders on carbamazepine alone
Lovett et al.[49]	3	Carbamazepine	Lithium	3/3 response	Carbamazepine added to lithium
Lerer et al.[50]	2	Carbamazepine	None	2/2 response	Double-blind trial vs lithium
von Zerssen and Emrich[36]	7	Valproate	Lithium	7/7 response	
Emrich et al.[55]	3	Valproate	Lithium	3/3 response	
Puzynski and Klosiewicz[53]	3	Valpromide	None	1/3 response	
Herridge and Pope[54]	1	Valproate	None	Response	Relapse with discontinuation or subtherapeutic levels
McElroy et al.[57]	5[b]	Valproate	2 lithium; 2 lithium + antidepressant; 1 lithium + neuroleptic	5/5 response	2 relapsed with discontinuation or subtherapeutic valproate levels
Keck[58]	1	Valproate	Neuroleptic	Response	Maintained in remission on valproate alone
Victor et al.[59]	1	Clonazepam	Lithium	Response	Received neuroleptic just prior to clonazepam
Zetin and Freedman[61]	1	Clonazepam	None	Response	Required antidepressant 1 year later

[a] *Response is scored if patient experienced a reduction >75% in frequency of affective episodes.*

[b] *This study actually presents six cases, but one of these is the case of Herridge and Pope listed immediately above; therefore, this case is deleted from those of McElroy et al.*

treatment of bipolar disorder and its rapid-cycling variant, a substantial literature, dating back to 1966, has suggested a similar role for valproate, or the closely related drug, valpromide.[56] (See Chapter 2 in this volume for a discussion of the relationship of valpromide to valproate.) The initial promise offered by this drug may have been dampened by reports of irreversible hepatotoxicity.[63] However, the risk of irreversible hepatotoxicity has recently been found to be associated with specific risk factors such as preexisting neurological deficits, age less than two years, and treatment with concomitant anticonvulsants.[63]

Six reports have described the response of 20 rapid-cycling bipolar patients to valproate in sufficient detail for tabulation (Table 1).[36,53-55,57,58] All patients received valproate on an open basis. Four received valproate alone and in all other cases valproate was added to preexisting psychotropic regimens. Eighteen (90%) of the 20 patients studied showed lasting improvement with valproate, although length of follow-up is not provided in the majority of reports. Three patients maintained on valproate alone after discontinuation of other agents exhibited prolonged remission.[57,58] Two (50%) of four patients treated acutely with valproate alone were described as responders.[53,54] In three cases, relapse followed promptly after discontinuation of the drug or a drop in blood level below the therapeutic range (less than 50 μg/ml).[54,57] Five patients who responded to valproate had failed previous trials of carbamazepine,[54,57] and two other valproate responders had been unable to tolerate carbamazepine because of side effects.[57,58] Eighteen (90%) of the 20 rapid cyclers tolerated valproate well without reports of adverse side effects or deleterious drug interaction. Two patients had valproate discontinued after developing asymptomatic hepatic transaminase elevations which gradually normalized upon discontinuation of the drug.[57]

This small series of reports suggests that valproate, like carbamazepine, is usually well tolerated and may represent a useful alternative or adjunctive treatment for rapid-cycling bipolar disorder.

CLONAZEPAM

Only two case reports have appeared to date describing clonazepam in the treatment of rapid-cycling bipolar patients (Table 1).[59,61] One patient with recurrent episodes of major depression punctuated by brief bouts of mania responded to clonazepam alone, although she required treatment with imipramine for recurrent mild depressive episodes one year later.[61] The response of the second patient to clonazepam is somewhat more equivocal, since the patient received trifluoperazine just prior to clonazepam, and follow-up data beyond the apparent acute response is lacking.[59]

PHENYTOIN

As previously noted, Post and colleagues described one rapid-cycling patient who failed to respond to phenytoin in a double-blind controlled trial.[44] No other reports, to our knowledge, of other anticonvulsants in the treatment of rapid-cycling bipolar disorder have appeared to date.

SUMMARY OF REPORTED CASES

In summary, reports of treatment of 79 patients with rapid-cycling bipolar disorder with anticonvulsant agents (carbamazepine, valproate, clonazepam, and phenytoin) have thus far appeared in the available scientific literature. Sixty patients (76%) among this group were described as responders. However, these optimistic results must be interpreted with a number of caveats. First, the vast majority of patients were studied under nonblind and uncontrolled conditions. Second, the apparent frequency of positive outcomes has been undoubtedly increased by the tendency of clinicians to report positive rather than negative results. Except for studies in which consecutive series of patients are treated, treatment failures may have gone unreported. Third, anticonvulsants were added to lithium salts, neuroleptics, antidepressants, or combinations of these agents in a majority of cases and may thus have exerted an adjuvant rather than a primary effect on treatment outcome. Fourth, although response represented a meaningful (greater than 75%) reduction in the frequency, and often, severity of affective episodes, many patients remained residually symptomatic.

On the other hand, the 79 patients described represent a demonstrably treatment-resistant population, and the marked reduction in morbidity in many cases often represented the difference between chronic or recurrent hospitalization and autonomous existence within the community. Thus, although lithium salts remain the drug of first choice in the treatment of rapid-cycling bipolar patients, carbamazepine and valproate, and possibly clonazepam, may represent second-line alternatives or adjunctive treatments in the partially responsive, lithium-refractory, or lithium-intolerant rapid-cycling patient.[13,62] These treatment alternatives, if successful, could also obviate the need for repeated or prolonged exposure to neuroleptics, thus reducing the risk of tardive dyskinesia, and possibly, of precipitating or exacerbating further depressive episodes.[64]

Moreover, it should be emphasized that failure to respond to one anticonvulsant did not predict failure to respond to another, as one rapid-cycling patient failing valproate but responding to carbamazepine,[44] as well as several patients failing carbamazepine but responding to valproate[45,57] were both reported. Therefore, failure to improve with one anticonvulsant should not preclude further trials with other agents.

POSSIBLE MECHANISMS OF ACTION

Emerging evidence of the efficacy of anticonvulsants in the treatment of major affective disorder has generated renewed interest in theories relating GABAergic transmission to the underlying pathophysiology of affective illness.[65-67]

Preclinical data suggest that some components of affective illness may be related to functional deficiencies in gamma-aminobutyric acid (GABA) activity at certain critical sites in the central nervous system (CNS). In learned helplessness paradigms, which are putative animal models of depression, the efficacy of tricyclic antidepressants is linked to their ability to increase GABA activity in the frontal neocortex and hippocampus.[68] Chronic lithium administration in rats induces increased GABA activity in the hypothalamus.[69] Carbamazepine,[66] valproate,[70] and ECT,[71] all reputed antimanic treatments, may decrease GABA turnover, possibly as a function of increased GABA activity. Similarly, clonazepam, a benzodiazepine with reputed antimanic activity, may enhance GABAergic transmission by binding to the GABA benzodiazepine-chloride ionophore macromolecular complex.[66] Finally, reduced plasma and cerebrospinal fluid (CSF) GABA levels have been reported in patients with major affective disorder, and lithium administration produced significant elevations in these levels.[72]

Lloyd and Morselli have reviewed data suggesting that both GABAergic and noradrenergic mechanisms are involved in the therapeutic action of thymoleptic drugs.[66] In animal models, $GABA_B$ receptor up-regulation and beta-adrenoreceptor down-regulation have been consistently demonstrated to result from repeated antidepressant drug adminstration.[66] Further support for joint involvement of thesc neurotransmitters comes from studies which suggest that GABAergic transmission modulates noradrenergic synaptic activity, as reflected by an increase in norepinephrine turnover induced by a variety of agents which enhance GABAergic transmission, including valproate.[66]

Noradrenergic mechanisms have long been hypothesized to play a critical role in the pathophysiology of mood disorders.[73] Alterations in urinary[74] and plasma[75] 3-methoxy-4-hydroxyphenylglycol (MHPG), a major norepinephrine metabolite, have been found to vary with mood state in rapid-cycling bipolar patients, leading to speculation that the pathophysiology of the switch process in bipolar disorder is correlated with changes in the activity of noradrenergic transmission.[76] Post and colleagues have observed that carbamazepine decreased elevated CSF norepinephrine in patients treated for mania.[48] (Carbamazepine exerts complex effects on noradrenergic transmission, including blockade of norepinephrine reuptake, weaker than that of imipramine, and increase of locus ceruleus firing without down-regulation of beta-adrenergic receptors.)[48] What role, if any, GABAergic transmission plays in this switch process remains unknown. However, it has been demonstrated that GABA, particularly at the $GABA_B$ receptor sites, modulates catecholaminergic activity.[66]

Interestingly, pivotal roles for noradrenergic[77] and GABAergic[78] neurotransmission have been suggested in the modulation of another potentially important physiologic process possibly involved in the pathogenesis of major affective disorder—the regulation of circadian rhythms. Patients with rapid-cycling bipolar disorder appear to have a profound desychronization of circadian rhythms.[79] These rhythms have been linked to coupled oscillators,[80] which include the suprachiasmatic nucleus of the ventromedial hypothalamus, a center richly innervated by GABAergic neurons.[81] Two distinct aberrations of circadian cycles may exist in bipolar patients: one group might have abnormally rapid (less than 24 hours) cycles, and a second group abnormally slow (greater than 25 hours) cycles.[29] One effect of chronic lithium administration in man is a significant lengthening of the sleep-wake and temperature cycles.[81] In their analysis of lithium response and circadian cycle length in bipolar patients, Kripke and colleagues found that patients with slow (greater than 25 hours) cycles tended to respond poorly to lithium.[29] Brennan and colleagues found that valproate exerts a reciprocal effect on circadian periodicity, often shortening sleep-wake cycles.[81] This reciprocal effect on circadian periodicity by valproate provides one possible explanation for the apparent efficacy of valproate, a GABAergic agent, in rapid-cycling bipolar patients, patients typically poorly responsive to lithium.[81] (For a more detailed discussion see Chapter 6 in this volume).

Finally, it should be mentioned that Post and others have postulated a limbic kindling model for bipolar disorder.[48] This model is based on the hypothesis that the progressive shortening of interepisodic euthymic periods typically seen in rapid cyclers might be due to progressive sensitization of neural structures to subthreshold stimuli (to which limbic and temporal lobe structures are most prone). Carbamazepine and valproate, both effective in temporal lobe and limbic seizures, have been reported to be the two most potent anticonvulsant compounds in their ability to inhibit the spread of amygdala-kindled after-discharges.[48] Direct electrophysiologic or metabolic studies of limbic and/or temporal lobe function in bipolar patients, to our knowledge, have not yet appeared in the literature to substantiate or refute this hypothesis.

CONCLUSIONS

Rapid-cycling bipolar disorder has been defined as a form of bipolar disorder in which four or more major affective episodes occur per year.[4] Estimates have placed up to 13% to 14% of bipolar patients in this category.[4,14,57] The disorder is often characterized by progressive shortening of interepisodic euthymic periods, sometimes culminating in continuous illness with rapid alternations between manic, depressed, and mixed affective states. The disorder is notoriously difficult to treat and often refractory or only minimally responsive to lithium salts and neuroleptics.[18,19]

A growing literature suggests that the anticonvulsants carbamazepine and valproate, and perhaps clonazepam, may offer an effective treatment for lithium-resistant patients with rapid-cycling bipolar disorder. Further studies are required to distinguish the effectiveness of these agents as primary or adjunctive treatments, to assess possible predictors of response, to clarify factors favoring response to one anticonvulsant over another, and to determine if concurrent use of anticonvulsants would provide synergistic action in certain patients. Finally, the putative efficacy of these agents in rapid-cycling bipolar disorder has important and exciting ramifications for understanding the pathogenesis of this debilitating illness.

REFERENCES

1. Kraepelin E. Manic-depressive insanity and paranoia. Edinburgh: E&S Livingstone, Ltd., 1921.
2. American Psychiatric Association, Task Force on Nomenclature and Statistics. Diagnostic and statistical manual of mental disorders. 3rd ed., revised. Washington, DC: American Psychiatric Association, 1987.
3. Zis AP, Goodwin FK. Major affective disorder as a recurrent illness. Arch Gen Psychiatry 1979; 36:835-9.
4. Dunner DL, Fieve RR. Clinical factors in lithium carbonate prophylaxis failure. Arch Gen Psychiatry 1974; 30:229-33.
5. Lundquist G. Prognosis and course in manic-depressive psychoses. Acta Neurol Scand 1945; 35:1S-96S.
6. Stenstedt A. A study in manic-depressive psychosis. Acta Psychiatr Scand 1952; 79:1S-111S.

7. Pollock HM. Recurrence of attacks in manic-depressive psychosis. Am J Psychiatry 1971; 11:568-73.
8. Bratfos I, Haug JO. The course of manic-depressive psychosis: a follow-up investigation of 215 patients. Acta Psychiatr Scand 1968; 44:89-122.
9. Astrup C, Fossum A, Holmboe R. A follow-up study of 270 patients with acute affective psychosis. Acta Psychiatr Scand 1959; 135:1S-65S.
10. Taschev T. The course and prognosis of depression on the basis of 652 patients deceased. In: Angst J, ed. Classification and prediction of outcome of depression. New York: Schattauer Verlag, 1974.
11. Bunney WE, Hartmann EL. Study of a patient with 48-hour manic-depressive cycles. Arch Gen Psychiatry 1965; 12:611-8.
12. Jenner FA, Gjessing LR, Cox JR, et al. A manic-depressive psychotic with a persistent forty-eight hour cycle. Br J Psychiatry 1967; 113:895-910.
13. McElroy SL, Pope HG, Jr, Keck PE, Jr, et al. Treatment of psychiatric disorders with valproate: a series of 73 cases. Psychiatr Psychobiol (in press).
14. Nurnburger JI, Guroff JJ, Hamovit J, et al. A family study of rapid-cycling bipolar illness. Presented at the American Psychiatric Association Annual Meeting, Chicago May 13, 1987. New Research abstract #155.
15. Dunner DL, Patrick V, Fieve RR. Rapid-cycling manic depressive patients. Compr Psychiatry 1977; 18:561-6.
16. Dunner DL, Patrick V, Fieve RR. Life events at the onset of bipolar affective illness. Am J Psychiatry 1979; 136:508-11.
17. Rosenthal NE, Rosenthal LN, Stallone F, et al. Toward the validation of RDC schizoaffective disorder. Arch Gen Psychiatry 1980; 37:804-10.
18. Roy-Byrne PP, Joffe RT, Uhde TW, et al. Approaches to the evaluation and treatment of rapid-cycling affective illness. Br J Psychiatry 1984; 145:543-50.
19. Alarcon RD. Rapid cycling affective disorders: a clinical review. Compr Psychiatry 1985; 26: 522-40.
20. Wehr TA, Goodwin FK. Rapid-cycling in manic-depressives induced by tricyclic antidepressants. Arch Gen Psychiatry 1979; 36:555-9.
21. Cowdry RW, Wehr TA, Zis AP, et al. Thyroid abnormalities associated with rapid cycling bipolar illness. Arch Gen Psychiatry 1983; 40:414-20.
22. Squillace K, Post RM, Savard R, et al. Life charting of the longitudinal course of recurrent affective illness. In: Post RM, Ballenger JC, eds. Neurobiology of mood disorders. Baltimore: Williams & Wilkins, 1984:38-59.
23. Cho JT, Boue S, Dunner DL, et al. The effect of lithium treatment on thyroid function in patients with primary affective disorder. Am J Psychiatry 1979; 136:115-6.
24. O'Shanick GJ, Ellinwood EH. Persistent elevation of thyroid-stimulating hormone in women with bipolar affective disorder. Am J Psychiatry 1982; 139:513-4.
25. Kellner CH, Post RM, Davenport Y, et al. Rapid-cycling bipolar disorder and multiple sclerosis. Am J Psychiatry 1984; 141:112-3.
26. Forrest D. Bipolar illness following right hemispherectomy. Arch Gen Psychiatry 1982; 39:817-23.
27. Himmelhoch J. Mixed states, manic-depressive illness and the nature of mood. Psychiatric Clin N A 1979; 2:449-59.
28. Healy D. Rhythm and blues. Neurochemical, neuropharmacological, and neurophysiological implications of a hypothesis of circadian rhythm dysfunction in the affective disorders. Psychopharmacology 1987; 93:271-85.
29. Kripke DL, Mullaney DJ, Atkinson M, et al. Circadian rhythm disorders in manic-depressives. Biol Psychiatry 1978; 13:335-50.
30. Wehr TA. Biological rhythms and manic-depressive illness. In: Post RM, Ballenger JC, eds. Neurobiology of mood disorders. Baltimore: Williams & Wilkins, 1984:190-205.
31. Wehr TA, Goodwin FK, Wirz-Justice A, et al. 48-hour sleep-wake cycles in manic-depressive illness. Arch Gen Psychiatry 1982; 39:559-68.
32. Stancer HC, Persad E. Treatment of intractable rapid-cycling manic-depressive disorder with levothyroxine. Arch Gen Psychiatry 1982; 39:311-2.

33. Potter WZ, Murphy DL, Wehr TA, et al. Clorgyline. Arch Gen Psychiatry 1982; 33:505-10.
34. Christodoulou GN, Malliaras DE, Lykouras EP, et al. Possible prophylactic effect of sleep deprivation. Am J Psychiatry 1978; 135:375-6.
35. Papadimitriou GN, Christodoulou GN, Trikkes GM, et al. Sleep deprivation prophylaxis in recurrent affective disorder. Bibliotheca Psychiatrica 1981; 160:56-61.
36. von Zerssen D, Emrich HM. New drugs for mania? Br J Psychiatry 1983; 142:532-3.
37. Okuma T, Inanaga K, Otsuki S, et al. Comparison of the antimanic efficacy of carbamazepine and chlorpromazine: a double-blind controlled study. Psychopharmacology 1979; 66:211-7.
38. Ballenger JC, Post RM. Carbamazepine in manic-depressive illness: a new treatment. Am J Psychiatry 1980; 137:782-90.
39. Lipinski JF, Pope HG, Jr. Possible synergistic action between carbamazepine and lithium carbonate in the treatment of three acutely manic patients. Am J Psychiatry 1982; 139:948-9.
40. Kishimoto A, Ogura C, Hazama H, et al. Long-term prophylactic effects of carbamazepine in affective disorder. Br J Psychiatry 1983; 143:327-31.
41. Nolen WA. Carbamazepine, a possible adjunct or alternative to lithium in bipolar disorder. Acta Psychiatr Scand 1983; 67:218-25.
42. Post RM, Uhde TW, Ballenger JC, et al. Prophylactic efficacy of carbamazepine in manic-depressive illness. Am J Psychiatry 1983; 140:1602-4.
43. Kanter GL, Yerevanian BI, Ciccone JR. Case report of a possible interaction between neuroleptics and carbamazepine. Am J Psychiatry 1984; 141:1101-2.
44. Post RM, Berrettini W, Uhde TW, et al. Selective response to the anticonvulsant carbamazepine in manic-depressive illness: a case study. J Clin Psychopharmacol 1984; 4:178-85.
45. Greil W, Kruger R, Rossnagl G, et al. Prophylactic therapy of affective disorders with carbamazepine: an open clinical trial. In: Emrich HM, Okuma T, Müller A, eds. Anticonvulsants in affective disorders. Amsterdam: Excerpta Medica, 1984:153-9.
46. Yerevanian B, Hodgman C. A haloperidol-carbamazepine interaction in a patient with rapid-cycling bipolar disorder. Am J Psychiatry 1985; 142:785-6.
47. Strömgren LS, Boller S. Carbamazepine treatment and prophylaxis of manic-depressive disorder. Psychiatr Dev 1985; 4:349-67.
48. Post RM, Ballenger JC, Uhde TW, et al. Efficacy of carbamazepine in manic-depressive illness: implications for underlying mechanisms. In: Post RM, Ballenger JC, eds. Neurobiology of mood disorders. Baltimore: Williams & Wilkins, 1984:777-816.
49. Lovett L, Watkins E, Shaw DM. The use of alternative drug therapy in nine patients with recurrent affective disorder resistant to conventional prophylaxis. Biol Psychiatry 1986; 21:1344-7.
50. Lerer B, Moore N, Meyerdorff E, et al. Carbamazepine versus lithium in mania: a double-blind study. J Clin Psychiatry 1987; 49:89-93.
51. Emrich HM, von Zerssen D, Kissling W, et al. On a possible role of GABA in mania. Therapeutic efficacy of sodium valproate. In: Costa E, DiChiara G, Gessa GL, eds. GABA and benzodiazepine receptors. New York: Raven Press, 1981:287-96.
52. Emrich HM, Altmann H, Dose M, et al. Therapeutic effect of GABAergic drugs in affective disorders. A preliminary report. Pharmacol Biochem Behav 1982; 19:369-72.
53. Puzynski S, Klosiewicz L. Valproic acid amide in the treatment of affective and schizoaffective disorder. J Affect Dis 1984; 6:115-21.
54. Herridge PL, Pope HG, Jr. Treatment of bulimia and rapid-cycling bipolar disorder with sodium valproate. J Clin Psychopharmacol 1985; 5:229-30.
55. Emrich HM, Dose M, von Zerssen D. The use of sodium valproate, carbamazepine, and oxcarbazepine in patients with affective disorders. J Affect Dis 1985; 9:243-50.
56. McElroy SL, Keck PE, Jr, Pope HG, Jr. Sodium valproate: its use in primary psychiatric disorders. J Clin Psychopharmacol 1987; 7:16-24.
57. McElroy SL, Keck PE, Jr, Pope HG, Jr, et al. Valproate in the treatment of rapid-cycling bipolar disorder. J Clin Psychopharmacol (in press).
58. Keck PE, Jr. Sodium valproate in rapid-cycling bipolar disorder. Mind (in press).
59. Victor BS, Link NA, Binder RL, et al. Use of clonazepam in mania and schizoaffective disorders. Am J Psychiatry 1984; 141:1111-2.

60. Freinhar JD, Alvarez WA. Clonazepam: a novel therapeutic adjunct. Int J Psychiatry Med 1986; 15:321-8.
61. Zetin M, Freedman MJ. Clonazepam in bipolar affective disorder (letter). Am J Psychiatry 1986; 143:1055.
62. Post RM, Uhde TW, Roy-Byrne PP, et al. Correlates of antimanic response to carbamazepine. Psychiatry Res 1987; 21:71-83.
63. Dreifuss FE, Santilli N, Langer DH, et al. Valproic acid hepatic fatalities: a retrospective review. Neurology 1987; 37:379-85.
64. Kukopulos A, Reginaldi D, Laddomada P, et al. Course of the manic-depressive cycle and changes caused by treatments. Pharmacopsychiatry 1980; 13:256-7.
65. Berrettini WH, Post RM. GABA in affective illness. In: Post RM, Ballenger JC eds. Neurobiology of mood disorders. Baltimore: Williams & Wilkins, 1984:673-85.
66. Lloyd KG, Morselli PL. Psychopharmacology of GABAergic drugs. In: Meltzer H, ed. Psychopharmacology: the third generation of progress. New York: Raven Press, 1987:183-95.
67. Post RM. Mechanism of action of carbamazepine and related anticonvulsants in affective illness. In: Meltzer H, ed. Psychopharmacology: the third generation of progress. New York: Raven Press 1987:567-76.
68. Sherman AD, Petty I. Neurochemical basis of the action of antidepressants on learned helplessness. Behav Neurol Biol 1980; 30:119-34.
69. Maggi A, Enna SJ. Regional alterations in rat brain neurotransmitter systems following chronic lithium treatment. J Neurochem 1980; 34:888-92.
70. Bernasconi R, Martin P. Effects of antiepileptic drugs on GABA turnover rate. Arch Pharmacol 1979; 307:251.
71. Green AR, Peralta E, Hong JS, et al. Alterations in GABA metabolism and met-enkephalin content in rat brain following repeated electroconvulsive shocks. J Neurochem 1978; 31:607-18.
72. Berrettini WH, Nurnberger JI, Hare TA, et al. Reduced plasma and CSF GABA in affective illness: effect of lithium carbonate. Biol Psychiatry 1983; 19:185-94.
73. Schildkraut JJ. Current status of the catecholamine hypothesis of affective disorder. In: Lipton MA, DiMascio A, Killam K, eds. Psychopharmacology: a generation of progress. New York: Raven Press, 1978:1223-34.
74. Post RM, Stoddard FJ, Gillin JC, et al. Alterations in motor activity, sleep, and biochemistry in a cycling manic-depressive patient. Arch Gen Psychiatry 1977; 34:470-7.
75. Ostrow D, Halaris A, Dyskeu M, et al. State dependence of noradrenergic activity in a rapid-cycling bipolar patient. J Clin Psychiatry 1984; 45:306-9.
76. Bunney WE, Wehr TA, Gillin JC, et al. The switch process in manic-depressive psychosis. Ann Intern Med 1977; 87:319-35.
77. Kripke DF. Does a weak REM-nonREM oscillator cause depression? In: Post RM, Ballenger JC, eds. Neurobiology of mood disorders. Baltimore: Williams & Wilkins, 1984:227-33.
78. Borsook D, Richardson GS, Moore-Ede MC, et al. GABA and circadian time-keeping: implications for manic-depression and sleep disorders. Med Hypoth 1986; 19:185-98.
79. Wehr TA, Goodwin FK. Desynchronization of circadian rhythms as a possible source of manic-depressive cycles. Psychopharmacol Bull 1980; 16:19-20.
80. Moore-Ede MC. The circadian timing system in animals: two pacemakers preside over many secondary oscillators. Fed Proc 1983; 43:2802-8.
81. Brennan MJW, Sandyk R, Borsook D. Sodium valproate in the management of affective disorders. Basic and clinical aspects. In: Emrich HM, Okuma T, Müller A, eds. Anticonvulsants in affective disorders. Amsterdam: Excerpta Medica, 1984:56-65.

CHAPTER 8

Anticonvulsants and Personality Disorders

David L. Gardner, M.D. *Rex William Cowdry, M.D.*
Bethesda, Maryland

INTRODUCTION

Personality disorders encompass a vast array of psychopathology and pose a conceptual paradox. On the one hand, they are characterized by enduring traits, deeply rooted in the developmental life of the organism and in its interaction with the environment. Thus, personality disorders are associated with specific enduring ego structures, defensive maneuvers, cognitive styles, and superego deficits. On the other hand, many personality disorders are particularly noteworthy for their dramatic and rapid state changes, commonly in response to events. Indeed, the state changes in some personality disorders are more frequent and in some sense more dramatic and "discontinuous" than state changes associated with classical DSM-III-R Axis I disorders such as major depression.[1] For personality disorders such as borderline personality, one of the most stable and enduring traits is the predisposition to rapidly changing states, captured in the phrase "stable instability".

The traditional approach to conceptualizing personality disorders has emphasized disturbances in the psychological development of the child and has regarded the rapidly shifting panoply of symptoms as a manifestation of the primary disturbance of ego structure and function. We believe that the development of theories of personality disorders may be advanced by inverting the traditional causal assumptions—that is, by assuming that affective lability and behavioral dyscontrol are primary components of labile personality disorders and that the enduring "traits", such as rigid cognitive and defensive styles and maladaptive interpersonal relations, represent secondary adaptations to an inner experience characterized by instability.

Whatever its validity, this approach has heuristic advantages. Emphasizing fundamental phenomenology may serve to highlight neglected features of the disorder, to facilitate comparisons with other psychiatric disorders, to identify possible biological underpinnings of these disorders, and to provide targets for symptom relief through pharmacotherapy. This approach may also have a therapeutic advantage, in that it may help diminish the propensity of many patients with personality disorders either to assign blame to significant others or alternately to view the self as "bad". Emphasizing possible biological underpinnings may help shift the focus from blame to understanding and from omnipotence or victimization to coping with a predisposition.

We believe that borderline personality is a paradigmatic disorder for this approach. In this chapter, we propose to trace the features of borderline personality disorder which suggest that anticonvulsants may have therapeutic effects, to review the literature supporting this proposition, and to review briefly the implications of this work for the developing psychobiology of borderline personality disorder.

BORDERLINE PERSONALITY DISORDER

One of the most striking aspects of the borderline syndrome is the complexity of its symptomatology. Profound disturbances are seen in most realms of feeling and behavior. These disturbances tend to be episodic and paroxysmal in nature, and the periods of emotional upheaval are often interspersed with periods of adequate functioning and productivity, suggesting that one of the primary difficulties in this disorder is dysregulation of mood and behavior, particularly under stressful conditions. The diagnostic criteria of DSM-III-R for borderline personality disorder, outlined in Table 1, encompass three main areas of dysfunction: affective dysregulation, behavioral dysregulation, and impaired ego function and object relatedness.

TABLE 1. DSM-III-R criteria for borderline personality disorder (see reference 1)

1. A pattern of unstable and intense interpersonal relationships characterized by alternating between extremes of overidealization and devaluation
2. Impulsiveness in at least two areas that are potentially self-damaging, e.g., spending, sex, substance use, shoplifting, reckless driving, binge eating
3. Affective instability: marked shifts from baseline mood to depression, irritability, or anxiety, usually lasting a few hours and only rarely more than a few days
4. Inappropriate, intense anger or lack of control of anger, e.g., frequent displays of temper, constant anger, recurrent physical fights
5. Recurrent suicidal threats, gestures, or behavior, or self-mutilating behavior
6. Marked and persistent identity disturbance manifested by uncertainty about at least two of the following: self-image, sexual orientation, long-term goals or career choice, type of friends desired, preferred values
7. Chronic feelings of emptiness or boredom
8. Frantic efforts to avoid real or imagined abandonment

Individuals with borderline personality have a rather distinctive and atypical affective disorder, characterized by intense negative mood states of relatively rapid onset and brief duration. In many instances, these mood states can best be characterized not as discrete depressive episodes but rather as dysphorias, rapidly escalating primitive states of affective arousal that involve a mixture of depression, anxiety, rage, and despair. These states are often triggered by real or imagined loss or rejection and are commonly associated with psychological and behavioral regression. The episodic negative mood states may also take the form of rage episodes, again commonly environmentally triggered, with rapid onset and brief duration. In addition to these dysphoric and rageful states, some borderline patients experience activated states during which they may appear hypomanic, and Akiskal has hypothesized that these patients have a cyclothymic or bipolar II disorder.[2]

This problem with episodic dyscontrol of affect is mirrored by a similar problem with episodic behavioral dyscontrol. While some episodes of self-injury and apparent suicide attempts may be planned in advance, such dyscontrol behaviors are more frequently impulsive responses to an overwhelming negative feeling state and represent frantic efforts to terminate dysphoria.[3] Indeed, one of the fundamental problems that these individuals face is learning to bind their dysphoric inner states with cognitive mechanisms, so that feelings do not erupt as uncontrolled self-destructive behavior.

Moreover, borderline individuals show a marked disturbance of ego function and object relatedness. Their internal experience is that of ego discontinuity. They have marked difficulty identifying a consistent "self" and frequently experience themselves (and others) as alternating between "good self" and "bad self". To defend against negative affects and impulses, these individuals frequently utilize projection, projective identification, and splitting, which are primitive defenses indicative of their markedly impaired ego function. In the realm of object relations, these individuals often have a profound "object hunger", which may lead either to intense, tumultuous, and ultimately disappointing relationships or to a protective withdrawal from other people.

It is almost axiomatic to suggest that biological mechanisms underlie some of the symptoms of borderline personality disorder, particularly the episodic symptoms, and that pharmacotherapy may be a useful adjunct in the overall treatment of the disorder. The rationale for the use of anticonvulsants in particular may be based on the identification of comorbid states or critical target symptoms that have been shown to be responsive to anticonvulsants in other studies. The patterns of clinical response to anticonvulsants can in turn further our understanding of the biological underpinnings of this disorder.

COMORBID STATES WHICH MAY RESPOND TO ANTICONVULSANTS

The most frequently identified comorbid state in patients with borderline personality is major affective disorder. Numerous small studies have demonstrated the occurrence of major depressive episodes in 40% to 75% of persons with borderline personality disorder.[4-11] Likewise, several investigators report an increased incidence of unipolar affective disorder in relatives of borderline patients compared with normal and psychiatric control groups.[4,12-14] The nature of affective symptoms has also led Akiskal to suggest that the labile mood seen in the syndrome is a variant of bipolar disorder and to classify many borderline patients as having "subaffective disorders".[2] These phenomenological links to affective illness are strengthened by reports of biological abnormalities in borderline personality disorder similar to those observed in major depression. These include abnormal dexamethasone suppression tests,[5,6,10] abnormal TSH response to TRH infusions,[15,16] and abnormal rapid eye movement latencies on sleep electroencephalograms (EEG's).[17-20] These findings suggest that antidepressants such as the tricyclics and the monoamine oxidase inhibitors may be efficacious for a number of borderline patients who are experiencing a steady autonomous depression. Although a retrospective chart review by Pope and colleagues[4] suggests beneficial results from antidepressants in patients with coexisting major depression, it is noteworthy that the only controlled studies did not find a significant association between current[21] or past[22] major depressive episodes and responsivity to antidepressant medications. Thus the degree of interrelatedness between primary affective disorder and the symptomatology of borderline personality disorder, and the implications of the interrelatedness for choice of pharmacologic agents remain uncertain.

A growing body of controlled and uncontrolled trials has shown that anticonvulsants such as carbamazepine and valproate are effective in treating episodes of major affective disorder. Carbamazepine has been shown to be effective in the treatment of acute mania[23-25] and in the prophylaxis of bipolar disorder, particularly in lithium-resistant cases.[26] The drug appears to have a lesser degree of efficacy in the treatment of acute depressive episodes.[26] Clinical response to carbamazepine in mania appears to be associated with severity of mania, dysphoria, and rapid cycling[26] (and see Chapter

1 in this volume). Similarly valproate has been reported to be effective in mania, schizoaffective disorder, and prophylaxis of bipolar disorder[27] (and see Chapter 2 in this volume). Thus, anticonvulsants appear to exhibit both mood-normalizing and mood-stabilizing activity. These anticonvulsants might therefore have a role in treating the prominent affective components of borderline personality disorder, either by relieving the depressive state per se or by reducing the dysregulation of mood and affect.

Neurological disorders represent another group of conditions that may display comorbidity with borderline personality disorder. This association has been reported by Andrulonis, who studied a group of inpatient adolescents at the Institute of Living.[14,28] He reported that 38% of this sample had a history of organicity, with 11% of the patients reporting a history of brain trauma, encephalitis, or epilepsy, and 27% reporting a history of minimal brain dysfunction or learning disability. This latter group was predominantly composed of males (53% of the males had histories suggestive of organicity versus 13.5% of the females). He also reported that a history of organicity was more likely to be associated with occurrences of acting-out behavior (including behavioral dyscontrol). While the majority of adult borderline patients do not have definite neurological disorders and lack evidence of clear-cut abnormalities on brain computed tomography scans (Lucas PB, Gardner DL, Cowdry RW, et al., manuscript in preparation) and electroencephalograms,[29] there may be an increased prevalence of nonspecific, nonlocalizing neurological "soft signs"[30] or nonspecific, nonlocalizing EEG abnormalities[31] in patients with borderline personality disorder.

Beyond these nonspecific indicators of subtle neurological dysfunction, more overt syndromes such as complex partial seizures may present as comorbid disorders with borderline personality disorder. The two disorders can be difficult to distinguish diagnostically because of the similarity of many of the presenting symptoms (mood lability, rage episodes, psychosensory phenomena). In our clinical experience, when individuals with coexisting clear-cut complex partial seizures and borderline personality are treated with and respond to carbamazepine, improvement occurs in the marked mood and behavioral disturbances. In addition, the stabilized patients do not exhibit the prominent character disturbances of emptiness, fear of abandonment, and identity disturbance, which are characteristic of patients with classical "uncomplicated" borderline personality disorder. Thus, the array of symptoms characteristic of borderline personality disorder may arise from diverse causes. Moreover, the character pathology, usually thought to be an entrenched trait relatively unresponsive to pharmacologic intervention, in some instances is found to be a secondary state phenomenon which remits with treatment of the predisposing primary condition.

IDENTIFICATION OF TARGET SYMPTOMS

Comorbidity alone may not provide an adequate rationale for initiating pharmacotherapy with anticonvulsants. The identification of critical target symptoms thought to respond to anticonvulsants may help provide an additional rationale for this approach to treatment.

Mood lability is perhaps the fundamental feature of affective disturbance in borderline personality disorder. The day-to-day and even hour-to-hour variability of mood can be quite striking. As noted in the discussion of comorbidity, mood swings which are autonomous and without precipitants may reflect comorbid bipolar II disorder or "emotionally unstable character disorder (EUCD)".[32] However, it is the environmentally triggered dysphoric reactions that are the hallmark of the borderline patient's affective instability. Such dysphoric mood states (described as rejection-sensitive dysphoria by Liebowitz and Klein[33]) are distinctly different from the autonomous steady depression observed in major affective disorder and from the frequently unprecipitated mood shifts observed in bipolar II disorder or EUCD. Given the efficacy of the mood-stabilizing agents lithium and carbamazepine in protecting against relatively autonomous mood shifts, the efficacy of these drugs in protecting against mood lability associated with precipitants certainly warrants further investigation.

Both the dysphorias and the rage episodes experienced by borderline patients are described as precipitated and rapidly escalating "uncontrollable" mood states. Like the dysphoria, the rage may be terminated by self-destructive behavior or outwardly directed violence. Such dramatic shifts in mood states have been characterized as "paroxysmal" or "epileptoid", leading to the suggestion that anticonvulsants such as carbamazepine may modulate both the frequency and intensity of the dysphoria and rage.

Perceptual and cognitive disturbances characteristic of borderline personality disorder also suggest a possible role for anticonvulsant medication. These symptoms may include a variety of dissociative experiences such as depersonalization, derealization, out-of-body experiences, or brief lapses of awareness. Although these symptoms may merely represent extensions of the patient's hysterical cognitive style, they also closely resemble symptoms described by patients with complex partial seizures. Post and colleagues have reported, however, that when compared to normal and medical controls, these symptoms are also encountered with increased frequency in other psychiatric disorders, such as major affective disorder and panic disorder.[34,35] Occurrence of these symptoms across several diagnostic groupings suggests that they are unlikely to reflect true ictal events, but may reflect the expression of excitable limbic structures in these disorders. Extensive speculation about the significance of these episodic psychosensory symptoms vis-a-vis etiology or even response to anticonvulsant medication in borderline personality disorder would be premature, particularly since the occurrence of these symptoms did not predict response to carbamazepine in affectively ill patients.[26] Nonetheless, the existence of psychosensory symptoms in both epileptic and borderline individuals provides a further rationale for trials of anticonvulsants in borderline personality disorder.

A long-standing controversy exists over whether distinctive interictal personality characteristics are seen in patients with temporal lobe epilepsy. Recent work by Bear and Fedio suggests that patients with temporal lobe epilepsy manifest heightened emotional responses—anger, sadness, dependence—and in some, a tendency to view themselves in severely harsh terms.[36] Bear and Fedio also reported an increased incidence of psychiatric disorders (including affective and thought disorders), suicide attempts, and violent crimes in patients with temporal lobe foci when compared to neurological and normal controls.[36] Other authors, however, dispute the existence of interictal traits associated with temporal lobe epilepsy. Given the contradictory data with regard to temporal lobe epilepsy, the parallels between Bear and Fedio's observations and characteristics of borderline personality disorder can provide only slight support for anticonvulsant treatment of borderline personality disorder. Nonetheless, they are mentioned because of their possible significance in linking limbic excitability to specific behavioral traits. Similarities can also be drawn between the behavioral dyscontrol of borderline personality disorder and the behavioral dyscontrol described by Monroe in his work on "episodic dyscontrol".[37] In his descriptions of the episodic dyscontrol syndrome, Monroe links rage and aggressive outbursts to limbic system "epileptoid" activity and reports responsivity to anticonvulsant medication.[37]

Behavioral dyscontrol in borderline personality disorder takes the form of both impulsive, poorly thought out actions and planned self-injury. Much of the behavioral dyscontrol occurs in conjunction with mounting dysphoria and represents an attempt to relieve inner tension and turmoil through action rather than thought. The most striking and puzzling example of this behavior is the self-mutilation used to terminate dysphoric feelings. Borderline patients commonly report that they can effectively stop the progression of dysphoria by cutting themselves with a razor or burning themselves with a cigarette.[3] Many of these patients report that they do not experience physical pain when performing these acts, but instead experience relief of the inner tension.

Interventions with pharmacological agents to decrease self-injury can be based on either (1) an improvement in mood or (2) an increase in impulse inhibition. The first assumes that treating the atypical depression will lessen the intensity of inner turmoil and the need to terminate or attenuate these feelings through self-destructive acts, i.e. the reduction in behavioral dyscontrol is secondary to the primary effects of improvement in mood. The second assumes that some classes of medications have a direct effect on the behavioral dyscontrol itself, raising arousal thresholds and reducing the likelihood of acting on impulses. Research assessing the efficacy of pharmacological intervention in inhibiting anger and behavioral dyscontrol has been limited in its scope and of necessity tentative in its conclusions. Studies to date have focused on the effects of medication on these symptoms in other disorders. Trials of phenytoin in neurotic outpatients,[38] carbamazepine in violent nonepileptic schizophrenics[39] and in patients with uncontrolled rage outbursts,[40] propranolol in patients with violent or self-injurious behavior associated with acute[41] and chronic[42] brain syndromes, and lithium in aggressive patients with character disorders[43,44] all suggest that pharmacologic agents may have beneficial effects in aggression and impulsivity, but the pharmacological actions which these drugs have in common are not readily apparent.

ANTICONVULSANTS IN BORDERLINE PERSONALITY DISORDER: THE NIMH STUDY

The identification of several common comorbid states and the multiplicity of possible target symptoms suggest an array of possible pharmacological interventions in borderline personality disorder. In clinical practice, most severely ill borderline patients receive trials of several medications in the course of their treatment, most commonly low-dose neuroleptics, antidepressants, and anxiolytics. Unfortunately, there are limited data from controlled trials of medication in borderline personality to guide these empirical clinical efforts, and the issue of long-term treatment with medication has not been rigorously studied.

The specific use of anticonvulsants in any of the personality disorders has received limited attention from psychiatric researchers, and only carbamazepine has been studied in a controlled trial. We included carbamazepine with tranylcypromine, alprazolam, and trifluoperazine in a placebo-controlled double-blind crossover study of medication effects in patients with borderline personality disorder at the National Institute of Mental Health.[22] Sixteen female outpatients participated in the study. We elected to study only females in order to control for the confounding effects of sex on biological studies. All met at least five of eight DSM-III criteria[45] for borderline personality, had a score of at least seven out of 10 on Gunderson's Diagnostic Interview for Borderlines (DIB),[46] had histories of extensive behavioral dyscontrol (including self-mutilation, multiple overdoses, or physical violence), and met Klein and Liebowitz's criteria for hysteroid (rejection-sensitive) dysphoria.[33] In addition, all had a duration of illness of at least two years since age 18 and did not have a current DSM-III diagnosis of schizophrenia, major affective disorder, alcohol abuse, or substance abuse, although many had received one or more of these diagnoses in the past. In particular, 50% of the patients had experienced major affective disorder in the past. The family histories were noteworthy for a high incidence of affective disorder, alcohol abuse, and physical violence.

After an initial evaluation, which included a complete physical and neurological examination, an EEG, a computed tomography (CT) scan of the cerebrum, psychological testing, a dexamethasone suppression test, and an EEG study of the effects of intravenous procaine hydrochloride (described later in this chapter), patients entered into a series of six-week-long medication trials. A full medication trial was composed of a two-week dosage adjustment period and four weeks of constant dosage, followed by a week of tapering the medication and at least a week off all medication before beginning the next trial. Assessment of medication effects focused on change from baseline in ratings of depression, anxiety, anger, loneliness, feelings of rejection, sense of unreality, and euphoria (mood states commonly experienced by borderline patients during the course of a week) and occurrences of episodes of dyscontrol. These episodes were classified as "mild" (e.g. angry outbursts, suicide threats), "moderate" (e.g. throwing an object, physical assault without intention of causing injury, head banging), or "serious" (e.g. overdoses, wrist or neck cutting, assaults with potential injury). Ratings were completed by both patients and blinded physicians.

The average final daily dosage of each medication was: alprazolam 4.7 mg, carbamazepine 820 mg, trifluoperazine 7.8 mg, and tranylcypromine 40 mg. Completion rates of the individual trials, in general, were low. Only carbamazepine and tranylcypromine had completion rates above 50%. Carbamazepine had the lowest incidence of early termination due to clinical worsening (6%) and tranylcypromine the second lowest (8%); both rates were significantly lower than that on placebo (54%). Side effects of medications were evenly distributed across all five agents, and no medication produced a statistically significant increase in physical symptoms over that seen with placebo. Six patients on carbamazpine developed allergic manifestations ranging from a pruritic rash to hives. Three of these reactions necessitated early termination of the trial. There were no cases of leukopenia (defined as white blood count less than 3,500 cells per ml) during the carbamazepine trials.

The diversity of responses to the various medications was striking. Each of the active medications was rated as the best medication in at least one patient. Nonetheless, several important patterns emerged from the comparison of placebo and carbamazepine trials. First, there was no evidence of a significant placebo effect on mood or behavioral dyscontrol when comparing placebo trials with the baseline period prior to beginning the medication trials. Second, during the carbamazepine trials, clear discrepancies emerged between the blind patient ratings and the blind physician ratings. The physicians rated statistically significant improvement on all but one measure of mood (global mood, depression, anxiety, anger, sensitivity to rejection, and euphoria, but not capacity for pleasure). On the other hand, patients rated only anxiety as significantly improved (Figure 1).

Similarly, physicians rated impulsivity and suicidality as significantly improved during the carbamazepine trials, but patients did not report this improvement. Finally, when looking at actual occurrences of behavioral dyscontrol, carbamazepine was the

FIGURE 1. Physician and patient ratings for placebo and carbamazepine trials (adapted from reference 22)

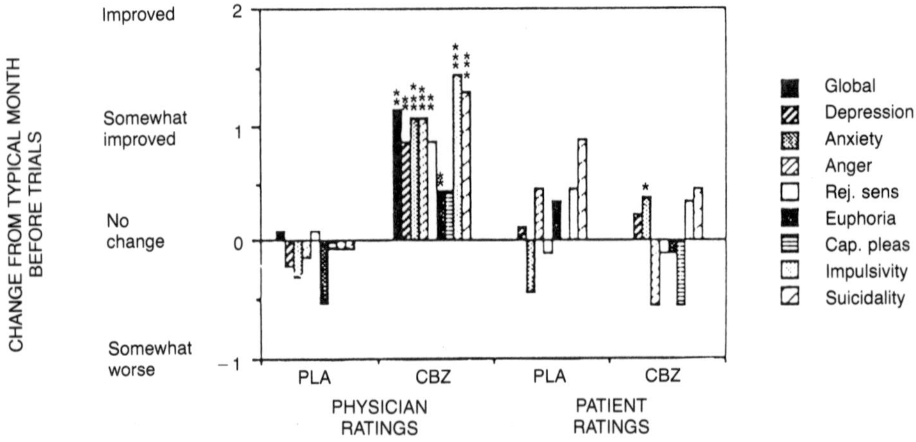

* Asterisks indicate significant improvement compared with placebo by Mann Whitney Test

*p<.05 **p<.01 ***p<.002

only active medication which showed dramatic and statistically significant improvement in the severity of behavioral dyscontrol when compared with placebo ($p = .0008$ by Mann-Whitney U test, one-tailed) (Table 2). There were no occurrences of serious dyscontrol and only one occurrence of moderate dyscontrol during the carbamazepine trials.

TABLE 2. Overall severity of behavioral dyscontrol during placebo versus carbamazepine trials (adapted from reference 22)

Severity of behavioral dyscontrol	Number of episodes of behavioral dyscontrol	
	Placebo	Carbamazepine
Severe	2	0
Moderate	6	1
Mild	5	9
None	0	5

Difference significant at $p = .0008$ by Mann-Whitney U test, one-tailed.

The results of the other trials showed that tranylcypromine produced the most consistent improvement in mood ratings by both patients and physicians, with particularly noteworthy improvement in depression, anxiety, and sensitivity to rejection. Physicians rated significant improvement in impulsivity and suicidality during the tranylcypromine trial, but patients' ratings showed only a nonsignificant trend towards decreased impulsivity and suicidality. Behavioral dyscontrol also showed a nonsignificant trend towards less severity.

Trifluoperazine produced significant improvement in anxiety on physician ratings. Patient ratings were variable but significant improvement was rated for depression, anxiety, and sensitivity to rejection for those who were able to tolerate a trial of three weeks or longer. Physicians rated significant improvement in suicidality during this trial, and there was a trend towards less severe behavioral dyscontrol.

Alprazolam trials produced only trends towards improvement in anxiety, reflected in both physician and patient ratings. The striking finding during this trial was that both physicians and patients rated significant worsening of suicidality. The incidence of "serious" dyscontrol episodes increased significantly on alprazolam, although the distribution of dyscontrol severity was not significantly different from placebo because of the high number of "moderate" dyscontrol episodes during placebo and the presence of two individuals who showed no behavioral dyscontrol on alprazolam.

At the end of each trial, physicians and patients were asked to make recommendations about possible continuation of the medication. The physicians were significantly more likely to recommend continuation of or return to carbamazepine and tranylcypromine compared to placebo. The patients did not show a significant preference for one agent above another, although individual patients had individual preferences.

Clearly, the two medications which demonstrated the most effectiveness in this study were carbamazepine and tranylcypromine, but these agents appeared to affect different aspects of the borderline syndrome. The beneficial effects of tranylcypromine were more evident in ratings of improved mood and decreased impulsivity than in actual decreases in behavioral dyscontrol. All mood ratings on tranylcypromine showed statistically and clinically significant improvement, suggesting that the mood response was generalized and not confined to specific symptom dimensions. The nonsignificant reduction in behavioral dyscontrol in these patients, contrasted with the significant decrease in affective symptoms, suggests that the behavioral improvement may have occurred as a secondary effect of the improved mood rather than as a primary effect of the monoamine oxidase inhibitor on impulse control.

Carbamazepine, on the other hand, produced a pattern of improvement qualitatively different from that of tranylcypromine. Even though improvement in mood was rated by physicians, patients did not report feeling significantly improved. In contrast, the severity of actual episodes of behavioral dyscontrol was clearly reduced during the carbamazepine trials. This is consistent with previous reports, emerging from uncontrolled or partially controlled trials of the drug in various other diagnostic groups, which have noted an effect of carbamazepine on impulsive or violent behavior.[39,40,47]

Clinically, we commonly observed a phenomenon best described as "reflective delay". Patients stated that their dysphoric episodes continued to occur, although to a somewhat attenuated degree, and that they still felt the impulses to act to relieve their dysphoric state. However, the patients experienced less urgency to act on the impulses to gain relief from the tension. Indeed, patients frequently reported that carbamazepine afforded them an increased ability to pause, to reconsider the situation and their reactions, to consider options, and to choose alternatives to impulsive self-destructive acts.

One of the puzzling aspects of behavioral dyscontrol, particularly self-mutilation, in borderline personality disorder, is that this behavior is often not viewed by the patients as ego-dystonic. The self-destructive behavior may not be identified as a problem by the patients, presumably because the behavior is so effective in terminating the dysphoria and inner tension that they experience. This observation may help to explain the discrepancy between patient and physician ratings of mood improvement for the carbamazepine trial. The improvement in behavioral dyscontrol was highly valued clinically and therapeutically by the physicians, who might, therefore, have imputed an underlying improvement in mood. However, our clinical involvement with these patients suggests that the mood effects of carbamazepine are not simply a matter of a "halo" effect in physician ratings. Rated mood improvement on carbamazepine seems to be clinically real but qualitatively different from the activating "antidepressant" effects of tranylcypromine, and thus is not as readily recognized or as highly valued by the patients.

IMPLICATIONS FOR UNDERLYING MECHANISMS

The differential effects of carbamazepine on mood and behavioral dyscontrol support a partial independence of the biological mechanisms modulating behavior from those modulating mood. A natural question arising from this observation is whether all anticonvulsants share this effect on behavioral dyscontrol, particularly since different anticonvulsants act through different mechanisms and have different effects on discharges in different central nervous system structures. We might note here that we administered phenytoin in open trials to several patients who could not complete trials of carbamazepine because of allergic reactions and who had shown initial improvement on the drug. None of the patients reported improvement in either their mood or their behavioral dyscontrol during the phenytoin trial, implying that the anticonvulsants may not be interchangeable in their efficacy for treating psychiatric symptoms, and that an understanding of their mechanisms of action, coupled with their differential effects on symptoms, may help elucidate our understanding of these disorders.

Carbamazepine appears to have neurophysiological effects which set it apart from classical cortical anticonvulsants such as phenytoin, since it preferentially reduces the likelihood of dischanges in limbic areas of the brain.[48] This anatomical locus of drug action, along with animal studies implicating the involvement of limbic sites in a variety of aggressive behaviors,[49,50] suggests that low thresholds for activiation of limbic structures (inherited or acquired) may be associated with a predisposition to behavioral dyscontrol.

Identification of biological mechanisms of dysphoria and behavioral dyscontrol in humans is difficult because of the episodic and variable nature of their occurrence. It is unclear whether studies conducted during baseline functioning will illuminate our understanding of underlying mechanisms. To explore the role of limbic system responsivity in psychiatric patients, we have been studying the effects of procaine hydrochloride, a local anesthetic which induces limbic seizures in animals when given in high doses.[51] In lower doses, procaine has been shown to have anticonvulsant properties in some seizure models.[51] We have administered procaine intravenously in increasing bolus doses to patients with borderline personality disorder, patients with major affective disorder, and normal volunteers, while simultaneously recording the EEG.[51] The majority of the borderline patients responded with a marked dysphoric reaction which some said was very similar to their spontaneously occurring dysphoria. The affectively ill patients had mixed responses, with some experiencing euphoria and others dysphoria. The normal volunteers generally had mild mood responses. Psychosensory phenomena and cognitive distortions suggestive of limbic system involvement (e.g. olfactory and gustatory hallucinations, expressive aphasia) were common in all three groups. However, the marked degree of dysphoria experienced by the borderline patients during procaine administration did not predict the degree of clinical response to carbamazepine. Further studies of this limbic system probe, perhaps coupled with cerebral blood flow studies or positron emission tomography, may help identify the mechanism of action of procaine-induced dysphoria.

We are not aware of any other controlled trials of anticonvulsants in patients with borderline personality disorder or other personality disorders. Two patients with borderline personality disorder were included in a retrospective review of psychiatric patients who had received open, uncontrolled trials of valproate[27] (and see Chapter 2 in this volume). Neither patient, including one who had evidence of left temporal lobe and occipital lobe slowing on EEG, showed improvement on this medication. This review reported improvement in 44% of patients (with predominantly major affective disorder and schizoaffective disorder) during valproate treatment. Despite the negative findings in the two borderline patients, further study of valproate in borderline personality disorder is indicated because of the small number of borderline patients treated, the drug's effectiveness in treating affective symptoms in other disorders, and the need to assess improvement in borderline patients on a variety of dimensions. Again, the differential activity of this anticonvulsant and its effect on dimensions of borderline personality disorder may provide further information for understanding this disorder.

Research is needed to examine whether anticonvulsants will prove to be a useful adjunct in the treatment of other personality disorders, particularly those which overlap with borderline personality disorder and the dyscontrol syndromes, such as the "dramatic cluster" of personality disorders (histrionic, narcissistic, antisocial, borderline). Antisocial personality disorder in particular has characteristics in common with borderline personality disorder and may provide another opportunity to study the effects of anticonvulsants in aggressive, labile, and impulsive disorders. It is likely that a number of men with borderline personality disorder end up in the criminal justice system, receiving the diagnosis of antisocial personality disorder, instead of being referred to the mental health system, largely because of their tendency to discharge dysphoric feelings in outwardly directed ways (assault, violence) rather than in self-directed ways (self-injurious behavior).

CONCLUSIONS

In summary, data from the only controlled study of an anticonvulsant, namely carbamazepine, in the treatment of borderline personality disorder suggest significant improvement in impulsivity and behavioral dyscontrol and significant but perhaps subtle effects on mood. This study is consistent with earlier findings of improvement in aggressive and dyscontrol states in response to anticonvulsants in other psychiatric disorders. Thus, carbamazepine (and possibly other anticonvulsants with similar spectra of action) may be of benefit specifically in the treatment of patients with borderline personality disorder, a particularly distressed and dysfunctional group of individuals. Furthermore, these results may have broader implications, suggesting that the mechanisms modulating behavior and impulse may be pharmacologically as well as biologically separable from those regulating mood.

REFERENCES

1. American Psychiatric Association, Task Force on Nomenclature and Statistics. Diagnostic and statistical manual of mental disorders. 3rd ed., revised. Washington, DC: American Psychiatric Association, 1987.
2. Akiskal H. Sub-affective disorders: dysthymic, cyclothymic and bipolar II disorders in the borderline realm. Psychiatr Clin N Am 1981; 4:25-46.
3. Gardner DL, Cowdry RW. Suicidal and parasuicidal behavior in borderline personality disorder. Psychiatr Clin N Am 1985; 8:389-403.
4. Pope HG, Jr, Jonas JM, Hudson JI, et al. Borderline personality disorder: a phenomenologic, family history, treatment response, and long-term follow-up study. Arch Gen Psychiatry 1983; 40:23-30.
5. Soloff PH, Anselm G, Nathan R, et al. Dexamethasone suppression test in patients with borderline personality disorder. Am J Psychiatry 1982; 139:1621-2.
6. Baxter L, Edell W, Gerner R, et al. Dexamethasone suppession test and axis I diagnosis of inpatients with DSM-III borderline personality disorder. J Clin Psychiatry 1984; 45:150-3.

7. Steiner M, Martin S, Wallace JE, et al. Distinguishing subtypes within the borderline realm: a combined psychoneuroendocrine approach. Biol Psychiatry 1984; 19:907-11.
8. Beeber AR, Kline M.D., Pies RW, et al. Dexamethasone suppression test in hospitalized depressed patients with borderline personality disorder. J Nerv Ment Dis 1984; 172:301-3.
9. Torgenson S. Genetic and nosological aspects of schizotypal and borderline personality disorder. Arch Gen Psychiatry 1984; 41:546-54.
10. Carroll BJ, Greden JF. Neuroendocrine evaluation of depression in borderline patients. Psychiatr Clin N Am 1981; 4:89-99.
11. Grunhaus L, Kling D, Greden JF, et al. Depression and panic in patients with borderline personality disorder. Biol Psychiatry 1985; 20:668-92.
12. Loranger AW, Oldham JM, Tulis EH. Familial transmission of borderline personality. Arch Gen Psychiatry 1982; 39:795-802.
13. Stone M. Contemporary shift of the borderline concept from a subschizophrenic to a subaffective disorder. Psychiatr Clin N Am 1979; 2:577-94.
14. Andrulonis PA, Glueck BC, Stroebel CF, et al. Organic brain dysfunction and the borderline syndrome. Psychiatr Clin N Am 1981; 4:47-66.
15. Garbutt JC, Loosen PT, Tipermas A, et al. The TRH test in patients with borderline personality disorder. Psychiatry Res 1983; 9:107-13.
16. Sternbach HA, Fleming J, Extein I, et al. The dexamethasone suppression test and thyrotropin-releasing hormone tests in depressed borderline patients. Psychoneuroendocrinology 1983; 8:459-62.
17. Akiskal H, Rosenthal TL, Haykal RF, et al. Characterlogical depressions: clinical and sleep electroencephalographic findings separating "subaffective dysthymias" from "character-spectrum disorders". Arch Gen Psychiatry 1980; 37:777-83.
18. Bell J, Lycaki H, Jones D, et al. Effect of preexisting borderline personality disorder on clinical and EEG sleep correlates of depression. Psychiatry Res 1983; 9:115-23.
19. McNamara E, Reynolds CF, Soloff PH, et al. EEG sleep evaluation of depression in borderline patients. Am J Psychiatry 1984; 141:182-6.
20. Reynolds CF, Soloff PH, Kupfer DJ, et al. Depression in borderline patients: a prospective EEG sleep study. Psychiatry Res 1985; 14:1-15.
21. Soloff PH, George A, Nathan S, et al. Progress in pharmacotherapy of borderline disorders. Arch Gen Psychiatry 1986; 43:691-7.
22. Cowdry RW, Gardner DL. Pharmacotherapy of borderline personality disorder: alprazolam, carbamazepine, trifluoperazine, and tranylcypromine. Arch Gen Psychiatry 1988; 45:111-9.
23. Ballenger JC, Post RM. Therapeutic effects of carbamazepine in affective illness: a preliminary report. Commun Psychopharmacol 1978; 2:159-78.
24. Ballenger JC, Post RM. Carbamazepine (Tegretol) in manic-depressive illness: a new treatment. Am J Psychiatry 1980; 137:782-90.
25. Okuma T, Inanaga K, Otsuki S, et al. Comparison of the antimanic efficacy of carbamazepine and chlorpromazine: a double-blind study. Psychopharmacology 1979; 66:211-7.
26. Post RM, Uhde TW. Anticonvulsants in non-epileptic psychosis. In: Trimble MR, Bolwig TG, eds. Aspects of epilepsy and psychiatry. New York: John Wiley and Sons Ltd., 1986:177-212.
27. McElroy SL, Keck PE, Jr, Pope HG, Jr. Sodium valproate: its use in primary psychiatric disorders. J Clin Psychopharmacol 1987; 7:16-24.
28. Andrulonis PA, Donnelly J, Glueck BC, et al. Preliminary data on ethosuximide and the episodic dyscontrol syndromes. Am J Psychiatry 1980; 137:1455-6.
29. Snyder S, Pitts WM. Electroencephalography of DSM-III borderline personality disorder. Acta Psychiatr Scand 1984; 69:129-34.
30. Gardner DL, Lucas PB, Cowdry RW. Soft sign neurological abnormalities in borderline personality disorder and normal controls. J Nerv Ment Dis 1987; 175:177-80.
31. Cowdry RW, Pickar D, Davies R. Symptoms and EEG findings in the borderline syndrome. Int J Psychiatry Med 1985-1986; 15:201-11.
32. Rifkin A, Levitan SJ, Galewski J, et al. Emotionally unstable character disorder: a follow-up study. Biol Psychiatry 1972; 4:65-79.

33. Liebowitz MR, Klein DF. Interrelationship of hysteroid dysphoria and borderline personality disorder. Psychiatric Clin N Am 1981; 4:67-87.
34. Silberman EK, Post RM, Nurnberger J, et al. Transient sensory, cognitive and affective phenomena in affective illness: a comparision with complex partial epilepsy. Br J Psychiatry 1985; 146:81-9.
35. Bierer LM, Uhde TW, Boulenger JP, et al. Panic attacks and psychosensory symptoms in patients with affective illness. Abstracts of the Society of Biological Psychiatry annual meeting, 1985.
36. Bear DM, Fedio P. Quantitative analysis of interictal behavior in temporal lobe epilepsy. Arch Neurol 1977; 34:454-67.
37. Monroe RR. Episodic behavior disorder. Cambridge: Harvard University Press, 1970.
38. Stephens J, Shaffer J. A controlled study of the effects of diphenylhydantoin on anxiety, irritability and anger in neurotic outpatients. Psychopharmacologia 1970; 17:169-81.
39. Luchins, DJ. Carbamazepine in violent non-epileptic schizophrenics. Psychopharmacol Bull 1984; 20:569-71.
40. Mattes, JA. Carbamazepine for uncontrolled rage outbursts. Lancet 1984; 2:1164-5.
41. Elliot, FA. Propranolol for the control of belligerent behavior following acute brain damage. Ann Neurol 1977; 1:489-91.
42. Yudofsky S, Williams D, Gorman J. Propranolol in the treatment of rage and violent behavior in patients with chronic brain syndromes. Am J Psychiatry 1981; 138:218-20.
43. Tupin J, Smith D, Clanon T, et al. The long-term use of lithium in aggressive prisoners. Compr Psychiatry 1973; 14:311-7.
44. Sheard M, Marini J, Bridges C, et al. The effect of lithium on impulsive aggressive behavior in man. Am J Psychiatry 1976; 133:1409-13.
45. American Psychiatric Association, Task Force on Nomenclature and Statistics. Diagnostic and statistical manual of mental disorders. 3rd ed. Washington, DC: American Psychiatric Association, 1980.
46. Gunderson J, Kolb J, Austin V. The diagnostic interview for borderline patients. Am J Psychiatry 1981; 138:896-903.
47. Neppe VM. Carbamazepine as adjunctive treatment in non-epileptic chronic inpatients with EEG temporal lobe abnormalities. J Clin Psychiatry 1983; 44:326-31.
48. Kobayashi K, Inverta Y, Mukawa J. Preferential action of Tegretol to limbic seizures. Brain and Nerve 1967; 19:199-205.
49. Koella WP, Levin P, Baltzer V. The pharmacology of carbamazepine and some other anti-epileptic drugs. In: Birkmeyer W, ed. Epileptic seizures-behavior-pain. Baltimore: University Park Press, 1975:32-48.
50. Valzelli L. Psychobiology of aggression and violence. New York: Raven Press, 1981.
51. Kellner CH, Post RM, Putnam F, et al. Intravenous procaine as a probe of limbic system activity in psychiatric patients and normal controls. Biol Psychiatry 1987; 22:1107-26.

CHAPTER 9

The Role of Anticonvulsants in the Treatment of Bulimia

James I. Hudson, M.D. *Harrison G. Pope, Jr., M.D.*
Belmont, Massachusetts

INTRODUCTION

Bulimia, the syndrome of compulsive binge eating, is a common disorder, particularly among young women in Western industrialized countries.[1-4] Although the cause of bulimia is unknown, it has long been theorized that specific biological disturbances may contribute to its etiology.[1,5,6] The response of bulimia to pharmacologic agents, particularly thymoleptic medications (i.e. agents effective in affective disorders), is one line of evidence supporting the hypothesis that primary neurophysiologic abnormalities are present in this disorder.[7]

Although thymoleptics are the medications most often used to treat bulimia, anticonvulsant agents have also been studied in this disorder. However, these studies have been less extensive, and have generally shown less success than those with thymoleptics. This chapter reviews the evidence for the efficacy of anticonvulsants in bulimia and discusses the possible mechanisms of action of these agents in the treatment of bulimic patients.

DEFINITIONS OF BULIMIA

Over the past 15 years, the term "bulimia" has been applied three different ways to describe overlapping but not identical syndromes. It is important to review the evolution of this diagnostic term, since studies of anticonvulsants in the treatment of bulimia have been performed in individuals with bulimia according to different diagnostic criteria, and thus the results of these various investigations may not be totally comparable.

Following Stunkard's description of binge eating in association with obesity in 1959,[8] and until about 1980, bulimia was generally used broadly to refer to individuals of all weight ranges who had frequent eating binges. These individuals may also have been described as "compulsive eaters"[5,9] or "binge eaters".[10]

In 1980, the third edition of the *Diagnostic and Statistical Manual of Mental Disorders*[11] defined bulimia as a syndrome characterized not only by recurrent episodes of binge eating, but also by other features, including awareness that the eating pattern is abnormal, fear of not being able to stop eating voluntarily, and depressed mood and self-deprecating thoughts following eating binges. In addition, at least three of the following five criteria had to be fulfilled: consumption of high-caloric, easily ingested food during a binge; inconspicuous eating during a binge; termination of such eating binges by abdominal pain, sleep, social interruption, or self-induced vomiting; repeated attempts to lose weight by severely restrictive diets, self-induced vomiting, or use of cathartics or diuretics; and frequent weight fluctuations greater than ten pounds due to alternating binges and fasts.

There are three important differences between the *DSM-III* definition and previous conceptions of bulimia: (1) in *DSM-III*, the syndrome was defined by specific operational criteria, rather than the less precise and varying conceptions of compulsive binge eating; (2) the *DSM-III* criteria were more exclusive, or narrow, because of the requirement of many features in addition to eating binges; and (3) whereas earlier conceptions of bulimia had been derived from reports of binge eating in association with the entire range of body weight, the *DSM-III* construct was influenced also by studies of binge eating in association with anorexia nervosa[12,13]—the syndrome of compulsive dieting and weight loss associated with an intense fear of obesity. Although the *DSM-III* criteria for bulimia excluded current anorexia nervosa, the individuals defined by the term "bulimia" had attitudes towards food and weight very similar to those of anorexic patients and, indeed, often had past histories of anorexia nervosa.[14]

The next step in the evolution of the term bulimia came in 1987, with the publication of the revised version of *DSM-III* (*DSM-III-R*).[15] The syndrome was defined even more narrowly, requiring all of the following criteria: (1) recurrent episodes of binge eating (rapid consumption of a large amount of food in a discrete period of time); (2) a feeling of lack of control over eating behavior during the eating binges; (3) regular self-induced vomiting, use of laxatives or diuretics, strict dieting or fasting or vigorous exercise in order to prevent weight gain; (4) a minimum average of two binge eating episodes a week for at least three months; and (5) persistent overconcern with body shape and weight. In addition, the name of the syndrome was changed from "bulimia" to "bulimia nervosa", a term coined by Russell to describe individuals of normal weight who had eating binges and who also exhibited purging behavior, together with attitudes toward food and weight similar to those seen in anorexia nervosa.[16] The changes in *DSM-III-R* produced criteria for bulimia nervosa more consistent with Russell's definition, which had been used since 1979 in the British Commonwealth. The term "bulimia" may now again be used more generally to describe compulsive binge eating without these other features. The deliberations resulting in these changes have been described elsewhere.[17]

In evaluating the studies presented in this chapter, the differences in diagnostic criteria used for bulimia at various points in time must be kept in mind. For example, compared with the *DSM-III* and *DSM-III-R* constructs, the earlier definitions of bulimia, which focused primarily on episodic eating binges and did not require specific psychological attitudes towards food and weight or attempts to prevent weight gain, may have included a larger number of individuals with what would now be called "atypical" eating disorders. Some of these individuals may have had a primary neurologic disorder. Such individuals, in turn, might be expected to respond to anticonvulsant agents better than individuals with "typical" bulimia meeting the narrower *DSM-III* or *DSM-III-R* criteria.

EFFICACY OF ANTICONVULSANT AGENTS IN BULIMIA

Studies have assessed the efficacy of three anticonvulsant agents—phenytoin, carbamazepine, and valproate—in the treatment of bulimia. These investigations are summarized in Table 1.

TABLE 1. Studies of anticonvulsants in the treatment of bulimia

Study	No. of patients	EEG characteristics	Study design	Response
Phenytoin				
Green and Rau[5,18-22]	47	64% abnormal, including 38% with ctenoids	Open[a]	57% good 17% equivocal 26% poor
Weiss and Levitz[23]	1	Mildly abnormal	Open	Poor
Greenway et al.[9]	4	1 mildly abnormal	PC/XO[b]	Drug equal to placebo
Wermuth et al.[24]	19	11% definitely abnormal; 21% questionably abnormal	PC/XO	Drug significantly, but only modestly, superior to placebo
Moore and Rakes[25]	1	Mildly abnormal	Open	Poor
Carbamazepine				
Pope et al.;[26] Hudson et al.[27]	2	1 markedly abnormal; 1 not assessed	Open[c]	1 remission; 1 poor
Kaplan et al.[30,31]	16	Not reported[d]	PC/XO	Drug equal to placebo
Valproate				
Herridge and Pope;[35] McElroy et al.[33,34,36]	3	3 mildly abnormal	Open[c]	3 marked

[a] *Open, uncontrolled trial.*
[b] *Placebo-controlled, double-blind, cross-over.*
[c] *One patient treated concomitantly with lithium.*
[d] *No abnormalities among first 6 subject[30]; EEG data for next 10 subjects not reported.[31]*

Phenytoin

In 1974, Green and Rau reported that nine of 10 patients with compulsive eating binges were successfully treated with phenytoin.[5] Four of the patients were underweight and were also diagnosed as having anorexia nervosa; two were of normal weight; and four were obese. Of particular interest was that nine of the patients exhibited electroencephalographic (EEG) abnormalities: six had 14 Hz and 6 Hz positive spikes, or ctenoids (a controversial pattern discussed later in this chapter in the section on electrophysiologic abnormalities in bulimia); and three displayed other abnormalities.

In the wake of this promising finding, several reports of phenytoin in the treatment of bulimia appeared over the next five years. Green and Rau continued their investigations[18-20] and ultimately expanded their series to 47 patients.[21,22] Of these, 27 (57%) showed a good response, eight (17%) an equivocal response, and 12 (26%) a poor response. Individuals with abnormal EEG's were significantly more likely to respond than those with normal EEG's. The presence of ctenoids, in particular, appeared to account for the differences between the two groups: 16 (89%) of 19 patients with ctenoids responded to phenytoin, compared to 11 (38%) of 29 patients without ctenoids. Of the 12 patients with abnormal EEG's but without ctenoids, only five (42%) responded—a rate similar to the 35% response rate found among patients with normal EEG's.

Although these results are impressive, the interpretation of the findings is limited by several considerations. First, the criteria for compulsive binge eating were broad, as discussed above, and the study may thus have included a heterogeneous group of patients with binge eating of differing etiologies. At the very least, one cannot assume that results obtained from this patient group would be similar to those found in patients meeting the *DSM-III* or *DSM-III-R* criteria for bulimia or bulimia nervosa. Second, the series did not appear to be consecutive; patients with EEG abnormalities may have been more likely to have received phenytoin. Third, the trials were uncontrolled and nonblind, and thus the effect of expectation alone is not taken into account. Fourth, there appears to have been a deterioration of response rate over time: nine (90%) of the first ten patients treated had a marked response to phenytoin, whereas only 18 (49%) of 37 subsequently treated patients achieved such a response.

Other investigators have generally failed to replicate the optimistic findings of Green and Rau. Weiss and Levitz reported a young woman with bulimia and a mildly abnormal EEG who was unsuccessfully treated with phenytoin.[23] Greenway and associates treated four obese bulimic women with phenytoin in a placebo-controlled double-blind crossover design.[9] Only one subject had a mildly abnormal EEG. None of the subjects responded markedly to phenytoin, and there were no significant differences between drug and placebo on any outcome measure.

The only controlled study of phenytoin involving more than four subjects was conducted by Wermuth and colleagues.[24] Prompted by Green and Rau's initial reports, together with their own observation that four of five bulimic patients had abnormal EEG's,[10] these investigators enrolled 20 subjects in a placebo-controlled double-blind crossover study (six weeks in each treatment). The criteria used for bulimia were very similar to those ultimately adopted by *DSM-III*: (1) impulsive, unpredictable, episodic, uncontrolled, and rapid ingestion of large quantities of food over a relatively short period of time; (2) termination of the episode only when a point of physical discomfort has been reached (e.g., abdominal pain and feelings of nausea or distention); self-induced vomiting supported but was not required for the diagnosis; and (3) subsequent feelings of guilt, remorse, or self-contempt.

Although phenytoin proved significantly superior to placebo in this study, the results were modest. Of the 19 subjects who completed the study, only one experienced a remission of bulimia on phenytoin, and only five others had a reduction of more than 75% in the frequency of binge eating episodes. Of the four marked responders followed long-term on phenytoin, two relapsed within two months despite continuing to take the drug. Of note also, in contrast to the reports by Green and Rau and their own pilot data, the authors found only three subjects with definitely abnormal EEG's, and four additional subjects who had "small sharp spikes"—a pattern deemed by the authors to be of questionable significance. However, the presence of ctenoids was not assessed, since the authors considered this pattern to be a normal variant (see discussion later in this chapter). Since the presence of ctenoids—regardless of their significance—was the only EEG pattern significantly associated with positive response in the studies of Green and Rau, it is unfortunate that this pattern was not sought in the study of Wermuth and colleagues.

Since 1979, there have not been any published studies of the use of phenytoin in the treatment of bulimia, with the exception of one case report, which described a young bulimic woman who had ctenoids on her EEG and was successfully treated long-term with phenytoin.[25] It is conceivable that phenytoin was commonly used in the late 1970's and early 1980's to treat bulimia, but that its use did not survive in the "marketplace" of clinical practice because of lackluster performance. Alternatively, it is possible that as attention was drawn more towards individuals meeting the narrower *DSM-III* and *DSM-III-R* definitions of bulimia and bulimia nervosa in the 1980's, other individuals with binge eating more broadly defined—and possibly more likely to respond to anticonvulsants—may not have been studied systematically.

Carbamazepine

Only two groups have reported on the efficacy of carbamazepine in the treatment of bulimia. Pope and colleagues described the results of their experience with carbamazepine in two patients with bulimia by *DSM-III* criteria.[26] One patient failed to respond; not mentioned in this report was that this patient had previously failed trials of imipramine, lithium, imipramine plus lithium, tranylcypromine, and trazodone. Of note, after her unsuccessful trial of carbamazepine, she ultimately achieved a marked response to magnesium pemoline (Pope HG, Jr, Hudson JI, unpublished observations).

The second patient reported by Pope and associates experienced a remission of binge eating on the combination of carbamazepine and lithium. In the course of her history, this patient also had episodes of cyclothymia and anorexia nervosa and was also described in a subsequent report on the efficacy of pharmacotherapy for anorexia nervosa.[27] Interestingly, the combination of carbamazepine and lithium was more effective than either medication alone—an observation which recalls reports of the synergistic action of these medications in the treatment of bipolar disorder.[28,29] Further relevant information on this patient is that her neurologic history and examination were normal, but her brain electrical activity monitoring (BEAM) study, which included visual and spectral analysis of EEG as well as topographic analysis of visual and auditory evoked responses, was markedly abnormal (Pope HG, Jr, Hudson JI, unpublished observations). The EEG showed diffuse background slowing bilaterally and paroxysmal bursts of slow-wave activity bitemporally. Spectral analysis confirmed excessive background slowing, revealing increases of delta and theta activity, more prominent in the right temporal region. Auditory evoked responses showed unusual components in the right frontal and right temporal areas and in the central-parietal areas bilaterally. In follow-up of her course of treatment, the patient was maintained on carbamazepine and lithium, with remission of symptoms of eating and affective disorders for two years. However, she had persistent anemia, which was felt possibly to be caused or exacerbated by the known bone marrow suppressant effects of carbamazepine. For that reason, she was switched from carbamazepine to valproate, while continuing on lithium. She continued in remission of symptoms. Shortly thereafter, lithium was withdrawn and she experienced a rapid relapse of eating and affective symptoms, which were ameliorated promptly by the reintroduction of lithium. Subsequently, she has been in remission of symptoms of eating and affective disorders for two years on valproate and lithium.

The only controlled trials of carbamazepine in the treatment of bulimia have been performed by Kaplan and associates,[30,31] who have reported preliminary data on the first 16 patients to complete a placebo-controlled double-blind crossover study.[30] The first six subjects were treated over 18 weeks in a placebo-carbamazepine-placebo or carbamazepine-placebo-carbamazepine sequence (six weeks for each trial). The 10 subsequent subjects were treated over 12 weeks in a placebo-carbamazepine or carbamazepine-placebo sequence. All patients had bulimia by *DSM-III* criteria and had at least one binge eating episode per week, without an interval of more than three weeks without binge eating during the year prior to study.

The results of this study were modest. One subject, with concomitant cyclothymic disorder, had a remission of bulimic and affective symptoms on carbamazepine. A second subject had a marked improvement of bulimic and affective symptoms on the drug. Three additional subjects improved on carbamazepine compared to baseline, but did not show a difference on drug as compared to placebo. Overall analysis of the response data did not show significant differences between drug and placebo.

In summary, although it is difficult to generalize from the small amount of data addressing the efficacy of carbamazepine in the treatment of bulimia, it tentatively appears that carbamazepine is effective in only a minority of patients with bulimia. However, the positive response reported in two patients with bulimia and concomitant cyclothymia is noteworthy, particularly since carbamazepine has been shown to be an effective treatment for bipolar disorder[32] (see also Chapter 1 in this volume). Thus, a trial of carbamazepine should perhaps be considered in bulimic patients with co-existing cyclothymic or bipolar disorder.

Valproate

Only one group has reported treatment of bulimia with valproate. McElroy and associates identified three patients with bulimia and bipolar disorder in a retrospective evaluation of a cohort of 73 patients with psychiatric disorders treated at McLean Hospital in Belmont, Massachusetts[33,34] (and see Chapter 2 in this volume). Details of one of these patients, with rapid-cycling bipolar disorder, have been published as a case report[35] and subsequently as part of a series of six patients with rapid-cycling bipolar disorder treated with valproate.[36]

All three patients were young women (two were 17 and one 20 years of age) hospitalized at McLean Hospital for treatment of bipolar disorder.[33,34] All had mildly abnormal EEG's. One patient showed generalized slowing, another showed left temporal slowing, and the third patient showed right posterior slowing. One patient had an abnormality on brain computerized tomography (CT), showing dilated temporal horns. All patients were previously unresponsive or only partially responsive to lithium and neuroleptics. Two patients were treated with valproate alone, and one was treated with valproate in combination with lithium. All patients had an excellent clinical response to the trial of valproate, with marked improvement of binge eating and affective symptoms. Of note is that in one case,[35] bulimic and affective symptoms recurred on two occasions when plasma valproate levels fell below 50 μg/ml (a figure generally quoted as the lower limit of the therapeutic range for valproate in the treatment of epilepsy[37]), with prompt remission of symptoms when valproate dosage was increased to bring plasma levels to above 50 μg/ml.

As in the case of carbamazepine, discussed above, it is of interest that valproate (either alone or in combination with lithium) was successful in the treatment of patients with concomitant bulimia and bipolar disorder, particularly since valproate appears to represent an effective treatment for bipolar disorder[33,34] (and see Chapter 2 in this volume). Thus, based on this encouraging preliminary data, a trial of valproate might be considered in bulimic patients with cyclothymic or bipolar disorder.

MECHANISM OF ACTION OF ANTICONVULSANTS IN THE TREATMENT OF BULIMIA

It is clear from the above discussion that anticonvulsants benefit at least some patients with bulimia and that they have been associated with long-term remissions of the syndrome in certain individuals. By what mechanisms do these agents act in the treatment of bulimia? The three major hypotheses that have been proposed are that they work via (1) anticonvulsant effects, implying that bulimia may be related to epilepsy; (2) thymoleptic effects, implying that bulimia may be related to major affective disorder; and (3) independent antibulimic effects, perhaps operating via neurotransmitter systems which regulate appetite and body weight. The evidence in favor of the first two hypotheses will be reviewed. The third hypothesis, although quite tenable, will not be discussed in detail, since it has not been formulated in specific terms. Also, a review of the effects of anticonvulsant agents on neurotransmitter systems and the evidence for disturbances in these systems in bulimia is beyond the scope of this chapter.

Evidence in favor of anticonvulsant effects: relationship of bulimia to seizure disorders

The fact that phenytoin, carbamazepine, and valproate are established as effective in the treatment of seizure disorders, and hence are classified primarily as "anticonvulsants", raises the possibility that these drugs may benefit bulimia via their anticonvulsant effects and that bulimia may be related in some manner to seizure disorders.

A possible relationship between bulimia and seizure disorders is supported by evidence of neurophysiologic abnormalities seen in at least some bulimic patients. Green and Rau, as discussed previously, noted that patients with "compulsive eating binges" often displayed EEG abnormalities.[5] In their summary report of a series of 59 patients (47 of whom received phenytoin, as discussed above), these investigators found that 38 (64%) had abnormal EEG's.[21] Furthermore, the presence of EEG abnormalities, particularly ctenoids, was significantly associated with response to phenytoin. However, several considerations limit interpretation of these data.

As discussed above, not all of these patients with compulsive binge eating would meet *DSM-III* or *DSM-III-R* criteria for bulimia or bulimia nervosa and hence cannot be compared to samples of patients meeting these latter criteria. Second, because of the investigators' interest in neurophysiologic abnormalities, patients may have been referred to them in a selective manner, leading to a higher than expected proportion of abnormal EEG's in their sample. The authors report a 41% rate of EEG abnormalities in unselected psychiatric patients in their own center and quote another study[38] that reports a 40% prevalence of abnormal EEG's in 1000 consecutive adult psychiatric inpatients. Thus, selection bias might account for a fair portion of the modest difference between the 64% rate of abnormal EEG's found by the investigators in their sample of bulimic patients and the expected 40% rate of abnormalities. Third, a large proportion of the 38 subjects with abnormal EEG's were rated as abnormal exclusively because of ctenoids. The authors note that 58% of the patients had ctenoids but do not specify how many of these patients also had other EEG abnormalities. Of importance, it is not clear whether ctenoids represent an abnormal pattern or whether they are a normal variant in adolescents and young adults.[39-41] The authors argue, however, that although ctenoids may be normal variants in adolescence and young adulthood, many of the compulsive binge eaters were older patients in whom ctenoids would not normally be expected. Fourth, the highest rate of EEG abnormalities was observed in the subgroup of patients who were less than 75% of expected body weight, and as discussed below, it is unclear to what extent weight loss alone may cause EEG abnormalities.

Other investigators have not generally found high rates of abnormal EEG's among bulimic patients. Greenway and colleagues found an abnormal EEG in only one of seven obese patients with compulsive eating.[9] Although their pilot study found that four of five bulimic patients had EEG abnormalities,[10] Wermuth and associates[24] found that only three of 20 subsequently evaluated patients had definite abnormalities (see preceding discussion). Three additional patients had a questionably abnormal pattern consisting of small sharp spikes. Furthermore, response to phenytoin in their study was not significantly correlated with the presence of EEG abnormalities.

Three centers have reported EEG findings in patients meeting *DSM-III* criteria for bulimia. Mitchell and associates performed sleep and awake EEG's with nasopharyngeal leads in 25 women outpatients with bulimia by *DSM-III* criteria, all of whom were greater than 75% of ideal body weight.[42] Readings of the recordings were done blind to the patient's diagnosis. Only four (16%) of the EEG's were abnormal. Kaplan noted that, of 38 bulimic patients at his center on whom an EEG was obtained, only three (8%) showed clear abnormalities, with a fourth patient displaying a questionably abnormal pattern.[31]

To look at the prevalence of EEG abnormalities in bulimic patients seen at our center, we reviewed retrospectively the records of all patients hospitalized at McLean Hospital between 1977 and 1987 who met *DSM-III-R* criteria for bulimia nervosa.[43] An age- and sex-matched group of individuals with major depression, who had never been described as having bulimic symptoms, was obtained as a control group. We identified 107 bulimic patients, of whom 41 had an EEG recorded, and 64 depressed patients, of whom 41 had an EEG recorded. Abnormal EEG's were found in 11 (27%) of the bulimic patients and in 15 (37%) of the depressed control patients. These rates are similar to the 41% rate of abnormal EEG's reported by Rau and associates[21] in general psychiatric patients and to the 40% rate reported by Gibbs and Novick[38] in private psychiatric inpatients. It should be noted that the rate of abnormal EEG's found in our patients is probably greater than the true rate in patients with bulimia, since (1) our patients were all hospitalized, and (2) EEG's were only ordered on 38% of these patients; and presumably, an EEG would more likely be ordered on patients suspected of having an abnormality.

In evaluating the overall literature on EEG abnormalities in bulimia, several considerations must be kept in mind. First, mild EEG abnormalities of several different types have been reported. None of these abnormalities is specific for bulimia; all occur in other medical and psychiatric conditions, as well as occasionally in normal individuals.

In addition, it is unclear to what extent the EEG abnormalities seen in bulimic patients may be a consequence of the abnormal eating behavior itself, such as weight loss and purging. Weight loss, in particular, has profound effects on neuroendocrine and metabolic function.[44,45] Patients with anorexia nervosa, who invariably show these neuroendocrine and metabolic abnormalities as well,[44,46] also appear to have somewhat higher rates of EEG abnormalities than normal-weight patients with bulimia. Green and Rau found the highest rates of abnormal EEG's in their low-weight bulimic patients, and similarly high rates of EEG abnormalities in patients with anorexia nervosa, with and without bulimic symptoms, have been reported by other investigators.[47-49] Furthermore, normal-weight patients with bulimia often show evidence of metabolic and neuroendocrine dysfunction similar to that seen in mild starvation, suggesting that due to restricting calories by dieting, these patients may be in a physiologic state of semi-starvation even though they are in the normal weight range by population norms.[44,46,50,51] Thus, it is very likely that abnormal eating behavior itself causes some degree of electrophysiologic disturbance.

Finally, there is a 40% to 50% false negative rate for abnormal EEG's in patients with documented grand mal epilepsy,[52] and presumably this rate would be expected to be even higher when assessing more subtle neurophysiologic dysfunction, especially in the limbic cortex and diencephalon which are far removed from scalp electrodes.

In summary, electrophysiologic abnormalities are present in a sizable proportion of patients with bulimia. However, the significance of this observation is unclear, mainly because similar abnormalities are also commonly present in patients with major affective and other psychiatric disorders as well as in many individuals without psychiatric disorders. Further studies, using more sophisticated neurophysiologic techniques, such as computerized EEG and 24-hour EEG monitoring, or functional brain imaging techniques, such as positron emission tomography, may help resolve this issue. Thus, pending these further investigations, the evidence for a relationship between bulimia and seizure disorders remains equivocal.

Evidence in favor of thymoleptic effects: relationship between bulimia and major affective disorder

Given the equivocal evidence for an increased prevalence of electrophysiologic abnormalities in bulimia, one must consider the possibility that phenytoin, carbamazepine, and valproate may benefit bulimia not via their anticonvulsant effect but via a thymoleptic effect. In favor of the latter possibility are (1) the large body of evidence suggesting a close relationship between bulimia and major affective disorder and (2) the observation that these medications may have thymoleptic properties in addition to their anticonvulsant properties.

Several lines of evidence suggest that bulimia is closely related to major affective disorder (reviewed in detail elsewhere[53]). Phenomenologic studies have found high rates of major affective disorder among patients with bulimia.[53-57] Also, studies of family history have found high rates of major affective disorder in the relatives of patients with bulimia.[53,58-60] Additionally, controlled studies have demonstrated the efficacy of thymoleptic medications from several different classes, including tricyclics,[61-64] monoamine oxidase inhibitors,[65-67] bupropion,[68] and trazodone,[69] in the treatment of bulimia. Over twenty uncontrolled reports have supported further the efficacy of these and other thymoleptic agents in bulimia.[7,70] Conversely, although some agents not traditionally classified as thymoleptics, such as opiate antagonists[71-73] or sympathomimetics and anorexiants,[26,74,75] have been reported effective in the treatment of bulimia, all of these types of agents have been shown to possess thymoleptic properties.[76-79]

In keeping with the latter observation, phenytoin, carbamazepine, and valproate —although generally classified as anticonvulsant agents—all appear to possess thymoleptic properties. Carbamazepine has been shown in controlled studies to be an effective treatment for bipolar disorder[32] and major depression[80] (and see Chapter 1 in this volume). Valproate also appears effective in bipolar disorder, although controlled data are limited[33,34] (and see Chapter 2 in this volume). And phenytoin may possess thymoleptic properties, although studies of this agent in patients meeting modern diagnostic criteria for major affective disorder have not been performed[81-83] (and see Chapter 4 in this volume).

Thus, in view of these considerations, it is possible that anticonvulsant medications benefit bulimia primarily via their thymoleptic properties, or more accurately stated, via the same mechanism by which they benefit major affective disorder. Clearly, however, further testing of this hypothesis must await a more sophisticated understanding of the pathophysiology of both bulimia and major affective disorder and an understanding of the mechanism by which more classical thymoleptic agents act in these conditions.

CONCLUSIONS

1. Anticonvulsant agents appear to benefit only a minority of patients with bulimia. Thus, pending studies demonstrating greater efficacy of these medications, their routine use in bulimic patients would not be advised.

2. Carbamazepine or valproate (alone or in combination with lithium) may be useful treatments in patients with bulimia and concomitant bipolar disorder or cyclo-

thymia. The appropriate doses and blood levels to be maintained appear to be the same as those for treatment of bipolar disorder or cyclothymia (see other appropriate chapters in this volume).

3. The mechanisms by which anticonvulsants benefit bulimia are unknown: anticonvulsants may ameliorate bulimic symptoms as a direct result of their anticonvulsant properties, they may act as a result of their thymoleptic properties, or they may possess independent anti-bulimic properties. The first hypothesis is supported by the established anticonvulsant properties of these agents and evidence of neurophysiologic abnormalities in some patients with bulimia. The second hypothesis is supported by the relatively recent demonstration that these agents have thymoleptic properties, as well as evidence that bulimia and major affective disorder are closely related on a number of indices.

4. Future research on the use of anticonvulsants in the treatment of bulimia should not be confined to patients meeting the narrow *DSM-III* or *DSM-III-R* criteria. Rather, all patients with the symptom of compulsive binge eating should be studied, and comparisons in response to treatment should be made among various types of bulimic patients, for example, those of different weight categories, those with and without certain neurophysiologic abnormalities, and those with and without specific concomitant psychiatric or neurologic disorders. Such a broad strategy may help to identify subgroups for which anticonvulsant therapy is particularly useful.

REFERENCES

1. Pope HG, Jr, Hudson JI. New hope for binge eaters. New York: Harper and Row, 1984.
2. Pope HG, Jr, Hudson JI, Yurgelun-Todd D. Anorexia nervosa and bulimia among 300 suburban women shoppers. Am J Psychiatry 1984; 141:292-4.
3. Szmukler GI. The epidemiology of anorexia nervosa and bulimia. J Psychiatr Res 1985; 19:143-53.
4. Cooper PJ, Charnock DF, Taylor MJ. The prevalence of bulimia nervosa: a replication study. Br J Psychiatry 1987; 151:684-6.
5. Green RS, Rau JH. Treatment of compulsive eating disturbances with anticonvulsant medication. Am J Psychiatry 1974; 131:428-31.
6. Pope HG, Jr, Hudson JI. Is bulimia a heterogenous disorder? Lessons from the history of medicine. Int J Eat Dis 1988; 7:155-66.
7. Pope HG, Jr, Hudson JI. Antidepressant drug therapy of bulimia: current status. J Clin Psychiatry 1986; 47:339-45.
8. Stunkard AJ. Eating patterns and obesity. Psychiatr Q 1959; 33:284-95.
9. Greenway FL, Dahms WT, Bray GA. Phenytoin as a treatment of obesity associated with compulsive eating. Curr Ther Res 1977; 21:338-42.
10. Davis KL, Qualls B, Hollister L, et al. EEGs of "binge" eaters (letter). Am J Psychiatry 1974; 131:1409.
11. American Psychiatric Association, Task Force on Nomenclature and Statistics. Diagnostic and statistical manual of mental disorders. 3rd ed. Washington, DC: American Psychiatric Association, 1980.
12. Garfinkel PE, Moldofsky H, Garner DM. The heterogeneity of anorexia nervosa: bulimia as a distinct subgroup. Arch Gen Psychiatry 1980; 37:1036-40.
13. Casper RC, Eckert ED, Halmi KA, et al. Bulimia: its incidence and clinical importance in patients with anorexia nervosa. Arch Gen Psychiatry 1980; 37:1030-5.
14. Garner DM, Garfinkel PE, O'Shaughnessy M. The validity of the distinction between bulimia with and without anorexia nervosa. Am J Psychiatry 1985; 142:581-7.
15. American Psychiatric Association, Task Force on Nomenclature and Statistics. Diagnostic and statistical manual of mental disorders. 3rd ed., revised. Washington, DC: American Psychiatric Association, 1987.

16. Russell GFM. Bulimia nervosa—an ominous variant of anorexia nervosa. Psychol Med 1979; 9:429-48.
17. Pope HG, Jr, Hudson JI, Spitzer RL, et al. Revisions to the DSM-III criteria for bulimia nervosa. In: Garner DM, Garfinkel PE, eds. Diagnostic issues in anorexia nervosa and bulimia nervosa. New York: Brunner/Mazel (in press).
18. Rau JH, Green RS. Compulsive eating: a neuropsychologic approach to certain eating disorders. Compr Psychiatry 1975; 16:223-31.
19. Green RS, Rau JH. The use of diphenylhydantoin in compulsive eating disorders: further studies. In: Vigersky RA, ed. Anorexia nervosa. New York: Raven Press, 1977:377-82.
20. Rau JH, Green RS. Soft neurological correlates of compulsive eaters. J Nerv Ment Dis 1978; 166:435-7.
21. Rau JH, Struve FA, Green RS. Electroencephalographic correlates of compulsive eating. Clin Electroenceph 1979; 10:180-9.
22. Rau JH, Green RS. Neurological factors affecting binge eating: body over mind. In: Hawkins RC, Fremouw WJ, Clement PF, eds. The binge-purge syndrome: diagnosis, treatment, and research. New York: Springer Verlag, 1984:23-43.
23. Weiss T, Levitz L. Diphenylhydantoin treatment of bulimia (letter). Am J Psychiatry 1976; 133:1093.
24. Wermuth BM, Davis KL, Hollister LE, et al. Phenytoin treatment of the binge-eating syndrome. Am J Psychiatry 1977; 134:1249-53.
25. Moore SL, Rakes SM. Binge eating—therapeutic response to diphenylhydantoin: case report. J Clin Psychiatry 1982; 43:385-6.
26. Pope HG, Jr, Hudson JI, Jonas JM. Antidepressant treatment of bulimia: preliminary experience and practical recommendations. J Clin Psychopharmacol 1983; 3:274-81.
27. Hudson JI, Pope HG, Jr, Jonas JM, et al. Treatment of anorexia nervosa with antidepressants. J Clin Psychopharmacol 1985; 5:17-23.
28. Lipinski JF, Pope HG, Jr. Possible synergistic action between carbamazepine and lithium carbonate in the treatment of three acutely manic patients. Am J Psychiatry 1982; 139:948-9.
29. Keisling R. Carbamazepine and lithium carbonate in the treatment of refractory affective disorders (letter). Arch Gen Psychiatry 1983; 40:223.
30. Kaplan AS, Garfinkel PE, Darby PL, et al. Carbamazepine in the treatment of bulimia. Am J Psychiatry 1983; 140:1225-6.
31. Kaplan AS. Anticonvulsant treatment of eating disorders. In: Garfinkel PE, Garner DM, eds. The role of drug treatments for eating disorders. New York: Brunner/Mazel, 1987:96-123.
32. Ballenger JC, Post RM. Carbamazepine in manic-depressive illness: a new treatment. Am J Psychiatry 1980; 137:782-90.
33. McElroy SL, Keck PE, Jr, Pope HG, Jr. Sodium valproate: its use in primary psychiatric disorders. J Clin Psychopharmacol 1987; 7:16-24.
34. McElroy SL, Keck PE, Jr, Pope HG, Jr, et al. Treatment of psychiatric disorders with valproate: a series of 73 cases. Psychiatr Psychobiol (in press).
35. Herridge PL, Pope HG, Jr. Treatment of bulimia and rapid-cycling bipolar disorder with sodium valproate. J Clin Psychopharmacol 1985; 5:229-30.
36. McElroy SL, Keck PE, Jr, Pope HG, Jr, et al. Valproate in the treatment of rapid-cycling bipolar disorder. J Clin Psychopharmacol (in press).
37. Rimmer E, Richens A. An update on sodium valproate. Pharmacotherapy 1985; 5:171-84.
38. Gibbs FA, Novick RG. Electroencephalographic findings among adult patients in a private psychiatric hospital. Clin Electroenceph 1977; 8:79-88.
39. Lombroso CT, Schwartz IH, Clark DM, et al. Ctenoids in healthy youths: controlled study of 14- and 6-per second positive spiking. Neurology (Minneapolis) 1968; 16:1152-8.
40. Wegner JT, Struve FA. Incidence of the 14- and 6-per second positive spike pattern in an adult clinical population: an empirical note. J Nerv Ment Dis 1977; 164:340-5.
41. Maulsby RL. EEG patterns of uncertain diagnostic significance. In: Klass DW, Daly DD, eds. Current practice of clinical electroencephalography. New York: Raven Press, 1979:411-9.
42. Mitchell JE, Hosfield W, Pyle RL. EEG findings in patients with the bulimia syndrome. Int J Eat Dis 1983; 2(3):17-23.

43. Pope HG, Jr, McElroy SL, Keck PE, Jr, et al. Electrophysiologic abnormalities in bulimia and their implications for pharmacotherapy. Int J Eat Dis (in press).
44. Hudson JI, Hudson MS. Endocrine dysfunction in anorexia nervosa and bulimia: comparision with abnormalities in other psychiatric disorders and disturbances due to metabolic factors. Psychiatr Dev 1984; 4:237-72.
45. Fichter MM, Pirke K-M, Holsboer F. Weight loss causes neuroendocrine disturbances: experimental study in healthy starving subjects. Psychiatry Res 1986; 17:33-9.
46. Pirke K-M, Pahl J, Schweiger, et al. Metabolic and endocrine indices of starvation in bulimia: a comparision with anorexia nervosa. Psychiatry Res 1985; 15:51-72.
47. Crisp AH, Fenton GW, Scotton L. A controlled study of the EEG in anorexia nervosa. Br J Psychiatry 1968; 114:1149-60.
48. Neil JF, Merikangas JR, Foster FG, et al. Waking and all-night sleep EEG's in anorexia nervosa. Clin Electroenceph 1980; 11:9-15.
49. Grebb JA, Yingling CD, Reus VI. Electrophysiologic abnormalities in patients with eating disorders. Compr Psychiatry 1984; 25:215-24.
50. Pirke K-M, Schweiger U, Laessle R, et al. Metabolic and endocrine consequences of eating behavior and food composition in bulimia. In: Hudson JI, Pope HG, Jr, eds. The psychobiology of bulimia. Washington, DC: American Psychiatric Press, 1987:129-43.
51. Pirke K-M, Schweiger U, Fichter MM. Hypothalamic-pituitary-ovarian axis function in bulimia. In: Hudson JI, Pope HG, Jr, eds. The psychobiology of bulimia. Washington, DC: American Psychiatric Press, 1987:13-28.
52. Gibbs FA, Gibbs EL. Atlas of electroencephalography. Vol 3. Neurological and psychiatric disorders. Reading, MA: Addison-Wesley, 1965.
53. Hudson JI, Pope HG, Jr. Depression and eating disorders. In: Cameron OG, ed. Presentations of depression: depression in medical and other psychiatric disorders. New York: John Wiley & Sons, 1987:33-66.
54. Hudson JI, Pope HG, Jr, Jonas JM, et al. Phenomenologic relationship of eating disorders to major affective disorder. Psychiatry Res 1983; 9:345-54.
55. Herzog DB. Are anorexic and bulimic patients depressed? Am J Psychiatry 1984; 141:1594-7.
56. Walsh BT, Roose SP, Glassman AH, et al. Bulimia and depression. Psychosom Med 1985; 47:123-31.
57. Hudson JI, Pope HG, Jr, Yurgelun-Todd D, et al. A controlled study of lifetime prevalence of affective and other psychiatric disorders in bulimic outpatients. Am J Psychiatry 1987; 144: 1283-7.
58. Hudson JI, Pope HG, Jr, Jonas JM, et al. Family history study of anorexia nervosa and bulimia. Br J Psychiatry 1983; 142:133-8.
59. Stern SL, Dixon KN, Nemzer E, et al. Affective disorder in the families of women with normal weight bulimia. Am J Psychiatry 1984; 141:1224-7.
60. Hudson JI, Pope HG, Jr, Jonas JM, et al. A controlled family history study of bulimia. Psychol Med 1987; 17:883-90.
61. Pope HG, Jr, Hudson JI, Jonas JM, et al. Bulimia treated with imipramine: a placebo-controlled, double-blind study. Am J Psychiatry 1983; 140:554-8.
62. Mitchell JE, Groat R. A placebo-controlled, double-blind trial of amitriptyline in bulimia. J Clin Psychopharmacol 1984; 4:186-93.
63. Hughes PL, Wells LA, Cunningham CJ, et al. Treating bulimia with desipramine: a placebo-controlled double-blind study. Arch Gen Psychiatry 1986; 43:182-6.
64. Agras WS, Dorian BG, Kirkley BG, et al. Imipramine in the treatment of bulimia: a double-blind controlled study. Int J Eat Dis 1987; 6:29-38.
65. Walsh BT, Stewart JW, Roose SP, et al. Treatment of bulimia with phenelzine: a double-blind, placebo-controlled study. Arch Gen Psychiatry 1984; 41:1105-9.
66. Walsh BT, Gladis M, Roose SP, et al. A controlled trial of phenelzine in bulimia. Psychopharmacol Bull 1987; 23:49-51.
67. Kennedy SH, Piran N, Garfinkel PE. Isocarboxazid in the treatment of bulimia (letter). Am J Psychiatry 1986; 143:1495-6.

68. Horne RL, Ferguson JM, Pope HG, Jr, et al. Treatment of bulimia with bupropion: a multicenter controlled trial. J Clin Psychiatry (in press).
69. Pope HG, Jr, Keck PE, Jr, McElroy SL, et al. Treatment of bulimia nervosa with trazodone: a placebo-controlled double-blind study. Presented at the Third International Conference on Eating Disorders. New York, April 24, 1988.
70. Hudson JI, Pope HG, Jr. Newer antidepressants in the treatment of bulimia nervosa. Psychopharmacol Bull 1987; 23:52-7.
71. Jonas JM, Gold MS. Naltrexone reverses bulimic symptoms (letter). Lancet 1986; 1:807.
72. Jonas JM, Gold MS. Opiate antagonists as clinical probes in bulimia. In: Hudson JI, Pope HG, Jr, eds. The psychobiology of bulimia. Washington, DC: American Psychiatric Press, 1987:115-27.
73. Mitchell JE, Laine DE, Morley JE, et al. Naloxone but not CCK-8 may attenuate binge-eating behavior in patients with the bulimia syndrome. Biol Psychiatry 1986; 21:1399-406.
74. Ong YL, Checkley SA, Russell GFM. Suppression of bulimia symptoms with methylamphetamine. Br J Psychiatry 1983; 143:288-93.
75. Robinson PH, Checkley SA, Russell GFM. Suppression of eating by fenfluramine in patients with bulimia nervosa. Br J Psychiatry 1985; 146:169-76.
76. Costa E, Garattini S, eds. International symposium on amphetamines and related compounds. New York: Raven Press, 1970.
77. Judd LL, Janowsky DS, Segal DS, et al. Naloxone-induced behavioral and physiological effects in normal and manic subjects. Arch Gen Psychiatry 1980; 37:583-6.
78. Klein DF, Gittelman R, Quitkin F, et al. Diagnosis and drug treatment of psychiatric disorders: adults and children. 2nd ed. Baltimore: Williams and Wilkins, 1980.
79. Lechin F, Van der Dijs B, Gomez F, et al. Distal colon motility as a predictor of antidepressant response to fenfluramine, imipramine, and chlorimipramine. J Affect Dis 1983; 5:27-35.
80. Post RM, Uhde TW, Roy-Byrne PP, et al. Antidepressant effects of carbamazepine. Am J Psychiatry 1986; 143:29-34.
81. Bogoch S, Dreyfus J. The broad range of use of diphenylhydantoin: bibliography and review. Vol I. New York: Dreyfus Medical Foundation, 1970.
82. Stephen JH, Shaffer JW. A controlled replication of the effectiveness of diphenylhydantoin in reducing irritability and anxiety in selected neurotic outpatients. J Clin Pharmacol 1973; 13:351-6.
83. Bogoch S, Dreyfus J. DPH, 1975, a supplement to the broad range of use of diphenylhydantoin: bibliography and review. Vol II. New York: Dreyfus Medical Foundation, 1975.

Chapter 10

Anticonvulsants in Anxiety and Withdrawal Syndromes: Hypotheses for Future Research

Peter P. Roy-Byrne, M.D.
Seattle, Washington

INTRODUCTION

This chapter will explore the possibility that various anticonvulsant medications may have some efficacy in the treatment of certain anxiety states as well as withdrawal syndromes occurring after the discontinuation of sedative-hypnotic drugs and alcohol. These two conditions have been selected and addressed together for several reasons. First, the clinical phenomenology observed in both alcohol/sedative-hypnotic withdrawal and human anxiety states, although variable, is highly similar, with tachycardia, sweating, dizziness, nausea, tremulousness, hypertension, hyperventilation, and nervousness occurring prominently in both conditions. Second, the same drugs (i.e. benzodiazepines and barbiturates) can be used to treat both anxiety and sedative-hypnotic withdrawal, and even alcohol has short-term anxiolytic properties. However, alcohol has actions in multiple brain areas not affected by other sedative-hypnotics, resulting in additional clinical properties that may attenuate or reverse its anxiolytic effects after short periods of time. Third, emerging evidence from basic animal studies now suggests that alcohol[1] as well as barbiturates[2] acts at the GABA benzodiazepine-chloride ionophore macromolecular complex to facilitate GABAergic transmission, and that withdrawal syndromes resulting from discontinuation of these agents may be related to transient loss or reduction of the action of GABA.[3] Additional studies in primates[4] and humans[5] have also demonstrated that administration of novel compounds with structural similarities to the benzodiazepines, but which retard rather than enhance GABAergic neurotransmission, produces robust anxiety in both species. Thus, the GABA benzodiazepine-chloride ionophore macromolecular complex provides a common neurochemical mechanism that might explain both certain forms of anxiety and sedative-hypnotic withdrawal syndromes.

It should be noted, however, that other neuronal systems may also be implicated in both types of syndromes. For example, overactivity of central noradrenergic neurons has been implicated in the pathophysiology of panic anxiety, and attenuation of central noradrenergic neurotransmission with clonidine has been found to reduce both anxiety and the anxiety-like symptoms of opiate withdrawal.[6] Clonidine may also attenuate sedative-hypnotic withdrawal in some patients,[7] although one study disputes this.[8]

CURRENT CONCEPTS OF "ANXIETY"

In the last decade evidence has accumulated validating the existence of two major types of anxiety which were recognized decades, even centuries, earlier by various clinicians.[9] In one type (termed "panic") the anxiety occurs in discrete, often unpredictable, burst-like attacks accompanied by prominent somatic symptoms and, usually, profound terror and feelings of impending doom. In the other (termed "generalized"), anxiety occurs more chronically, at a somewhat lower level of intensity, often with an admixture of somatic and cognitive (i.e. worry and rumination) symptoms. Of note, this clinical-descriptive distinction is now supported by evidence that individuals with these two syndromes have distinctive biological responses[10,11] and family histories.[12] However, many patients have both forms of anxiety, although there seem to be more patients with "pure" panic than with "pure" generalized anxiety. In addition, there is a frequent co-occurrence of depressive syndromes in anxious patients,[13] especially in primary care populations[14] in which patients appear with mixed "anxious-depressive" syndromes that depart considerably from the ideal syndromal definitions offered by *DSM-III-R*.[15] Therefore, several investigators have questioned whether these clinical syndromes should be considered separate diagnoses or disorders.[16] In light of this controversy, we will not review the various diagnoses listed in the *DSM-III-R* section on anxiety disorders but will instead focus on the two forms of anxiety: panic and generalized.

RATIONALE: DO WE NEED MORE ANTI-ANXIETY DRUGS?

A number of reviews have recently suggested that both panic and generalized forms of anxiety are among the most treatment-responsive syndromes in psychiatry. Nonetheless, between 5% and 20% of individuals with these syndromes may fail to respond optimally to conventional treatment.[17] Because the combined yearly prevalence of both types of anxiety may approach 5% in this country of 245 million,[18] even an 8% nonresponse rate could affect as many as a million individuals in the United States alone. In addition, conventional treatments are associated with unacceptable side effects in some individuals. For example, a number of patients suffering from panic anxiety often cannot tolerate either the stimulatory effects of some cyclic antidepressants or the insomnia, weight gain, and dietary restrictions associated with monoamine oxidase (MAO) inhibitors.[17] Also, while benzodiazepines are highly effective and usually well tolerated in patients with both types of anxiety, some problems may preclude their use in certain individuals.[19] These include a coexistent problem with alcohol and/or drug abuse, a "dependent" personality, the need for long-term use (which greatly increases problems with dependence and withdrawal), and side effects of psychomotor and/or cognitive impairment. The latter, although not typically problematic, may be intolerable for individuals in certain jobs requiring fine motor control, rapid psychomotor reaction, or high-level cognitive or computational performance.

Thus, the pragmatic rationale for exploring alternative drug therapies in anxiety disorders is similar to that which prompted initial trials of anticonvulsants in bipolar disorder, i.e. the existence of "treatment-resistant" or "treatment-intolerant" patient subgroups. The analogy is not perfectly apt, however, since the proportion of such patients is probably smaller for anxiety syndromes and the disability associated with these syndromes, although not to be minimized, is usually less severe.

WHICH ANTICONVULSANTS?

This chapter will discuss primarily two anticonvulsants often reported to have psychotropic properties in humans: carbamazepine and valproate. These two drugs are unlike phenytoin and phenobarbital, in that they have been shown in double-blind placebo-controlled studies to be effective in the treatment of major affective disorder.[20,21] There is still controversy as to whether this psychotropic efficacy relates to their ability to suppress amygdala-kindled seizures in animals.[22,23] For example, valproate, although second to carbamazepine in potency in suppressing amygdala-kindled after-discharges, is only slightly more effective in this seizure model than other anticonvulsants.[23] Nonetheless, the kindling model of psychopathology is attractive and can explain the progressive symptomatic deterioration that occurs in certain psychiatric syndromes. Clonazepam, another anticonvulsant demonstrated in controlled studies to be effective in major affective and anxiety disorders, will also be discussed briefly, but as this drug is also a benzodiazepine anxiolytic, it is more difficult to attribute its psychotropic efficacy to its anticonvulsant properties (see Chapter 3 in this volume).

Unfortunately, there is a paucity of controlled data on the efficacy of anticonvulsant drugs in homogeneous populations of patients with anxiety disorders or withdrawal states. Hence, this chapter must rely heavily on information derived from other sources to formulate hypotheses that remain to be empirically investigated. This information will include evidence for anxiolytic properties of these drugs in other populations, the anticonvulsant properties of benzodiazepines, some neuroanatomic similarities between ictal fear and panic attacks, and the known neurochemical effects of carbamazepine and valproate, respectively, as these relate to neural mechanisms of anxiety.

PRELIMINARY EVIDENCE

Anxiolytic effects in other populations

A number of studies and anecdotal reports document reductions in anxiety with the use of carbamazepine in epileptic and affectively ill patient populations. This phenomenon has not been reported for valproate, although its use has been less widespread. While several examples will be cited for carbamazepine, this brief review will not be exhaustive since these studies do not involve the population of interest and serve only to establish one factor needed to build an hypothesis. Furthermore, there is often confusion between effects on anxiety and depression, with studies often reporting effects on "dysphoria", an obvious mixture of depression and anxiety.

Puente reported on the use of carbamazepine in children with "behavioral disorders".[24] Of 47 children with prominent symptoms of anxiety, 34 showed good to excellent response (i.e. reduction of anxiety). Silanepa reviewed the results of two additional studies examining the efficacy of carbamazepine in childhood behavioral disorders.[25] Of 20 symptoms in 66 children, anxiety was the third most affected. Robertson compared the psychotropic effects of carbamazepine with that of other anticonvulsants in an epilepsy clinic.[26] In addition to demonstrating that patients treated with carbamazepine had less severe depression compared with patients treated with other anticonvulsants, the author also found that carbamazepine dose and blood level was inversely correlated with anxiety level as measured by the Spielberger Trait Anxiety Scale. Thus, patients with the highest doses and blood levels were least anxious. Post and Uhde, reviewing their group's studies of the efficacy of carbamazepine in major affective disorder, noted a reduction in ratings of anxiety and agitation that paralleled reductions in depression level.[27] Several patients with severe agitated depression showed robust reductions in agitation and anxiety. In a different population, Klein and colleagues showed that carbamazepine substantially reduced both the anxiety and tension factors on the BPRS ratings of patients with schizoaffective disorder.[28] Again, these findings do not represent an exhaustive list, but serve to highlight the anxiolytic efficacy of carbamazepine when used to treat other disorders in which anxiety may be a prominent symptom.

Controlled studies of valproate in human anxiety disorders have not been performed. However, basic research, which will be reviewed subsequently, suggests that in animal conflict models, anxiolytic effects of valproate occur at *higher* doses than anticonvulsant effects and can paradoxically be antagonized by benzodiazepines.[29] It is possible, therefore, that epileptic patients are receiving too little drug to show anxiolysis or that concurrent use of the sedative-hypnotic anticonvulsant phenobarbital might paradoxically attenuate such effects in the same manner that benzodiazepines do.

Anticonvulsant effects of benzodiazepines

The benzodiazepines are among the most clinically potent anxiolytics available. Although intravenous benzodiazepines such as diazepam and lorazepam are often used for acute control of seizures, oral benzodiazepines are not typically employed as anticonvulsant agents. Exceptions are clonazepam, the most potent benzodiazepine, and clorazepate dipotassium, sometimes used in the treatment of partial complex seizures. These drugs, however, are usually added to existing anticonvulsant regimens rather than used alone. A number of studies have demonstrated a direct correlation between anxiolytic and anticonvulsant potencies and between both of these and receptor binding affinity.[30-32] However, not all anxiolytic drugs are anticonvulsant, nor are all anticonvulsants anxiolytic. (For an excellent review of this see Pellow.[33])

However, if, as Haefely (as cited in reference 33) has proposed, anxiety may in some cases be caused by abnormal activity of neuronal circuits in the limbic system (excessive response to normal inputs as might occur when the septo-hippocampal circuits are overloaded), such a state might be associated with mild epileptiform activity. Thus, benzodiazepines may possibly control anxiety by enhancing recurrent inhibition or decreasing repetitive neuronal activity.

Neuroanatomy of anxiety

There are numerous case reports documenting the occurrence of panic-like episodes secondary to organic lesions or disease in limbic brain areas. For example, Brodsky and colleagues described ten cases in which anxiety was part of a masked epileptiform disorder and responded to conventional anticonvulsants, including phenytoin.[34] Other reports have described panic and fear as clear-cut ictal phenomena, occurring either as a direct manifestation[35] or as part of the prodrome[36] of complex partial seizures. Recently, Weilberg and associates also noted that concurrent epilepsy and panic may or may not be related.[37] In some cases alprazolam is insufficient when given alone and more formal anticonvulsants are required.[37] Moreover, Edlund and colleagues reported on a subgroup of panic disorder patients with "atypical" attacks who displayed electroencephalogram (EEG) abnormalities.[38] These patients had severe derealization and evidence of impulsive behavior following attacks. While all of these studies were able to document EEG abnormalities, there are cases where surface electrodes might not effectively pick up these abnormalities.

These findings have been complimented by the work of Gloor and colleagues, in which neurosurgical patients have undergone stereotaxic stimulation of certain brain areas while awaiting brain surgery.[39] Fear was the most commonly encountered phenomenon and was most specifically associated with stimulation of, or after-discharge spread to hippocampus, amygdala, and parahippocampal gyrus. Although it can be argued that the brains of these individuals are affected with complex partial epilepsy and may not be reflective of the norm, these findings have been reinforced by animal studies in which the anxiolytic effects of benzodiazepines are reproduced by lesions of the septo-hippocampal circuit.[40] These structure-function relationships have been further reinforced by the recent position emission tomography (PET) scan studies of Reiman and colleagues, who found that patients with panic disorder who were vulnerable to panic attacks following infusions of sodium lactate had a characteristic asymmetry in cerebral blood flow and oxygen metabolism in the parahippocampal gyrus.[41] This area contains all of the major input and output of the hippocampus and projects by way of the amgydala to hypothalamus and brainstem areas that affect various hormonal, autonomic, and cardiovascular responses to stress.

BASIC STUDIES OF VALPROATE AND CARBAMAZEPINE: FURTHER CLUES TO POSSIBLE ANXIOLYTIC EFFICACY

Valproate

Evidence that benzodiazepines exert their anxiolytic effects by potentiating GABA neurotransmission, together with studies clarifying the nature of the GABA benzodiazepine-chloride ionophore macromolecular complex (including evidence that these discrete sites mutually influence each other's binding characteristics), has prompted numerous studies in animals, and some in humans, to explore the anxiolytic efficacy of various GABAergic drugs.[42] While the evidence for anti-conflict effects of muscimol, THIP, and progabide is weak and contradictory, valproate stands alone in mirroring the actions of benzodiazepines in a variety of animal models. Valproate reduces the electroshock suppression of reinforced responding in rats[43] as well as the behavioral inhibition induced by novelty.[44] These two models are benzodiazepine-responsive and are frequently used to test for anxiolytic effects. In addition, valproate antagonizes the stimulus properties of pentylenetetrazol,[45] another effect associated with benzodiazepine anxiolytics. Although valproate facilitates GABA transmission and might thus be expected to raise GABA levels, there is no appreciable elevation of forebrain GABA levels at anti-conflict doses.[46] In fact, two studies have demonstrated that picrotoxin, which acts at the chloride channel, blocks the anti-conflict actions of valproate.[44,47] Furthermore, the competitive antagonism demonstrated in the study by Shephard and associates[44] (in which higher doses of valproate overrode the effect of picrotoxin) has been reinforced by another study showing that valproate can actually displace receptor-bound dihydropicrotoxin, which binds to a site on the chloride channel.[48] Thus, it is possible that valproate may work at the chloride ionophore to exert its anxiolytic effect.

Evidence that valproate and the benzodiazepines do not potentiate each other in conflict models, however, seems to contradict their individual anxiolytic actions, both of which are mediated through the same macromolecular complex. There is, in addition, a mutual antagonism on neophobia effects.[49] Finally, RO15-1788, a benzodiazepine antagonist, has been shown to antagonize valproate's anti-conflict effects in a dose-related manner.[47] To explain these anomalous results, Shephard proposed an hypothesis postulating that an "optimal" amount of activity at the benzodiazepine receptor is required for valproate to be maximally effective.[29] This proposition has not been tested, but the apparently discrepant interaction between valproate and benzodiazepines at the GABA benzodiazepine-chloride ionophore macromolecular complex is only one of several paradoxes involving this complex. Resolution of these paradoxes will depend on better elucidation of the nature and function of this complex.

Despite these contradictions, valproate seems to be quite active in animal models of anxiety. According to Shephard,[29] the finding that valproate is as effective as, although of lower potency than, benzodiazepines in animal models stands in contrast to the lower efficacy of serotonergic agents, such as buspirone, which are now known to be effective anxiolytic drugs. Consistent with this presumed efficacy, Petraglia and colleagues have recently shown that valproate is as effective as diazepam in inhibiting the increases in beta-endorphin, beta-lipotropin, and cortisol that are induced by hypoglycemic stress in humans.[50] Because stress-induced endocrine increases have been used as a model to study human anxiety, these findings are intriguing and should prompt further studies with valproate in pathologically anxious patients.

Carbamazepine

Although carbamazepine does not have any effects at the GABA benzodiazepine-chloride ionophore macromolecular complex, it has interesting actions at both central noradrenergic neurons (i.e. locus ceruleus) and the "peripheral" benzodiazepine receptor, which is known also to be present in various brain areas, and may, according to recent reports, be altered in patients with pathologic anxiety as well as in animals withdrawing from ethanol. (For a review of carbamazepine's mechanism of action, including the above issues, see Post.[51])

Carbamazepine decreases stimulus-induced release of norepinephrine in animals[52] and has been found to decrease elevated levels of cerebrospinal fluid norepinephrine in patients with bipolar disorder.[53] Furthermore, carbamazepine's efficacy in blocking amygdala-kindled seizures is partially reversed by the alpha-2 antagonist yohimbine, a drug which augments central norepinephrine release.[51] This finding suggests that a reduction in central norepinephrine activity may be an important mechanism in the limbic anticonvulsant effects of carbamazepine—effects which are also thought to play some possible role in its psychotropic properties. These findings, however, are at odds with the drug's ability to increase locus ceruleus firing, and hence central noradrenergic activity. In contrast, benzodiazepines, tricyclic antidepressants, and clonidine, all of which are effective anxiolytic and antipanic drugs, decrease locus ceruleus firing.[51] Interestingly, this ability to increase locus ceruleus firing is shared by buspirone, an effective drug for generalized anxiety, but not necessarily for panic.

The "peripheral" benzodiazepine receptor site was originally observed in tissues other than brain. Although now known to be found also in brain, the peripheral receptor differs from the central receptor in both its neuroanatomic distribution and in the absence of any link to GABA or the chloride ion channel. Classical benzodiazepines differ in their affinity for this receptor, with clonazepam having none and diazepam having some. Recently, animal studies have suggested an anxiogenic role for this receptor.[54] Interestingly, acute stress in rats has been shown to increase the number of these sites in both kidney and olfactory bulb.[55] Moreover, studies of the peripheral benzodiazepine receptor on the platelets of anxious patients show lowered receptor densities which increase with diazepam treatment.[56] This suggests that an increase in the density of this receptor might be an adaptive mechanism to handle stress, with some anxious patients perhaps not able to increase their receptors when stressed and requiring anxiolytic drugs to accomplish this. Carbamazepine appears to have a similar effect in epileptic patients, increasing the numbers of peripheral benzodiazepine receptors.[57] The drug's anticonvulsant effects on amygdala-kindled seizures have also been shown to be mediated through the peripheral receptor.[58] These findings suggest that the peripheral receptor might account for carbamazepine's anxiolytic effects. Despite these considerations, however, carbamazepine's lack of action at the central benzodiazepine receptor or GABA benzodiazepine-chloride ionophore macromolecular complex, and its paradoxically "anxiogenic-like" actions at central noradrenergic synapses, suggests it is less likely to be an effective treatment in "typical" cases of pathologic anxiety.

THE CLINICAL EVIDENCE

Clonazepam

Because the anxiolytic properties of this drug are discussed in depth in Chapter 3, we will only briefly discuss the finding that clonazepam may be effective in patients with panic disorder. Since other benzodiazepines are also effective, evidence of the efficacy of clonazepam in panic might seem redundant. However, a significant number of patients refractory to alprazolam treatment have been reported to show a robust response to clonazepam.[59] This finding is provocative and difficult to explain. Is it due to clonazepam's longer half-life? Is it due to clonazepam's higher potency and greater affinity for the central benzodiazepine receptor? Or is it possibly due to the drug's anticonvulsant efficacy, which may be greater than that of alprazolam, although this might merely reflect its greater potency? It is difficult to understand why comparably potent doses of alprazolam would not be effective in some patients, nor why daily administration on a QID schedule should not obviate the problem of rebound anxiety due to short half-life (for alprazolam, half-life is estimated to be 8 to 18 hours). Recent published proceedings of a symposium contain a good deal of information about clonazepam's utility in anxiety and panic but do not address the issue of whether its anticonvulsant potency may account for some of its antipanic or anxiolytic effects.[60]

Carbamazepine in anxiety

The most extensive research with carbamazepine and anxiety disorders has been performed by Uhde, Post, and collaborators at the National Institute of Mental Health. Uhde and associates reported early findings suggesting antipanic efficacy in three of the first four patients given the drug in a double-blind placebo-controlled study.[61] Interestingly, the greatest effect appeared to be on help-seeking behavior as measured by "distress" telephone calls patients made to the treating psychiatrist. Because panic attack frequency was less affected, these calls appeared to be more a manifestation of anticipatory anxiety. However, it should be noted that such behavior has been regarded by Klein and colleagues in their original descriptions as an actual indicator of attacks themselves.[62] Subsequently, analysis of data in a larger sample (Uhde TW, personal communication, September, 1987) has revealed that, on the average, the drug does not show more antipanic efficacy than placebo. However, four of the ten patients in this study showed significant decreases in panic attacks after failing to improve during an initial placebo period. Thus the possibility remains that certain patients might improve on the drug. As might be expected, patients with panic attacks *and* EEG abnormalities have been shown to respond well to carbamazepine.[38]

Carbamazepine in sedative-hypnotic and alcohol withdrawal

In a double-blind placebo-controlled study by Bjorkquist and colleagues, carbamazepine attenuated symptoms of mild-to-moderate alcohol withdrawal.[63] This effect was manifested in the first two days, and patients in the active drug group were noted to return to work faster. In two other controlled reports of the drug in the treatment of alcohol withdrawal, carbamazepine compared favorably with clomethiazole[64] and tiapride.[65] In addition, one group reports open use with favorable results in over 2,500 alcoholics.[66] (The entire area has been recently reviewed by Ballenger and Post[67] and Butler and Messiha.[68])

Another report notes that in Sweden and Switzerland, carbamazepine has also been used effectively to attenuate symptoms of benzodiazepine withdrawal in benzodiazepine-dependent patients.[69] Curiously, none of these reports had been followed up until recently, when Klein and colleagues reported that three patients with panic disorder, unable to be blindly tapered from alprazolam because of severe rebound symptoms of anxiety and panic, were able to discontinue the drug following addition of carbamazepine.[70] Doses of 400 mg to 600 mg were given for several days before again attempting to taper the alprazolam.

The following case, seen recently at the University of Washington Center for Anxiety and Depression in Seattle, was treated similarly, with equivalent success.

> A 33-year-old male with an eight-year history of panic disorder was treated intermittently with benzodiazepines for the first four years, with variable success, until he developed a severe major depression. Treatment with alprazolam resolved both the depression and panic attacks, although daily doses of 12 mg were required to achieve this effect. After two years without symptoms, the patient tried unsuccessfully to taper his alprazolam. Admission to a hospital for this purpose was also unsuccessful. At this point, severe depression recurred despite alprazolam. During the next year, his mother died, his panic attacks increased to a daily frequency, and he missed progressively more days of work because of the attacks. He finally lost his job and went on disability. Treatment was initiated with carbamazepine at a dose of 200 mg QHS and increased to 400 mg QHS and 200 mg QAM over five days. At this point alprazolam was tapered 0.5 mg every two to three days with minimal generalized anxiety but no change in panic attack frequency. One week after withdrawal was complete, carbamazepine was discontinued and phenelzine begun. The patient responded well with resolution of depression and panic attacks over five weeks.

Because carbamazepine does not have an effect on the GABA benzodiazepine-chloride ionophore macromolecular complex, it is hard to understand how it can attenuate alcohol and benzodiazepine withdrawal syndromes. It is possible that the peripheral benzodiazepine receptor may be involved, since ethanol treatment in rats increases peripheral benzodiazapine sites[71] and withdrawal further increases them transiently before receptor density returns to its baseline value. Since diazepam treatment also increases the number of peripheral benzodiazepine receptor sites[56] and carbamazepine has a similar action,[57] carbamazepine may in some way "substitute" for the withdrawn compound during the withdrawal process. However, if this is the explanation, it is not clear why discontinuation of carbamazepine does not produce further withdrawal symptoms. One possibility is that peripheral benzodiazepine receptor dysfunction is necessary to allow central receptor changes to be expressed, but not itself sufficient to induce withdrawal without central receptor abnormalities.

The hypothalamic-pituitary-adrenal axis might provide another mechanism by which carbamazepine could attenuate withdrawal symptoms. Benzodiazepines are known to inhibit release of cortisol by an action at the hypothalamic and/or pituitary level.[72] During benzodiazepine withdrawal, there is "rebound" hypercortisolemia, which is likely due to hypersecretion of hypothalamic CRH.[73] Recent evidence (Gold P, personal communcation, December, 1987) suggests that carbamazepine augments the ACTH response to CRH, implying an increased sensitivity to CRH at pituitary CRH receptors which might be due to attenuation of CRH release. It is possible that the vasopressin agonist effects of carbamazepine are responsible for this,[51] since vasopressin itself stimulates the hypothalamic-pituitary-adrenal axis,[74] and hence vasopressin agonist-like effects could "substitute" for CRH. This hypothesis could be tested most directly by administering a compound during withdrawal which would directly block the effects of, or itself reduce, hypercortisolemia.

Valproate in anxiety

There have been no double-blind placebo-controlled trials investigating the efficacy of valproate in panic disorder. Primeau and colleagues recently reported the results of a seven-week open-label study in which 10 patients with panic disorder were treated with valproate following a seven-day placebo washout.[75] Patients took 500 mg/day initially and increased their dose gradually to 2,250 mg/day as tolerated. Overall, a significant improvement was noted on the Clinical Global Impression Scale for panic severity ($p<.001$), the Hamilton Anxiety Scale ($p<.001$), and the panic factor of the SCL-90 ($p<.05$). Six patients were judged to be at least moderately improved. However, no measure of panic attack *frequency* was provided. Greatest improvement was noted in the first week of the trial. The drug was fairly well tolerated by patients with many side effects appearing to be dose-related.

In addition to this as yet unpublished study, a case of panic disorder responsive to valproate was noted in a recent study of this drug's efficacy in primary psychiatric disorders.[76] The details of this case, not included in the original reference, have been kindly provided by the authors (McElroy SL, personal communication, October, 1987).

> A 24-year-old male had a five-year history of panic attacks. For two and one-half years, attacks were infrequent and caused little dysfunction. At that point, however, attacks increased, and there was accompanying dysphoria and generalized anxiety. After imipramine was unsuccessfully tried, phenelzine eliminated both the attacks and depression. Because of side effects, the dose of phenelzine was reduced after several months and attacks returned. Alprazolam was tried unsuccessfully. Depression and suicidality developed; the patient was briefly hospitalized two times in the ensuing five months. Because of lability of mood, hostility, anxiety, depression, suicidality, and various interpersonal disturbances, an Axis II diagnosis of borderline personality disorder was also made. Although the patient's EEG was normal, a brain electrical activity mapping (BEAM) study revealed an increase in slow activity in left posterior temporal and occipital regions and abnormal visual and auditory evoked responses, also on the left. The patient was unable to tolerate a trial of carbamazepine, but valproate, 1,000 mg daily, resulted in total elimination of panic attacks and a decrease in generalized anxiety and dysphoria after one week. There has been no recurrence at one-year follow-up. Valproate blood levels were not obtained.

These findings suggest that this anticonvulsant, perhaps because of effects at the GABA benzodiazepine-chloride ionophore macromolecular complex not shared by carbamazepine, may have more efficacy in panic. It should be noted, however, that carbamazepine's antipanic efficacy, initially reported by Udhe and associates, was not confirmed by controlled clinical trials. Therefore, until controlled studies of valproate's antipanic efficacy are performed, these results must be taken cautiously. Furthermore, Primeau and colleagues have also reported frequent EEG abnormalities in their panic patients. This, along with the abnormal BEAM study in the previous case, may imply some subclinical epileptiform activity in these responsive patients.

Valproate in alcohol withdrawal

There is only one report discussing the use of valproate in alcohol withdrawal.[77] Forty-eight alcoholics were randomly allocated to receive either valproate 400 mg or nothing, along with conventional drug therapy (clomethiazole and/or tranquilizers) as needed. Fewer patients in the valproate group required additional medication for withdrawal symptoms, which *appeared* to decrease more quickly in the valproate group. However, no statistical analysis was provided, and although allocation was random, it is unclear whether severity of alcoholism at baseline was equal in the two groups. Thus, valproate's use in alcohol withdrawal is less well supported than carbamazepine's, and further studies are needed before definitive recommendations regarding clinical use can be made.

CONCLUSIONS

The evidence presented here is not meant to demonstrate that the anticonvulsants are effective anxiolytics, but to serve more of a heuristic, hypotheses-generating purpose. Controlled studies, using both placebo and active drugs as controls, need to be done to explore the comparative efficacy of these drugs in the treatment of pathologic states of anxiety. It is possible that some treatment-resistant patients with panic disorder may respond well to trials of certain anticonvulsants, although it is less likely that the "garden-variety" panic disorder patient will respond. It is also possible that some patients in the heterogeneous generalized anxiety disorder category may respond, particularly in light of the similarity between this type of anxiety and the symptoms of alcohol/sedative-hypnotic withdrawal.

REFERENCES

1. Allen AM, Harris RA. Involvement of neuronal chloride channels in ethanol intoxication, tolerance and dependence. In: Galanter M, ed. Recent developments in alcoholism. Vol. 5. New York: Plenum Press, 1986:313-25.
2. William SM. Molecular aspects of the action of benzodiazepine and non-benzodiazepine anxiolytics: a hypothetical allosteric model of the benzodiazepine receptor complex. Prog Neurol Psychopharmacol Biol Psychiatry 1984; 8:209-47.
3. Cowne PJ, Nutt DJ. Abstinence symptoms after withdrawal of tranquilizing drugs: is there a common neurochemical mechanism? Lancet 1982; 2:360-2.
4. Ninan PT, Insel TM, Cohen RM, et al. Benzodiazepine receptor-mediated experimental anxiety in primates. Science 1982; 218:1332-4.
5. Dorrow R, Horowski R, Pashelke G, et al. Severe anxiety induced by FG 7142, a beta-carboline ligand for benzodiazepine receptors. Lancet 1983; 2:98-9.
6. Uhde TW, Siever LJ, Post RM. Clonidine: acute challenge and clinical trial paradigms for the investigation and treatment of anxiety disorders, affective illness and pain syndromes. In: Post RM, Ballenger JC, eds. Neurobiology of mood disorders. Baltimore: Williams and Wilkins, 1984:554-71.

7. Kesharan MS, Crammer JL. Clonidine in benzodiazepine withdrawal. Lancet 1985; 1:1325-6.
8. Goodman WK, Charney DS, Price LH, et al. Ineffectiveness of clonidine in the treatment of the benzodiazepine withdrawal syndrome. Report of 3 cases. Am J Psychiatry 1986; 143:900-3.
9. Barlow DH. The dimensions of anxiety disorders. In: Tuma AH, Maser JD, eds. Anxiety and the anxiety disorders. Hillsdale, New Jersey: Lawrence Erlbaum, 1985:479-500.
10. Cowley DS, Dager SR, Foster SI, et al. Clinical characteristics and response to sodium lactate in patients with infrequent panic attacks. Am J Psychiatry 1987; 144:795-8.
11. Cowley DS, Dager SR, McClellan J, et al. Response to lactate infusion in generalized anxiety disorder. Biol Psychiatry (in press).
12. Noyes R, Clarkson C, Crowe RR, et al. A family study of generalized anxiety disorder. Am J Psychiatry 1987; 144:1019-24.
13. Breier A, Charney DS, Heninger GR. Major depression in patients with agoraphobia and panic disorder. Arch Gen Psychiatry 1984; 41:1129-35.
14. Von Korff M, Shapiro S, Burke JD, et al. Anxiety and depression in a primary care clinic. Arch Gen Psychiatry 1987; 44:152-6.
15. American Psychiatric Association, Task Force on Nomenclature and Statistics. Diagnostic and statistical manual of mental disorders. 3rd ed., revised. Washington, DC: American Psychiatric Association, 1987.
16. Tyrer P. Neurosis divisible. Lancet 1984; 1:685-8.
17. Ballenger JC. Pharmacotherapy of panic disorders. J Clin Psychiatry 1986; 47:27S-32S.
18. Weissman MM, Merikangas KR. The epidemiology of anxiety and panic disorders: an update. J Clin Psychiatry 1986; 47:11S-17S.
19. Swanson RP, Pecknold JC, Kirby ME. Benziodiazepine dependence. J Affect Dis 1987; 13: 109-18.
20. Post RM, Ballenger JC, Uhde TW, et al. Efficacy of carbamazepine in manic-depressive illness: implications for underlying mechanisms. In: Post RM, Ballenger JC, eds. Neurobiology of mood disorders. Baltimore: Williams & Wilkins, 1984:777-816.
21. Emrich HM, von Zerssen D, Kissling W, et al. Effect of sodium valproate in mania. The GABA-hypothesis of affective disorders. Arch Psychiatr Nervenkr 1980; 229:1-16.
22. Post RM, Uhde TW. Are the psychotropic effects of carbamazepine in manic-depressive illness mediated through the limbic system? Psychiatr J Univ Ottawa 1985; 10:205-18.
23. Albright PS, Burnham WM. Development of a new pharmacological seizure model: effects of anticonvulsants on cortical- and amygdala-kindled seizures in the rat. Epilepsia 1980; 21: 681-9.
24. Puente RM. The use of carbamazepine in the treatment of behavorial disorders in children. In: Birkmeyer W, ed. Epileptic seizures-behavior-pain. Bern: Hans Huber, 1976:243-51.
25. Silanepa M. Carbamazepine—pharmacology and clinical uses. Acta Neurol Scand 1981; 64: 1S-202S.
26. Robertson MM. Depression in patients with epilepsy. In: Proceedings of the 15th Epilepsy International Symposium. Washington, DC, September 27, 1983.
27. Post RM, Uhde TW. Carbamazepine in the treatment of mood and anxiety disorders. In: Trimble M, Zariffian E, eds. Psychopharmacology of the limbic system. New York: John Wiley and Sons, 1983:134-47.
28. Klein E, Bentil E, Lever B, et al. Carbamazepine and haloperidol vs. placebo and haloperidol in excited psychosis. Arch Gen Psychiatry 1984; 41:165-70.
29. Shephard RA. Behavioral effects of GABA agonists in relation to anxiety and benzodiazepine action. Life Sci 1987; 40:2429-36.
30. Lippa AS, Nash PA, Greenblatt EN. Preclinical neuropsychopharmacological testing procedures for anxiolytic drugs. In: Fielding S, Lal H, eds. Anxiolytics. Mount Kisco, New York: Futura, 1979:41-81.
31. Mohler H, Okada T. Benzodiazepine receptors: demonstration in the CNS. Science 1977; 198:849-51.
32. Paul SM, Syapin PJ, Paugh BA, et al. Correlation between benzodiazepine receptor occupation and anticonvulsant effects of diazepam. Nature 1979; 281:688-9.

33. Pellow S. Can drug effects on anxiety and convulsions be separated? Neurosci Biol Behav Rev 1985; 9:55-73.
34. Brodsky L, Zunidga J, Casenas E, et al. Refractory anxiety: a masked epileptiform disorder. Psychiatr J Univ Ottawa 1983; 8:42-5.
35. Henriksen GF. Status epilepticus partialis with fear as clinical expression: report of a case and ictal EEG findings. Epilepsia 1973; 14:39-46.
36. Stern TA, Murray GB. Complex partial seizures presenting as a psychiatric illness. J Nerv Ment Dis 1984; 172:625-7.
37. Weilberg JB, Bear DM, Sachs G. Three patients with concomitant panic attacks and seizure disorder: possible clues to the neurology of anxiety. Am J Psychiatry 1987; 144:1053-6.
38. Edlund MJ, Swann AC, Clothier J. Patients with panic attacks and abnormal EEG results. Am J Psychiatry 1987; 144:508-9.
39. Gloor P, Olivier A, Quesney LF, et al. The role of the limbic system in experimental phenomena of temporal lobe epilepsy. Ann Neurol 1982; 12:129-43.
40. Gray JAG. The neuropsychology of anxiety: an inquiry into the functions of the septo-hippocampal system. New York: Oxford University Press, 1982.
41. Reiman EM, Raichle ME, Robins E, et al. The application of positron emission tomography to the study of panic disorder. Am J Psychiatry 1986; 143:469-77.
42. Sanger DJ. Minireview: GABA and the behavioral effects of anxiolytic drugs. Life Sci 1985; 36:1503-13.
43. Lal H, Shearman GT, Fielding S, et al. Effect of valproic acid on anxiety-related behaviors in the rat. Brain Res Bull 1979; 4:711. abstract.
44. Shephard RA, Stevenson D, Jenkinson S. Effects of valproate on hyponeophagia in rats: competitive antagonism with picrotoxin and non-competitive antagonism with R015-1788. Psychopharmacology 1985; 86:313-7.
45. Lal H, Shearman GT, Fielding S, et al. Evidence that GABA mechanisms mediate the anxiolytic action of benzodiazepines: a study with valproic acid. Neuropharmacology 1980; 19:785-9.
46. Rasmussen KJ, Schneider HH, Peterson EN. Sodium valproate exerts anti-conflict activity in rats without any concomitant rise in forebrain GABA level. Life Sci 1981; 29:2163-70.
47. Liljequist S, Engle JA. Reversal of the anti-conflict action of valproate by various GABA and benzodiazepine antagonists. Life Sci 1984; 34:2525-33.
48. Ticku MK, Davis WC. Effect of valproic acid on [3H]- diazepam and [3H]-dihydropicrotoxin binding sites at the benzodiazepine-GABA receptor ionophore complex. Brain Res 1981; 223:218-22.
49. Shephard RA, Estall LB. Effects of chlordiazepoxide and of valproate on hyponeophagia in rats. Neuropharmacology 1984; 23:677-81.
50. Petraglia F, Bakalakis S, Facchinetti F. Effects of sodium valproate and diazepam on beta-endorphin, beta-lipotropin and cortisol secretion induced by hypoglycemic stress in humans. Neuroendocrinology 1986; 44:320-5.
51. Post RM. Mechanisms of action of carbamazepine and related anticonvulsants in affective illness. In: Meltzer HY, ed. Psychopharmacology: the third generation of progress. New York: Raven Press, 1987:567-76.
52. Purdy RC, Jahen RM, Fairhurst AS, et al. Effect of carbamazepine on the *in vitro* uptake and release of norepinephrine in adrenergic nerves of rabbit aorta and in whole brain synaptosomes. Epilepsy 1977; 18:251-7.
53. Post RM, Ballenger JC, Uhde TW, et al. Effect of carbamazepine on cyclic nucleotides in CSF of patients with affective illness. Biol Psychiatry 1982; 17:1037-45.
54. Mizoule J, Ganthier A, Uzan A, et al. Opposite effects of two ligands for peripheral type benzodiazepine binding sites, PK 11195 and RO5-4864, in a conflict situation in the rat. Life Sci 1985; 36:1059-68.
55. Novas ML, Medina JH, Calvo D, et al. Increase of peripheral type benzodiazepine binding sites in kidney and olfactoy bulb in acutely stressed rats. Eur J Pharmacol 1987; 135:243-6.
56. Weizman R, Tanne Z, Granek M. Peripheral benzodiazepine binding sites on platelet membranes are increased during diazepam treatment of anxious patients. Eur J Pharmacol 1987; 138: 289-92.

57. Weizman R, Tanne Z, Karp L, et al. Carbamazepine up-regulated the binding of [3H]-PKU195 to platelets of epileptic patients. Eur J Pharmacol 1987; 141:471-4.
58. Weiss SRB, Post RM, Patel J, et al. Differential mediation of the anticonvulsant effects of carbamazepine and diazepam. Life Sci 1985; 36:2413-7.
59. Spier SA, Tesar GE, Rosenbaum JF, et al. Treatment of panic disorder and agoraphobia with clonazepam. J Clin Psychiatry 1986; 47:238-42.
60. Rosenbaum JF, ed. New uses of clonazepam in psychiatry. J Clin Psychiatry 1987; 48:3S-56S.
61. Uhde TW, Ballenger JC, Post RM. Carbamazepine: treatment of affective illness and anxiety syndromes. In: Pichot P, Berner P, Wolf R, et al., eds. Psychiatry: state of the art. Vol. 3. New York: Plenum Press, 1985:479-84.
62. Klein DF. Anxiety reconceptualized. In: Klein DF, Rabkin JG, eds. Anxiety: new research and changing concepts. New York: Raven Press, 1981:235-64.
63. Bjorkquist SE, Isohanni M, Makela R, et al. Ambulant treatment of alcohol withdrawal symptoms with carbamazepine: a formal multicare double-blind comparison with placebo. Acta Psychiatr Scand 1976; 53:333-42.
64. Ritola E, Malinen L. A double-blind comparison of carbamazepine and clomethiazole in the treatment of alcohol withdrawal syndrome. Acta Psychiatr Scand 1981; 64:254-9.
65. Agricola R, Mazzarind M, Urani R. Treatment of acute alcohol withdrawal syndrome with carbamazepine: a double- blind comparison with tiapride. J Int Med Res 1982; 10:160-5.
66. Sternebring B, Holm R, Wadstein J. Reduction in early alcohol abstinence fits by administration of carbamazepine syrup instead of tablets. Eur J Clin Pharmacol 1983; 24:611-3.
67. Ballenger JC, Post RM. Carbamazepine in alcohol withdrawal syndromes and schizophrenic psychoses. Psychopharmacol Bull 1984; 20:572-84.
68. Butler D, Messiha FS. Alcohol withdrawal and carbamazepine. Alcohol 1986; 3:113-29.
69. Kuhn R. The psychotropic effect of carbamazepine in non-epileptic adults, with particular reference to the drug's possible mechanism of action. In: Birkmeyer W, ed. Epileptic seizures-behavior-pain. Bern: Hans Huber, 1976:268-74.
70. Klein E, Uhde TW, Post RM. Preliminary evidence for the utility of carbamazepine in alprazolam withdrawal. Am J Psychiatry 1986; 143:235-6.
71. Tambourska E, Morangos PJ. Brain benzodiazepine binding sites in ethanol dependent and withdrawal states. Life Sci 1985; 38:465-72.
72. Grandison L. Actions of benzodiazepines on the neuroendocrine system. Neuropharmacology 1983; 22:1505-10.
73. Mellman TA, Uhde TW. Withdrawal syndrome with gradual tapering of alprazolam. Am J Psychiatry 1986; 143:1464-6.
74. Lutz-Bucker B, Koch B, Mialhe C. Comparative *in vitro* studies on corticotropin releasing activity of vasopressin and hypothalamic median eminence extract. Neuroendocrinology 1977; 23:181-2.
75. Primeau F, Beauclair L, Fontaine R, et al. An open-label study of valproic acid in the treatment of panic disorder. Presented at the Society of Biological Psychiatry Annual Meeting, Chicago, May, 1987.
76. McElroy SL, Keck PE, Jr, Pope HG, Jr. Sodium valproate: its use in primary psychiatric disorders. J Clin Psychopharmacol 1987; 7:16-24.
77. Lambie DG, Johnson RH, Vijayasenan MG, et al. Sodium valproate in the treatment of the alcohol withdrawal syndrome. Aust NZ J of Psychiatry 1980; 14:213-5.

CHAPTER 11

Anticonvulsant Drug Therapy of Neuropsychiatric Disorders in Mentally Retarded Persons

Robert Sovner, M.D.
Watertown, Massachusetts

INTRODUCTION

The pharmacological treatment of mental disorders in developmentally handicapped persons has only recently begun to emerge as a distinct psychiatric subspecialty.[1] As the idea that the mentally retarded suffer from the full range of psychiatric disorders gains acceptance, the use of antidepressants, benzodiazepines, and lithium in this population has increased. However, the diagnosis and treatment of behavioral problems in the mentally retarded still remains problematic.

Despite a lack of demonstrated efficacy, antipsychotics remain the most commonly prescribed drug class for developmentally handicapped persons.[2] This is due, in large part, to the mistaken assumption that behavioral problems in the mentally retarded are a reflection of a psychotic process or a manifestation of the patient's developmental disabilities.[3-5]

These erroneous beliefs also reflect the fact that adequate diagnostic evaluations are rarely carried out with symptomatic mentally retarded persons. Even though the importance of psychiatric diagnosis in the choice of a specific psychotropic agent (or, for that matter, any treatment modality) is a basic tenet of psychiatric medicine, it is frequently ignored when prescribing for mentally retarded persons. As a result, clinicians have prescribed medication for so-called "behavior disorders", i.e. severe and often chronic maladaptive behavior. However, maladaptive behavior can be the nonspecific expression of conditions ranging from hiatal hernia (i.e. physical distress) to classic bipolar disorder. It is usually a symptom and not the problem.

Therefore, the purpose of rational psychotropic drug therapy is not to treat behavior *per se*.[6] Instead, rational psychotropic drug therapy seeks to alter the neurobiochemical and neurophysiological substrates of psychopathology and modifies behavior only secondarily. Drug selection, then, must be based upon a rigorous diagnostic assessment to identify the presence of a drug-responsive syndrome, as well as a treatment formulation which includes syndrome-associated target behaviors and a hypothesis for why these problems should be treatment-responsive.

As these controversies are debated in the clinical arena, the use of anticonvulsants with psychotropic effects is a mode of therapy currently being promoted for mentally retarded persons with emotional and behavioral problems. An examination of the significant clinical and theoretical issues surrounding the use of this novel psychotropic drug class may serve to refine and resolve many of the etiological, diagnostic, and treatment issues related to the management of psychiatric disorders in these often mismanaged patients.

RATIONALE FOR THE USE OF ANTICONVULSANTS

Mentally retarded persons suffer from anticonvulsant-responsive psychiatric disorders.

Since mentally retarded persons suffer from the full range of psychiatric disorders,[7-10] the already recognized psychotropic effects of anticonvulsants (discussed in other chapters in this volume) are applicable to treating symptomatic handicapped individuals. In particular, clinical observation suggests that the mentally retarded may be prone to atypical and treatment-resistant forms of affective disorder, especially rapid-cycling bipolar disorder.[11] Neurological dysfunction may mediate both phenomena,[12] with the atypical presentations representing subictal and anticonvulsant drug-responsive forms of epilepsy.[13]

In addition, the high incidence of central nervous system (CNS) impairments in mentally retarded persons with moderate or greater handicaps may predispose them to a variety of anticonvulsant-sensitive organic brain syndromes. Reid has strongly advocated this position. He comments, "It is my view that many of the gross personality and behavioural problems encountered in mentally retarded patients will also turn out, in the course of time, to be organically determined by subtle abnormalities of brain structure or by neurochemical, neurophysiological or neuroendocrine disorders."[14]

The clinical expression of these disorders in adult mentally retarded persons represents a complex interaction among: (1) the evolution of the pathological process producing the dysfunction; (2) the direct effects of central nervous system dysfunction on mood, affect regulation, and motor activity; (3) the onset of the CNS insult in relation to the affected person's developmental process; and (4) the quality of the person's environment.

These disturbances can best be viewed as organic personality disorders, given their chronicity and the influence which they have on the mentally retarded patient's interpersonal relationships. Affected individuals very much resemble nonretarded adults with frontal lobe dysfunction who also manifest affective lability, irritability, aggression, and decreased need for sleep.[15]

There is a very high incidence of seizure disorders in mentally retarded populations.

Anywhere from one-fifth to one-half of all mentally retarded children have a seizure disorder, with the highest incidence found in severely handicapped individuals.[16-18] Since antipsychotics, antidepressants, and lithium salts lower the seizure threshold,[19,20] the use of a drug with both anticonvulsant and psychotropic properties avoids the problem of a psychotropic drug-induced exacerbation of a coexistent seizure disorder or the unmasking of a previously quiescent one.

In addition, since many mentally retarded persons are already receiving anticonvulsant therapy, it is reasonable to use a drug with combined anticonvulsant-psychotropic properties which can replace several other co-prescribed psychotropic and anticonvulsant agents (see Case #3, later in this chapter). This reduces the risk of side effects and drug interactions. Indeed, anticonvulsant monotherapy has been demonstrated as a safe and effective practice with mentally retarded epileptics.[21]

Anticonvulsants reduce the risk of tardive dyskinesia.

Mentally retarded persons are at significant risk for developing tardive dyskinesia when antipsychotic agents are prescribed.[22,23] This makes the search for alternatives to antipsychotic drugs, the most commonly prescribed drug class in this population, a key therapeutic issue.[2] Therefore, the side-effect profiles of carbamazepine and valproate make them rational alternatives to more traditional psychotropic drug therapy.

Akathisia

Antipsychotic-induced akathisia or involuntary motor restlessness is an intensely uncomfortable experience that has been reported to produce an exacerbation of the symptoms being treated and to cause suicide attempts.[24] This side effect is not always diagnosable by physical examination and is based upon the patient's self-report of distress.[25]

Amphetamine reaction

An amphetamine-like reaction to heterocyclic and monamine oxidase (MAO) inhibitor antidepressants can produce a marked behavioral deterioration in mentally retarded persons.

Incontinence

Lithium-induced diabetes insipidus often presents in mentally retarded persons as urinary incontinence. High-dose antipsychotic drug therapy can also produce incontinence.[26]

Carbamazepine and valproate may have less impact upon the rehabilitation process than classic psychotropic agents

Carbamazepine and valproate are relatively nonsedating,[27] have minimal anticholinergic effects (which can impair short term memory), and have minimal effects on cognition and performance.[28-30]

USE OF SPECIFIC ANTICONVULSANTS

Carbamazepine

The psychotropic effects of carbamazepine in mentally retarded persons have been studied more than those of any other anticonvsulant.

Affective disorder

The antidepressant,[31] antimanic,[32] and lithium potentiating[33] effects of carbamazepine may be used to treat affectively ill mentally retarded persons. In the presence of a seizure disorder (other than absence), carbamazepine may be the drug of first choice. Although only one case report of the successful treatment of bipolar disorder with carbamazepine in a mentally retarded person has been published to date,[34] the following previously unpublished cases (obtained from the author's experience) further illustrate the use of carbamazepine with mentally retarded patients who have affective disorders.

Case #1

The first case represents treatment of major depression in an autistic woman. The patient was a 25-year-old woman with mild developmental disabilities who had been diagnosed as suffering from an autistic disorder when she was two years of age. She had lived at home until she was 16, at which time she moved into a community residence. An older brother had attempted suicide.

She was referred for evaluation because of an increase in skin picking and anxiety which had begun approximately 18 months earlier. She presented with two types of problems. The first related to behaviors consistent with autism, i.e. compulsive orderliness, a need for sameness, inappropriate water play, verbal perseveration, and picking at sores. In addition, she had marked anxiety, mood lability, mild insomnia, premenstrual temper tantrums, and intermittent tearfulness. At the time of her evaluation, she was drug-free and without significant medical problems. A 16-hour dexamethasone suppression test (DST), carried out according to the protocol of Carroll and colleagues,[35] was positive with a 4:00 P.M. cortisol of 16.9 μg/ml.

The patient was initally started on nortriptyline but had a major motor seizure. The drug was discontinued and carbamazepine was started. The daily dose was titrated to achieve a blood level of 8.7 μg/ml. There was a dramatic decrease in anxiety and dysphoria with a remission of her sleep disturbance. The severity of skin picking decreased. When interviewed, she seemed much more relaxed and happy. A follow-up DST was not carried out due to the false positive effect of carbamazepine on this test.[36]

Case #2

The second case represents augumentation of lithium response in a mentally retarded man with chronic mania. The patient was a 21-year-old man with idiopathic mild mental retardation who was referred for an assessment of aggressive behavior. He was in good health at the time of the assessment. His mother had been diagnosed as being "manic-depressive".

The patient had been intermittently hospitalized on psychiatric units because of his aggressive behavior. He had been predominantly manic for several years. When interviewed, he was moderately euphoric and extremely gregarious. His speech was moderately pressured and tangential. Speech content was grandiose (he was going to become a Little League coach). Staff reported that he was sleeping only three to four hours per night.

A review of his medical records indicated that he had been tried on both lithium (highest blood level achieved was 1.1 mEq/l) and carbamazepine (highest blood level was 11 μg/ml) but had never received the drugs in combination.

A combined trial of lithium (blood level 0.75 mEq/l) and carbamazepine (10.6 μg/ml) was initated. Over a four-week period, this regimen produced a marked reduction in his manic symptomatology. His sleep disorder and aggressiveness remitted, but he remained slightly euphoric and extroverted.

Atypical indications

Donner and Frisk treated seven mentally retarded children with severe epilepsy and an "organic psychosyndrome" or "neurotic symptoms" with carbamazepine.[37] They reported that three of the children demonstrated improvement of their psychological and behavioral symptoms in response to treatment. Kanjilal treated 38 mentally retarded epileptics with behavioral problems (restlessness, excitability, temper outbursts, aggression, and/or self-injury).[38] His subjective impression was that 14 of his patients had improved behavior during the carbamazepine trial. The patients' diagnoses were not provided, and it is difficult to assess his results. Also, blood level data were not reported.

Rapport and colleagues reported treatment of a 13-year-old girl with mental retardation secondary to measles encephalitis.[39] She also displayed a seizure disorder and aggressive behavior. The combination of carbamazepine (blood level not provided) and behavior therapy produced a remission in her aggressive behavior.

Buck and Havey reported treatment of a 23-year-old man with mild developmental handicaps with a history of chronic and treatment-resistant behavior problems, including aggressive outbursts and talking incoherently to himself in the second person.[40] He had nonspecific slowing on his EEG. There was a dramatic response to carbamazepine (blood level 10 μg/ml).

Reid and associates have presented evidence that carbamazepine may be effective in organic affective disorders in severely or profoundly handicapped persons.[41] They treated 12 institutionalized adults with marked disabilities who manifested life-long, treatment-resistant hyperactivity. Five also had a history of epilepsy. The patients were treated in a double-blind crossover trial in which carbamazepine and placebo were each prescribed for three months. Prior to the initiation of treatment, study subjects were divided into two groups based upon a classification scheme developed by Reid and colleagues.[42] In group A, hyperactivity was associated with mood elevation and distractability. In group B, hyperactivity was associated with behavioral problems such as self-injury, irritability, yelling, disrobing, stereotypies, and feeding problems. Outcome was measured using a nurses' rating scale that included a bipolar scale for symptom severity (+3 to −3). Carbamazepine blood levels were maintained between 5.5 and 9.9 μg/ml.

In group A, the mean weekly symptom severity rating was significantly less for five of six study completers. In group B, two patients significantly worsened and one significantly improved. Age and history of seizure disorder did not discriminate responders from nonresponders. The authors noted that the best treatment response was observed in patients whose features were consistent with "chronic mania".

Dalby, reviewing earlier studies on the use of carbamazepine in mentally retarded persons, cited evidence for its efficacy in the management of overactivity, impulsivity, and irritability.[43] Also, d'Hollander found a significant psychotropic response to carbamazepine in 35 mentally retarded and epileptic girls with behavioral disturbances.[44]

The following case (from the author's experience) illustrates the use of carbamazepine in a patient with an organic personality disorder.

Case #3

The patient was a 27-year-old woman with severe mental retardation, bilateral cataracts, cardiac valvular defects, bilateral neural hearing deficits, and complex partial seizures secondary to a congenital rubella infection. She was referred for evaluation of chronic behavioral problems including self-injurious behavior, irritability, intermittent hyposomnia, disrobing, and negativism. She had to be restrained up to 60 times per month. There was no evidence of overactivity or elated mood. Her symptoms did not demonstrate a biphasic course.

At the time of assessment she was taking chlorpromazine 300 mg per day, haloperidol 20 mg per day, phenytoin 200 mg per day, and phenobarbital 90 mg per day.

It was felt that her primary problem was a severe organic personality disorder with the primary features of irritability and hyposomnia. Her self-injurious behavior and negativism were viewed as secondary features which served a demand-avoidance function.

Carbamazepine was added to her drug regimen and the daily dose titrated to achieve a blood level of 8.5 μg/ml. There was a dramatic change in the patient's behavior with carbamazepine therapy. (See Sovner for presentation of behavioral response data.[1]) Her sleep normalized and the number of restraints per month dropped to less than seven. Staff found her to be significantly less irritable, and she was able to engage in a greater degree of rehabilitative programming.

In addition, the chlorpromazine, haloperidol, phenobarbital, and phenytoin were all discontinued without any loss of positive psychotropic effects or increase in seizure frequency.

Discussion

The study by Reid and colleagues demonstrates the utility of prospectively classifying subjects according to a diagnostic system.[41] It is difficult to make sense of the other reports because of the global nature of the claimed response and the failure to present a diagnostic hypothesis.

The available evidence, though limited, suggests that carbamazepine responsiveness appears to be associated with the presence of an organic affective disorder or the presence of irritability. It is intriguing to note that maladaptive behavior associated with frontal lobe dysfunction in nonretarded patients has also been reported to be responsive to carbamazepine.[43,45] However, it is doubtful that irritability or overactivity alone will predict response to carbamazepine. Other defining features such as a sleep disturbance or elated mood may also be necessary.

Adverse effects

In general carbamazepine is well tolerated by mentally retarded persons,[46] and agranulocytosis is a rare but serious adverse reaction.[47] However, behavioral side effects can develop. Silverstein and colleagues found that seven (3.5%) of 200 children treated with carbamazepine had adverse behavioral reactions to the drug.[48] Four of the children were mentally retarded (ranging in age from six to 18 years). Agitation or irritability were the most common adverse reactions in these cases. The authors noted the structural resemblance of carbamazepine to imipramine and postulated that the few instances of behavioral deterioration seen with carbamazepine may have occurred via a mechanism similar to that underlying the amphetamine-like reactions to heterocyclic antidepressants occurring in other mentally retarded persons.

Toxic carbamazepine blood levels have been implicated in producing a schizophreniform psychosis[49] and reversible dystonia[50] in mentally retarded children with epilepsy. The combination of lithium and carbamazepine can produce a neurotoxic syndrome, even when the blood levels of both drugs are within the therapeutic range.[51] Central nervous system dysfunction appears to be a mediating factor in all of these idiosyncratic reactions.[50,51]

Comments

Carbamazepine appears to be a promising psychotropic agent in mentally retarded persons, particularly those with affective disorder. With respect to atypical indications, the available data are inconclusive, but lend themselves to the hypothesis that the maladaptive behavior of some disturbed mentally retarded persons represents the expression of an organic affective disorder or an organic personality disorder. In general, carbamazepine blood levels between 8.5 μg/ml and 12 μg/ml are required to produce complete therapeutic effects.

Clonazepam

Anxiety and affective disorders

Mentally retarded persons can develop panic disorder, and panic attacks may account for some cases of intermittent self-injurious or aggressive behavior.[52] Thus, clonazepam with its antipanic effects may prove to be useful in such cases.[53] Furthermore, because clonazepam has been reported to have antimanic activity,[54] it may also prove to be a useful adjunct in the treatment of mania in mentally retarded persons, particularly those with tardive dyskinesia.

Atypical indications

Freinhar reported a case of a mildly retarded woman treated successfully with clonazepam (3 mg QID) for agitation and violent behavior associated with crying and hostility.[55] She had previously demonstrated a poor response to chlorpromazine. Her neurological status was not given, and there was no discussion of possible psychiatric diagnoses.

Adverse effects

Clonazepam is a sedating benzodiazepine and may produce clinically significant psychomotor dysfunction, aggression, and overactivity.

Comments

Based upon the presence of clonazepam-sensitive psychopathology in mentally retarded persons, the drug may be used for typical indications. The role of clonazepam in the treatment of organic brain syndromes in mentally retarded persons has not been explored. However, there is the distinct danger that, should clonazepam become a fashionable pharmacological treatment for mentally retarded persons, it will be used indiscriminately for chemical restraint.

Valproate

To date, there have not been any published reports of the treatment of psychiatric disorders in mentally retarded persons with valproate. However, the apparently beneficial psychotropic effects of this drug in the treatment of bipolar disorder and schizoaffective disorder suggest that it may prove useful in the treatment of developmentally handicapped persons with such disorders.[56]

Adverse effects

Severe liver dysfunction and blood dyscrasias are rare but serious side effects with valproate.[57] It is important to note that risk factors for development of valproate-induced fatal hepatotoxicity have been identified in epileptics and include: age equal to or less than two years, use of multiple anticonvulsants, and presence of neurologic disease in addition to a seizure disorder.[58] The drug has also been reported to cause nocturnal enuresis in children,[59,60] and hyperammonemia in mentally retarded adults.[61] However, valproate seems to have few adverse effects on learning in this population.[29]

Comments

Valproate may prove to be a reasonable alternative or adjuvant to lithium salts in the treatment of affective disorders in mentally retarded persons. Its role in the treatment of organic brain syndromes has not as yet been explored.

Hydantoins

Goldberg and Kurland carried out a double-blind placebo-controlled study with phenytoin in 47 nonepileptic mentally retarded boys.[62] They ranged in age from nine to 14 years and were diagnosed to have "cultural-familial" retardation. No specific behavioral problems were selected for treatment. Phenytoin-treated subjects were significantly improved on a measure of distractiblity, but there were no significant differences on measures of self-control and social interactions. Study subjects did not have serious behavioral problems prior to treatment, which makes it difficult to interpret drug response.

Adverse reactions

Hydantoin-induced gingival hyperplasia and the coarsening of facial features can be a significant problem in mentally retarded persons.[27,63]

Comments

The negative cosmetic effects of the hydantoins coupled with the lack of evidence for significant psychotropic effects argues against the use of this drug class to treat behavioral disturbances in mentally retarded persons.

Barbiturates and primidone

Barbiturate anticonvulsants and primidone (of which phenobarbital is a metabolite) do not appear to have any specific positive psychotropic effects. The risk of paradoxical excitement in severely retarded and self-injurious individuals,[64] significant impairments in cognitive function compared to other classes of anticonvulsants,[29,30] and their potent hepatic enzyme-inducing ability[65] would suggest that this class of anticonvulsants be avoided in psychiatrically impaired persons with developmental handicaps. Reported behavioral side effects of these drugs include phenobarbital-induced depression in epileptic children[66] and primidone-induced catatonia in a mentally retarded woman.[67]

Patients on multiple anticonvulsant medications, especially those with only one type of seizure, can often be taken off phenobarbital without adverse consequences and with an improvement in behavior.[68]

Comments

Barbiturates should not be used for their sedative effects in mentally retarded persons. Barbiturate-treated patients who present with self-injurious behavior should be tapered off the drug before other psychotropic interventions for this problem are considered.

Sulthiame

Sulthiame, a sulfonamide derivative unavailable in the United States, is a weak anticonvulsant which has been reported to have psychotropic effects. Moffat and colleagues carried out a double-blind placebo-controlled crossover trial of sulthiame for the treatment of behavioral problems in 42 mentally retarded adults.[69] All other psychotropic agents had been discontinued. It was found that sulthiame significantly reduced the overall incidence of maladaptive behavior without affecting any other behavior differentially.

Al-Kaisi and McGuire carried out a double-blind placebo-controlled study of sulthiame in the treatment of "disturbed" mentally retarded patients, half of whom had seizure disorders.[70] All psychotropic medications were withdrawn prior to study treatment. Subjects were treated for 14 weeks. At the end of the trial, the drug-treated group had a statistically significant decrease in aggressiveness and hyperactivity.

Adverse effects

In one long-term study of sulthiame in 45 treatment-refractory epileptics (30% of whom were mentally retarded), the most common side effects were ataxia (11%) and drowsiness (8%).[71] In this study, 37 (82%) of 45 patients lost weight, with 30 (67%) of 45 losing in excess of five pounds.

Comments

Although the presented studies suggest that sulthiame had significant psychotropic effects in individuals with severe disabilities, subsequent trials have not been published. It is also unclear what specific behavioral problems would respond to this drug.

Beclamide

Beclamide, an acetylurea derivative with anticonvulsant properties, not marketed in the United States, has been found to have psychotropic properties in mentally retarded persons with behavioral disturbances. Price and Spencer administered beclamide in a double-blind crossover design to 22 inpatients with behavioral problems such as tantrums, aggressiveness, destructiveness, restlessness, overactivity, and self-injury.[72] Nineteen subjects displayed a significant response to treatment. Unfortunately, there have been no other case reports or clinical trials with beclamide so that its clinical effectiveness as a psychotropic agent is unclear.

CONCLUSIONS

In work with developmentally disabled persons with severe behavioral problems, the psychiatrist faces a dilemma. These disturbances are often treatment resistant, even in optimal environments with the best available behavioral programming.[73] The presence of overactivity, hyposomnia, and irritability, or the signs of an affective disorder argue for psychotropic drug therapy, yet there are few "standard" treatments to chose from.

Antipsychotic drug therapy is not "conservative" treatment, despite the fact that some drugs from this class have labelled indications for use in mentally retarded persons. The possibility of drug-induced parkinsonism, akathisia, tardive dyskinesia, sedation, and performance impairments argues against their use for symptomatic mentally retarded persons, except in cases in which a classic psychotic disorder is present. In addition, lithium and antidepressants have a host of clinically significant side effects and may be only partially effective.

From a clinical perspective, carbamazepine and valproate represent rational therapeutic choices when mentally retarded persons require certain types of psychotropic drug therapy.

The absence of definitive research should not prevent their use. In carefully selected individuals, these drugs can produce dramatic improvement in the quality of life. The focus of future investigations should not be on justifying the use of anticonvulsants, but on defining those clinical criteria which predict a therapeutic response.

REFERENCES

1. Sovner R. Behavioral psychopharmacolgy. In: Stark J, Menolascino FJ, Albarielli M, et al., eds. Mental retardation and mental health: classification, diagnosis, treatment, services. New York: Springer Verlag, 1988:229-42.
2. Aman MG. Psychoactive drugs in mental retardation. In Matson JL, Andrasik F, eds. Treatment issues and innovations in mental retardation. New York: Plenum Press, 1983:455-513.
3. Aman M. Drugs in mental retardation: Treatment or tragedy? Aust NZ J Devel Dis 1985; 10:215-26.
4. Sovner R. Limiting factors in the use of DSM-III criteria with mentally ill/mentally retarded persons. Psychopharmacol Bull 1986; 22:1055-9.
5. Sovner R. Clonazepam in the treatment of mentally retarded persons (letter). Am J Psychiatry 1986; 143:1324.
6. Sheard MH. Clinical pharmacology of aggressive behavior. Clin Neuropharmacol 1984; 7:173-83.
7. Reid AH. Psychoses in adult mental defectives. I. Manic-depressive psychosis. Br J Psychiatry 1972; 120:203-12.
8. Reid AH. Psychosis in adult mental defectives. II. Schizophrenic and paranoid psychoses. Br J Psychiatry 1972; 120:213-8.
9. Sovner R, Hurley AD. Do the mentally retarded suffer from affective illness? Arch Gen Psychiatry 1983; 40:61-7.
10. Menolascino FJ, Levitas A. Nature and types of mental illness in the mentally retarded. Psychopharmacol Bull 1986; 22:1060-71.
11. Naylor GJ, Donald JM, Le Poidevin D, et al. A double-blind trial of long-term lithium therapy in mental defectives. Br J Psychiatry 1974; 124:52-7.
12. Himmelhoch JM, Neil JF, May ST, et al. Age, dementia, dyskinesias, and lithium response. Am J Psychiatry 1980; 137:941-5.
13. Himmelhoch JM. Major mood disorders related to epileptic changes. In: Blumer D, ed. Psychiatric aspects of epilepsy. Washington, DC: American Psychiatric Press, 1984:271-94.
14. Reid AH. The psychiatry of mental handicap. London: Blackwell Scientific Publications, 1982:88.
15. McAllister TW, Price TRP. Aspects of behavior of psychiatric inpatients with frontal lobe damage: some implications for diagnosis and treatment. Compr Psychiatry 1987; 28:14-21.
16. Corbett JA, Pond DA. Epilepsy and behaviour disorders in the mentally handicapped. In: Jame FE, Snaith RP, eds. Psychiatric illness and mental handicap. London: Gaskell Press, 1979:37-44.
17. Lewis MH, MacLean WE, Jr. Issues in treating emotional disorders. In: Matson JL, Barrett RP, eds. Psychopathology in the mentally retarded. New York: Grune & Stratton, 1982:1-36.
18. Richardson SA, Koller H, Katz M. Seizures and epilepsy in a mentally retarded population over the first 22 years of life. Appl Res Ment Retard 1980; 1:123-38.
19. Itil TM, Soldatos C. Epileptogenic side effects of psychotropic drugs. JAMA 1980; 244:1460-3.
20. James DH. Neuroleptics and epilepsy in mentally handicapped patients. J Ment Defic Res 1986; 30:185-9.
21. Bennet HS, Dunlop T, Ziring P. Reduction of polypharmacy for epilepsy in an institution for the retarded. Dev Med Child Neurol 1983; 25:735-7.
22. Gualtieri CT, Schroeder SR, Hicks RE, et al. Tardive dyskinesia in young mentally retarded individuals. Arch Gen Psychiatry 1986; 43:335-40.
23. Sprague RL. An analysis of institutionalized retarded residents using DIS-CO. Psychopharmacol Bull 1982; 18:60-1.
24. Drake RE, Ehrlich J. Suicide attempts associated with akathisia. Am J Psychiatry 1985; 142:499-501.
25. Van Putten T, May PRA, Marder SR. Akathisia with haloperidol and thiothixene. Arch Gen Psychiatry 1984; 41:1036-9.
26. Ambrosini PJ. A pharmacological paradigm for urinary incontinence and enuresis. J Clin Psychopharmacol 1984; 4:247-53.

27. Schain RJ. Problems with the use of conventional anticonvulsant drugs in mentally retarded individuals. Brain Dev 1979; 2:77-82.
28. Aman MG, Werry JS, Paxton JW, et al. Effect of sodium valproate on psychomotor performance in children as a function of dose, fluctuations in concentration, and diagnosis. Epilepsia 1987; 28:115-24.
29. Gay PE. Effects of antiepileptic drugs and seizure type on operant responding in mentally retarded persons. Epilepsia 1984; 25:377-86.
30. Vining EPG, Mellits ED, Dorsen MM, et al. Psychologic and behavioral effects of antiepileptic drugs in children: a double-blind comparison between phenobarbital and valproic acid. Pediatrics 1987; 80:165-74.
31. Post RM, Uhde TW, Roy-Byrne PP. Antidepressant effects of carbamazepine. Am J Psychiatry 1986; 143:29-34.
32. Post RM, Uhde TW. Carbamazepine in bipolar illness. Psychopharmacol Bull 1985; 21:10-7.
33. Post RM, Kramlinger KG, Uhde TW. Carbamazepine-lithium combination: clinical efficacy and side effects. Int Drug Ther Newsletter 1987; 22:5-8.
34. Singer SF, Benson DF, Rudnick FD. Undetected affective disorder in the developmentally retarded (letter). Am J Psychiatry 1986; 143:259.
35. Carroll BJ, Feinberg M. Greden JF, et al. A specific laboratory test for the diagnosis of melancholia: standardization, validation, and clinical utility. Arch Gen Psychiatry 1981; 38:15-22.
36. Orivitera MR, Greden JF, Gardner RW, et al. Interference by carbamazepine with the dexamethasone suppression test. Biol Psychiatry 1982; 17:611-20.
37. Donner M, Frisk M. Carbamazepine treatment of epileptic and psychotic symptoms in children and adolescents. Ann Paediat Fenn 1965; 11:91-7.
38. Kanjilal DC. An evaluation of Tegretol in adults with epilepsy. In: Roberts FD, ed. Tegretol in epilepsy. Proceedings of an international meeting. London: Geigy Pharmaceuticals, 1977:55-7.
39. Rapport M.D., Sonis WA, Fialkov MJ, et al. Carbamazepine and behavior therapy for aggressive behavior. Behav Modification 1983; 7:255-65.
40. Buck OD, Havey P. Combined carbamazepine and lithium therapy for violent behavior (letter). Am J Psychiatry 1986; 143:1487.
41. Reid AH, Naylor GJ, Kay DSS. A double-blind, placebo-controlled crossover trial of carbamazepine in overactive severely mentally handicapped patients. Psychol Med 1981; 11:109-13.
42. Reid AH, Ballinger BR, Heather BB. Behavioural syndromes identified by cluster analysis in a sample of 100 severely and profoundly retarded adults. Psychol Med 1978; 8:399-412.
43. Dalby MA. Behavioral effects of carbamazepine. In: Penry JK, Daly DD, eds. Advances in neurology. Vol 11. New York: Raven Press, 1975:331-43.
44. d'Hollander L. Traitement au moyen de carbamazépine de l'épilepsie avec trouble du comportement chez des enfants arrierées mentales en institut médicopédagogique. Acta Psychiatr Belg 1979; 79:557-69.
45. McQuinston HL, Adler LA, Leong S. Carbamazepine in frontal lobe syndromes: two more cases (letter). J Clin Psychiatry 1987; 48:456.
46. Bird CAK, Griffin BP, Miklaszewski JM, et al. Tegretol (carbamazepine): a controlled trial of a new anticonvulsant. Br J Psychiatry 1966; 112:737-42.
47. Joffe RT, Post RM, Roy-Byrne PP, et al. Hematological effects of carbamazepine in patients with affective illness. Am J Psychiatry 1985; 142:1196-9.
48. Silverstein FS, Parrish MA, Johnston MV. Adverse behavioral reactions in children treated with carbamazepine (Tegretol). J Pediatrics 1982; 101:785-7.
49. Franks RD, Richter AJ. Schizophrenia-like psychosis associated with anticonvulsant toxicity. Am J Psychiatry 1979; 136:973-4.
50. Croslye CJ, Swender PT. Dystonia associated with carbamazepine administration: experience in brain-damaged children. Pediatrics 1979; 63:612-5.
51. Shukla S, Godwin CD, Long LEB, et al. Lithium-carbamazepine neurotoxicity and risk factors. Am J Psychiatry 1984; 141:1604-6.
52. Cole JO, Hardy PM, Marcel B, et al. Organic states. In: Schatzberg A, ed. Common treatment problems in depression. Washington, DC: American Psychiatric Press, 1985:80-100.

53. Pollack MH, Tesar GE, Rosenbaum JF, et al. Clonazepam in the treatment of panic disorder and agoraphobia: a one-year follow-up. J Clin Psychopharmacol 1986; 6:302-4.
54. Chouinard G. Antimanic effects of clonazepam. Psychosomatics 1985; 26:7S-12S.
55. Freinhar JP. Clonazepam treatment of a mentally retarded woman (letter). Am J Psychiatry 1985; 143:1513.
56. McElroy SL, Keck PE, Jr, Pope HG, Jr. Sodium valproate: its use in primary psychiatric disorders. J Clin Psychopharmacol 1987; 7:16-24.
57. Browne TR. Valproic acid. New Eng J Med 1980; 302:661-6.
58. Dreifuss FE, Santilli N, Langer DH, et al. Valproic acid hepatic fatalities: a retrospective review. Neurology 1987; 37:379-85.
59. Choonara IA. Sodium valproate and enuresis (letter). Lancet 1985; 1:1276.
60. Panayiotopoulos CP. Nocturnal enuresis associated with sodim valproate (letter). Lancet 1985; 1:980-1.
61. William CA, Tiefenback S, McReynolds JW. Valproic acid-induced hyperammonemia in mentally retarded adults. Neurology 1984; 34:550-3.
62. Goldberg JB, Kurland AA. Dilantin treatment of hospitalized cultural-familial retardates. J Nerv Ment Dis 1970; 150:133-7.
63. Herberg KP. Effects of diphenylhydantoin in 41 epileptics institutionalized since childhood. South Med J 1977; 70:119-24.
64. Barron J, Sandman CA. Paradoxical excitement to sedative-hypnotics in mentally retarded clients. Am J Ment Defic 1985; 90:124-9.
65. Reynolds EH. The pharmacological management of epilepsy associated with psychological disorders. Br J Psychiatry 1982; 141:549-57.
66. Ferrari M, Barabas G, Matthews WS. Psychologic and behavioral disturbance among epileptic children treated with barbiturate anticonvulsants. Am J Psychiatry 1983; 140:112-3.
67. Sher A, Andersen JM, Bhatia SC. Primidone-induced catatonic schizophrenia. Drug Intell Clin Pharm 1983; 17:551-2.
68. Albright P, Bruni J. Reduction of polypharmacy in epileptic patients. Arch Neurol 1985; 42:797-9.
69. Moffat WR, Siddiqui AR, Mackay DN. The use of sulthiame with disturbed mentally subnormal patients. Br J Psychiatry 1970; 117:673-8.
70. Al-Kaisi AH, McGuire RJ. The effects of sulthiame on disturbed behaviour in mentally subnormal patients. Br J Psychiatry 1974; 124:45-9.
71. Liu MC. Clinical experience with sulthiame (Osplot). Br J Psychiatry 1966; 112:621-8.
72. Price SA, Spencer DA. A trial of beclamide (Hydrane) in mentally subnormal patients with disorders of behaviour. J Ment Subnormality 1967; 13:75-9.
73. Reid AH, Ballinger BR, Heather BB, et al. The natural history of behavioural symptoms among severely and profoundly mentally retarded patients. Br J Psychiatry 1984; 145:289-93.